0110478

AF616110

Cerebral SPECT Imaging

Second Edition

Cerebral SPECT Imaging

Second Edition

Editors

Ronald L. Van Heertum, M.D.
Professor of Clinical Radiology
Vice-Chairman
Department of Radiology
Columbia University
College of Physicians and Surgeons
and
Columbia Presbyterian Medical Center
New York, New York

Ronald S. Tikofsky, PH.D.
Research Associate Professor of Radiology
Division of Nuclear Medicine
Medical College of Wisconsin
Milwaukee, Wisconsin

Raven Press New York

Raven Press Ltd., 1185 Avenue of the Americas, New York, New York 10036

Made in the United States of America

Library of Congress Cataloging-in-Publication Data

Cerebral SPECT imaging / editors, Ronald L. Van Heertum, Ronald S. Tikofsky. — 2nd ed.
p. cm.
Rev. ed. of: Advances in cerebral SPECT imaging. © 1989.
Includes bibliographical references and index.
ISBN 0-7817-0188-0
1. Brain—Tomography. 2. Tomography, Emission. I. Van Heertum, Ronald L. II. Tikofsky, Ronald S. III. Advances in cerebral SPECT imaging.
[DNLM: 1. Brain Diseases—diagnosis—atlases. 2. Tomography, Emission-Computed, Single-Photon—methods—atlases. WL 17 C414 1994]
RC386.T65C47 1994
616.8'047575—dc20
DNLM/DLC
for Library of Congress 94-7879
CIP

The material contained in this volume was submitted as previously unpublished material, except in the instances in which some of the illustrative material was derived. Portions of the text have been updated and expanded from the First Edition, *Advances in Cerebral SPECT Imaging: An Atlas and Guideline for Practitioners,* published in 1989 by Trivirum Publishing Co.

Great care has been taken to maintain the accuracy of the information contained in the volume. However, neither Raven Press nor the editors can be held responsible for errors or for any consequences arising from the use of the information contained herein.

9 8 7 6 5 4 3 2 1

Contents

Contributing Authors

H. Branch Coslett, M.D., *Professor, Department of Neurology, Temple University School of Medicine, 3401 North Broad Street, Philadelphia, Pennsylvania 19140*

David L. Daniels, M.D., *Professor, Department of Radiology, Medical College of Wisconsin, 8700 West Wisconsin Avenue, Milwaukee, Wisconsin 53226*

Michael D. Devous, Sr., Ph.D., *Associate Professor, Department of Radiology, and Associate Director, Nuclear Medicine Center, The University of Texas Southwestern Medical Center, 5323 Harry Hines Boulevard, Dallas, Texas 75235*

Robert S. Hellman, M.D., *Associate Professor, Department of Radiology, Section of Nuclear Medicine, Medical College of Wisconsin, 8700 West Wisconsin Avenue, Milwaukee, Wisconsin 53226*

Leighton P. Mark, M. D., *Associate Professor, Department of Radiology, Medical College of Wisconsin, 8700 West Wisconsin Avenue, Milwaukee, Wisconsin 53226*

Charles R. Noback, Ph.D., *Professor Emeritus, Department of Anatomy, Columbia University College of Physicians and Surgeons, 222 West 168th Street, New York, New York 10032*

R. Anthony O'Connell, M.D., *Professor of Clinical Psychiatry, New York Medical College, Valhalla, New York; Clinical Director, Department of Psychiatry, St. Vincent's Hospital and Medical Center, 153 West 11th Street, New York, New York 10011*

Alan B. Rubens, M.D., *Professor and Head, Department of Neurology, University of Arizona College of Medicine, 1501 North Campbell, Tucson, Arizona 85724*

Ronald S. Tikofsky, Ph.D., *Research Associate Professor of Radiology, Department of Radiology, Section of Nuclear Medicine, Medical College of Wisconsin, 8700 West Wisconsin Avenue, Milwaukee, Wisconsin 53226*

Ronald L. Van Heertum, M.D., *Professor of Clinical Radiology and Vice-Chairman, Department of Radiology, Columbia University College of Physicians and Surgeons, 177 Fort Washington Avenue, New York, New York 10032*

Preface

Significant advances in functional brain imaging using single photon emission tomography (SPECT) have taken place since the original publication of *Advances in Cerebral SPECT Imaging: An Atlas and Guideline for Practitioners* in 1989. These advances include the introduction of new radiopharmaceuticals and instruments for performing SPECT brain imaging studies. As a result of these developments, members of the nuclear medicine community are increasingly being called upon to perform rCBF/SPECT studies.

In addition, there has been an explosion of papers focusing on the clinical applications of rCBF/SPECT. It is now nearly impossible to provide readers with a complete and comprehensive compilation of references pertaining to rCBF/SPECT brain imaging. Findings pertinent to the clinical application of rCBF/SPECT brain imaging are being published in an increasingly diverse range of scientific journals. This has led to greater awareness of the role of rCBF/SPECT brain imaging as a viable tool for the evaluation of patients with a wide range of neurologic and psychiatric disease states.

This new edition, while containing many of the original cases, has been greatly expanded. We have increased the number of cases to enable the imaging physician to see the variety of patterns that can occur within a given disease state. There is also a wide representation of imaging instruments and laboratories included in the text. Both color and black and white images are presented. Wherever possible, data pertinent to the method of image acquisition and processing is included with the case studies. Images obtained with single-head, multi-detector, and dedicated imaging systems are presented. Studies using IMP, HMPAO, and ECD (not yet FDA approved) are included. Interpretation of the studies are drawn from the reports provided by the contributing laboratories.

In addition to the greatly increased number of case studies included in Chapters 5-10, the text has also been expanded. A chapter on instrumentation, radiopharmaceuticals, and processing has been included. The chapters introducing the illustrations of the disease states have also been expanded. These emendations to the original text should provide those new to functional brain imaging, and the more experienced imaging clinician, with a broad-based foundation from which to approach the interpretation of rCBF/SPECT studies. This revised text should also provide nonimaging referring clinicians (neurologists, psychiatrists, neurosurgeons, physiatrists, and psychologists) with a better understanding of how they might better utilize this nuclear medicine procedure in their practice.

rCBF/SPECT brain imaging is a dynamic component of nuclear medicine practice and research. It is anticipated that developments in the area of receptor imaging, activation, and assessment of various forms of treatment will require future revisions of the present text. The authors hope that the present revision will serve to further enhance the practice and development of rCBF/SPECT brain imaging.

Ronald L. Van Heertum
Ronald S. Tikofsky

Acknowledgments

We would like to extend our appreciation to all those physicians, radiologists, and technicians who, in using SPECT, have contributed to its present state. Their continuing efforts—and those of the researchers advancing our knowledge in the field of functional brain imaging—will ensure the expanding clinical applications of this procedure.

We would also like to give special thanks to Dr. Robert S. Hellman of the Medical College of Wisconsin for his assistance in reviewing images and technical text, to Ms. Ann Voslar, CNMT at the Medical College of Wisconsin, for her work in processing many of the images in the text, to Robert J. Demarest for his outstanding artwork, and to Bridget Tamen and Rita Tikofsky for many hours of typing case histories and serving as contact person with manufacturers and contributing physicians. We would also like to acknowledge the cooperation of our colleagues who provided us with cases for this edition. Thanks too to Craig Percy of Raven Press for his assistance in producing this volume.

Finally to our wives, Jacqueline and Rita, and our children for their patience and forbearance. To them we dedicate this work.

Ronald L. Van Heertum
Ronald S. Tikofsky

Cerebral SPECT Imaging

Second Edition

SECTION I

General Aspects of SPECT Imaging

Cerebral SPECT Imaging, Second Edition,
edited by R.L. Van Heertum and R.S. Tikofsky.
Raven Press, Ltd., New York © 1995.

CHAPTER 1

Instrumentation, Radiopharmaceuticals, and Technical Factors

Michael D. Devous, Sr.

Functional brain imaging refers to that set of techniques used to derive images reflecting biochemical, physiologic, or electrical properties of the CNS. The most developed of these techniques are single-photon emission computed tomography (SPECT), positron emission tomography (PET), and topographic electroencephalography (TEEG). Of these three, SPECT has matured latest, but may offer the most widely available *and* widely applicable measure of neuronal behavior. Some recent reviews may be of interest to the reader (1–9).

Late maturation is likely the consequence of three factors. First, instrumentation for brain SPECT was initially substantially inferior to that of PET. Although PET still provides the highest resolution tomographic images of brain function, modern SPECT images have similar resolution, making any differences relatively inconsequential in clinical application. Second, radiopharmaceuticals for brain SPECT lagged behind those for PET. This is still true today, but the variety of both perfusion and receptor tracers for SPECT is expanding rapidly. The lack of a direct SPECT measure of metabolism is now the only significant difference between SPECT and PET tracers. Since perfusion and metabolism are tightly coupled in the CNS under most normal and pathologic circumstances, this difference may also be of no great clinical relevance. Furthermore, there are early reports of ^{123}I-labeled glucose analogs and of SPECT ligands that bind to hypoxic tissue. Should such tracers reach clinical utility, they would provide the currently missing metabolic markers. Third, the incorporation of SPECT brain imaging into clinical practice has been slow due to limited collaboration between the nuclear medicine and referent communities. Far greater collaboration will be required in the future to permit brain SPECT to achieve its full level of clinical utility.

This chapter provides an overview of the technical aspects of SPECT functional brain imaging, referring primarily to the most common SPECT brain function measure, regional cerebral blood flow (rCBF). SPECT images of rCBF are influenced by a number of factors separate from pathology, including (a) the quality of the tomographic device; (b) the radiopharmaceutical employed; (c) environmental conditions at the time of radiotracer administration; (d) characteristics of the subject (e.g., age, gender, handedness, etc.); (e) the format used for image presentation; and (f) image processing techniques. All but the last aspect are reviewed in this chapter. Image processing per se is not covered since the considerable variety in the details of various methods (e.g., filter choices, methods of reconstruction, attenuation and scatter correction schemes, etc.) is beyond the scope of this chapter. The reader is referred to available reviews (4, 10–14).

INSTRUMENTATION

Tremendous growth in instrumentation has resulted in commercially available, high-quality tomographs for SPECT brain imaging. SPECT instruments developed by university-based research paved the way for current devices. Once SPECT imaging emerged as a viable clinical entity, commercial involvement in tomograph development ensued. Cooperative ventures between academic centers and industry ultimately resulted in the excellent SPECT devices presently on the market. These fall into two categories: non-camera-based and camera-based systems.

M. D. Devous, Sr: Nuclear Medicine Center and Department of Radiology, The University of Texas Southwestern Medical Center, Dallas, Texas 75235.

Non-Camera-Based Systems

Non-camera-based systems include rotating detector arrays, multidetector scanners, and fixed rings. The rotating detector array group includes the Tomomatic two-, three-, and five-slice machines (Medimatic, Inc.) and the Hitachi four-head system. The Tomomatic's most characteristic attribute is that it is capable of ^{133}Xe SPECT, which requires very high sensitivity and the capacity for rapid dynamic imaging (i.e., complete tomographic studies every 10 sec)(11,15). Figure 1.1 shows two transverse slices from a normal volunteer ^{133}Xe SPECT study, with low flow in the cool end of the color scale increasing to high flow in the warm end. The advantage of ^{133}Xe SPECT is that it yields absolute quantitation of rCBF in ml/min/100 g tissue. The Tomomatic, by changing collimators, can also produce images of relatively high resolution (9–10 mm) using ^{99m}Tc hexamethylpropyleneamine-oxime (HMPAO) or ^{123}I *N*-isopropyl-*P*-iodoamphetamine (IMP). Collimator exchange is not difficult, permitting case-by-case selection between ^{133}Xe and high-resolution scans. The Hitachi rotating detector array system is also capable of both ^{133}Xe and high-resolution (8–10 mm; Fig. 1.2) static imaging (16).

Fixed-ring systems are also commercially available. The original fixed-detector research systems were the SPRINT (17), the HEADTOME (18), and the MUMPI (19). They were designed with fixed detectors or a circular annulus of sodium iodide with an internally rotating collimator. There are two commercially available versions. The Shimadzu (HEADTOME) system, available only in Japan, is capable of high-sensitivity ^{133}Xe studies and moderate resolution (10–12 mm) imaging using ^{123}I or ^{99m}Tc. The most widely available is the ASPECT (20), first of the fixed sodium-iodide annulus/rotating collimator machines to come to commercial production. It yields high-resolution images (8–10 mm), and may soon be capable of ^{133}Xe dynamic SPECT.

The original multidetector scanner was developed by Stoddart and colleagues (21). It was then called the Harvard multidetector scanner (22) and is now commercially available from Strichman, Inc. This is a slice-based tomograph, as are the Hitachi, Shimadzu, and Tomomatic, but it is built with very thick crystals that operate much like pinhole cameras as they traverse through space to obtain tomographic data. Hill and colleagues (23) have demonstrated that this device can image ^{18}F in a single-photon (not PET) mode, as well as ^{99m}Tc and ^{123}I. It cannot perform ^{133}Xe SPECT.

Gamma-Camera-Based Systems

Gamma-camera-based systems are more prevalent today than dedicated tomographs, primarily because they can do both head and body SPECT. There are two forms: single-head and multihead systems. Modern single-head tomographs have overcome many of the limitations of the original systems, such as poor head alignment, magnetic field aberrations, and inadequate uniformity and linearity for tomography. A few systems have also been designed to circumvent shoulders so that minimal radius scanning is possible. Most of these systems provide high-resolution

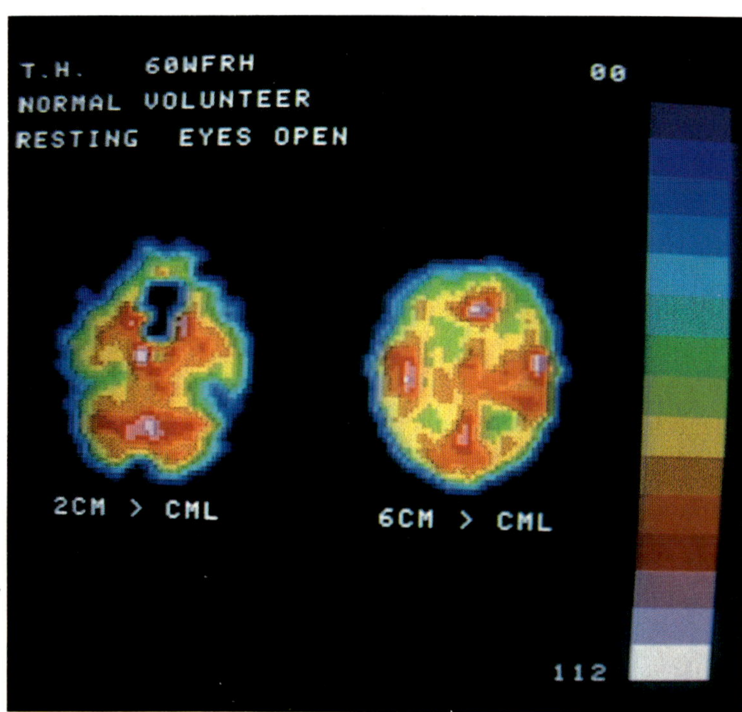

FIG. 1.1. Transverse rCBF images obtained by ^{133}Xe SPECT and the Tomomatic 64 (Medimatic A/S, Copenhagen). Images are obtained 2 and 6 cm above and parallel to the canthomeatal line (CML). The 16-shade color scale displays rCBF in ml/min/100 g. Images are displayed with the subject's left on the viewer's left, while images from all other scanners used in this chapter are in the more conventional left-on-right format.

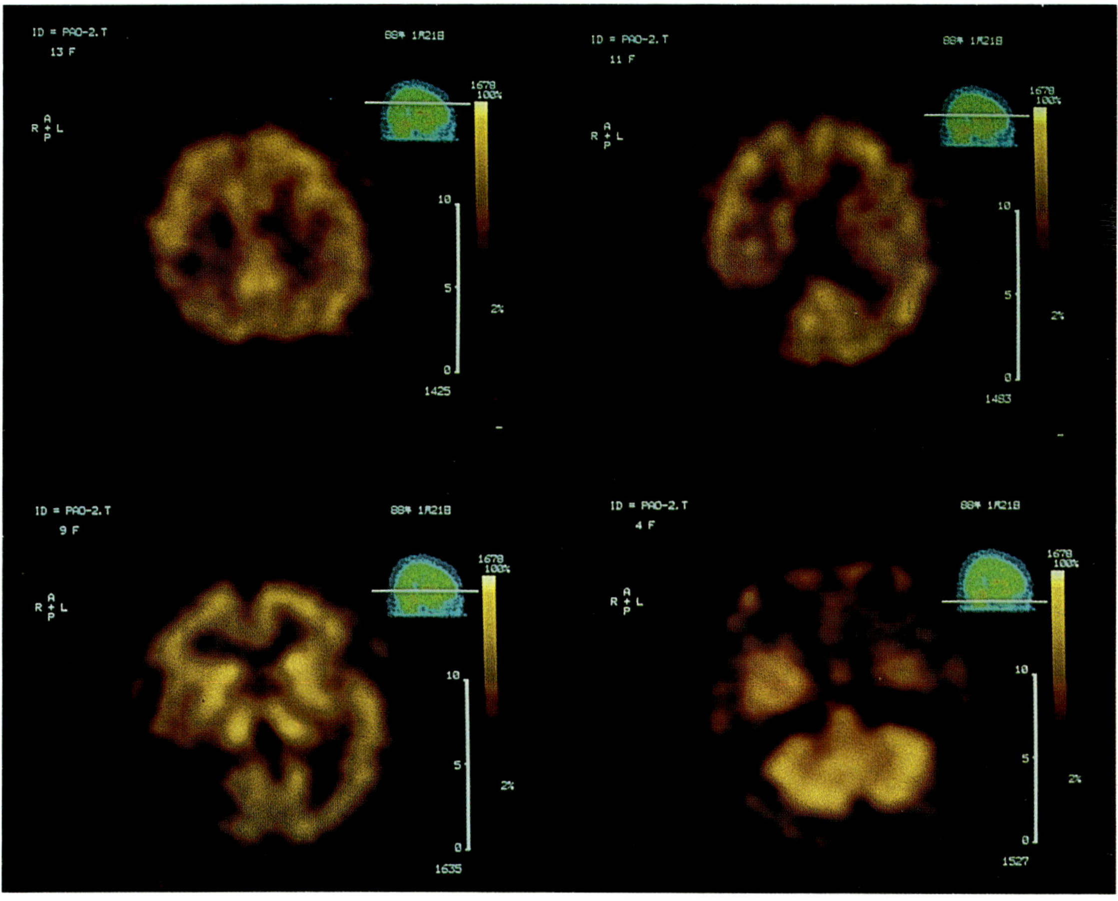

FIG. 1.2. High-resolution rCBF images obtained in a stroke patient with the Hitachi four-head dedicated SPECT unit using ^{99m}Tc HMPAO. (Images provided courtesy of Hitachi.)

images with static tracers (7–10 mm). Unfortunately, single-head systems suffer from poor sensitivity and prolonged imaging times.

A collaborative team from The University of Texas Southwestern Medical Center at Dallas and the nuclear engineering division of Technicare developed the first three-head gamma-camera-based SPECT system to address the limited sensitivity of single-head systems (24). This collaboration yielded a system capable of both head and body SPECT at high resolution with static tracers and with adequate sensitivity and rotation speed for dynamic tomography with ^{133}Xe (Fig. 1.3). The first three-head system (PRISM) was installed in Dallas in late 1987 under the sponsorship of Ohio Imaging, now a division of Picker. Additional three-head SPECT instruments have been produced by Trionix (also as a byproduct of the collaboration mentioned above), Toshiba, and General Electric. A prototype three-head instrument from Siemens is also under evaluation. Three-head SPECT systems currently are the most sophisticated instruments for brain SPECT. There are approximately 350 such units installed, indicating increasing acceptance of this technology. The tomographs from Picker and Trionix are coupled to sophisticated computer

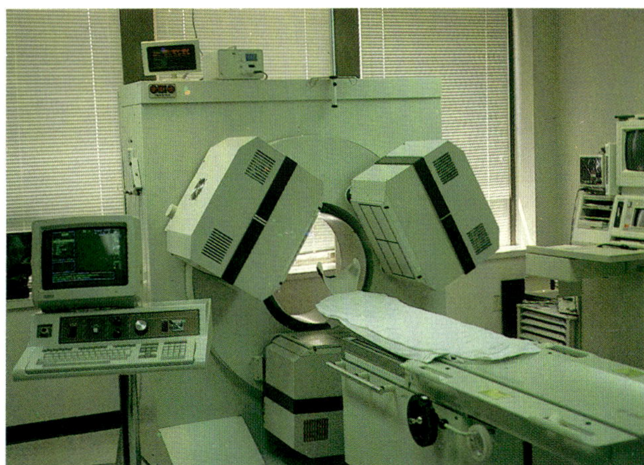

FIG. 1.3. The PRISM three-headed SPECT unit (Picker, Cleveland, OH) which can be used to obtain both high-resolution rCBF images with static tracers and fully quantitative rCBF images with ^{133}Xe.

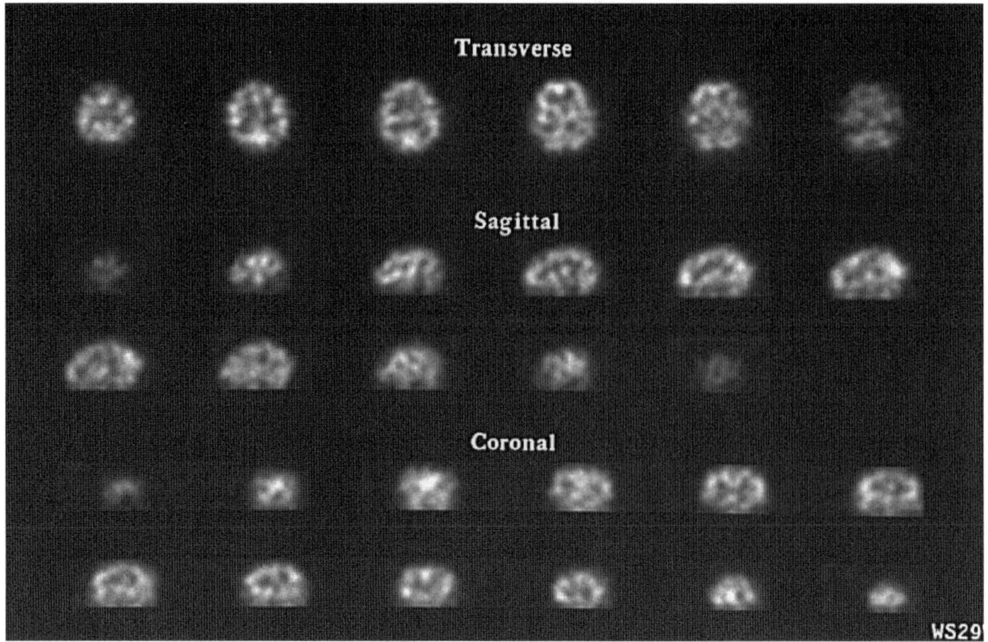

FIG. 1.4. Quantitative (ml/min/100 g) dynamic rCBF images obtained using ^{133}Xe and the PRISM 3000S. Images were obtained in 4 min, including 1 min of washin and 3 min of washout of the inert gas tracer.

systems facilitating image processing, analysis, and display. The first ^{133}Xe SPECT images in humans from a three-head system (PRISM) were produced in late 1992 by the Dallas group (Fig. 1.4).

State-of-the-art SPECT systems can be expected to provide high-resolution (6–9 mm) imaging of statically distributed brain radiopharmaceuticals with patient imaging times of 10–20 min (Fig. 1.5). Systems should also be capable of sequential image acquisitions, that is, it should be possible to acquire multiple short studies back to back and subsequently discard segments degraded by patient motion. Software should support dynamic filtering, multiple angle (oblique) reconstructions, surface-variable attenuation correction, and three-dimensional as well as conventional cross-sectional displays (Fig. 1.6). All of the currently available three-head systems offer excellent spatial resolution: 6-mm resolution in the cortex, and about 7 mm at the center of the brain, with appropriate collimators and ^{99m}Tc HMPAO. Unfortunately, the photon flux with ^{123}I IMP is reduced, requiring careful image processing to achieve equivalent spatial resolution.

Dual-Isotope Imaging

Finally, SPECT systems should have adequate energy resolution and multiple-energy-window capability in order to separate ^{99m}Tc and ^{123}I radiotracers in the same patient (Fig. 1.7). While typical gamma-camera energy resolution [12 to 15 percent full-width half-maximum (FWHM)]is insufficient to separate 140-keV (^{99m}Tc) from 159-keV (^{123}I) photopeaks, high-resolution multidetector SPECT units have substantially improved energy resolution. Our group examined the effect of dual-isotope imaging on isotope discrimination as a function of window width and position and on quantitative count recovery using the PRISM 3000 (Picker International) (25). Simultaneous dual-isotope imaging of phantoms separated isotope distributions for 10% asymmetric and for 15% or 10% centered ^{99m}Tc windows when combined with a 10% asymmetric ^{123}I window. Isotope concentrations were recovered as accurately from asymmetric dual-isotope windows as from conventional or asymmetric single-isotope windows.

We also applied this technique to the simultaneous measurement of resting rCBF and changes induced by vasodilation (1 g acetazolamide) in ten subjects with cerebrovascular disease (26). Resting and vasodilated ^{133}Xe SPECT images were compared with resting (^{99m}Tc HMPAO) and postacetazolamide [^{123}I IMP or *N,N,N′*-trimethyl-*N′*-(2 hydroxy-3-methyl-5-iodobenzyl)-1,3-propanediamine 2 HCl (HIPDM)]dual-isotope images (Fig. 1.8). Regression analyses demonstrated a linear relationship between ^{133}Xe SPECT and dual-isotope SPECT measurements of lesion/cerebellum ratios in baseline ($r = 0.92$), vasodilated ($r = 0.86$), and rest-minus-vasodilated data ($r = 0.85$). A further advantage of the dual-isotope technique is that ^{99m}Tc and ^{123}I images obtained through dual-isotope imaging are by definition in perfect anatomic registration.

In summary, this technique permits simultaneous imaging of ^{99m}Tc- and ^{123}I-labeled brain radiopharmaceuticals

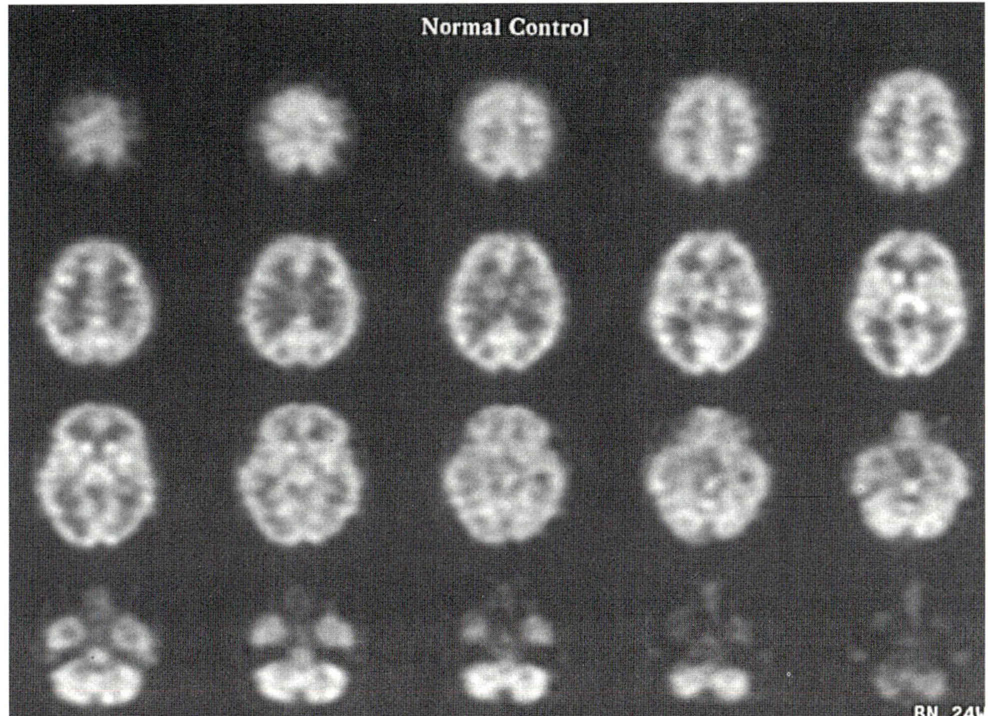

FIG. 1.5. Typical high-resolution rCBF SPECT images obtained using ^{99m}Tc HMPAO and the PRISM 3000S tomograph in a normal volunteer.

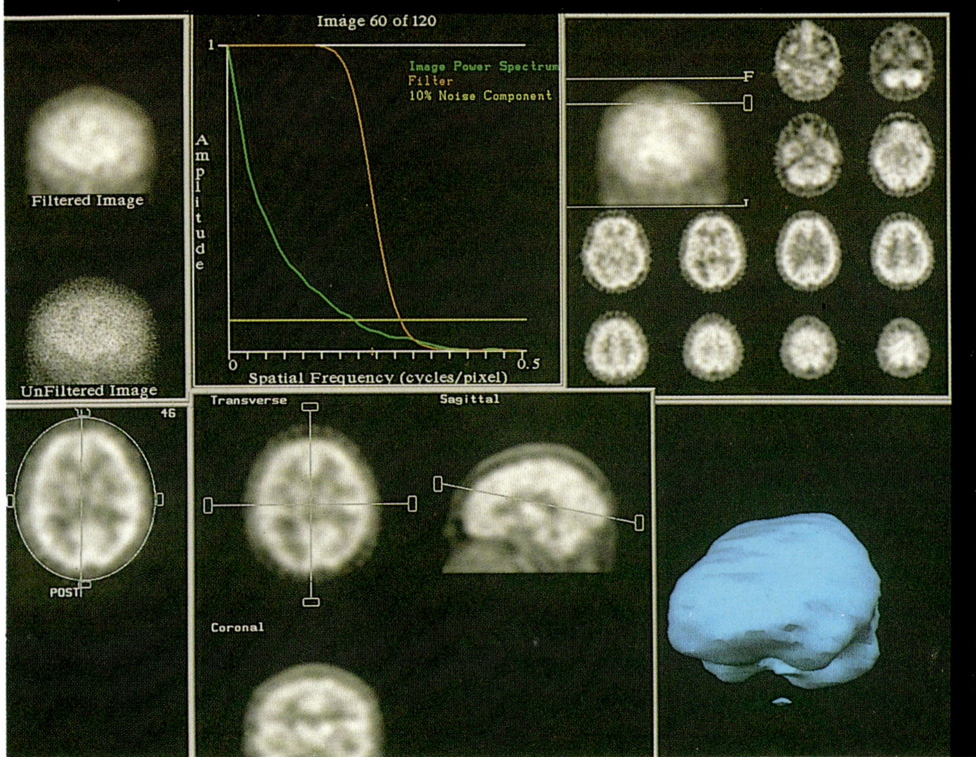

FIG. 1.6. Typical image processing applications that should be available on all SPECT instruments. **Upper row: left:** Fourier-space filtering; **center:** patient-specific filter design; **right:** back-projection reconstruction. **Lower row: left:** adjustable attenuation correction; **center:** oblique angle reconstruction; **right:** three-dimensional display.

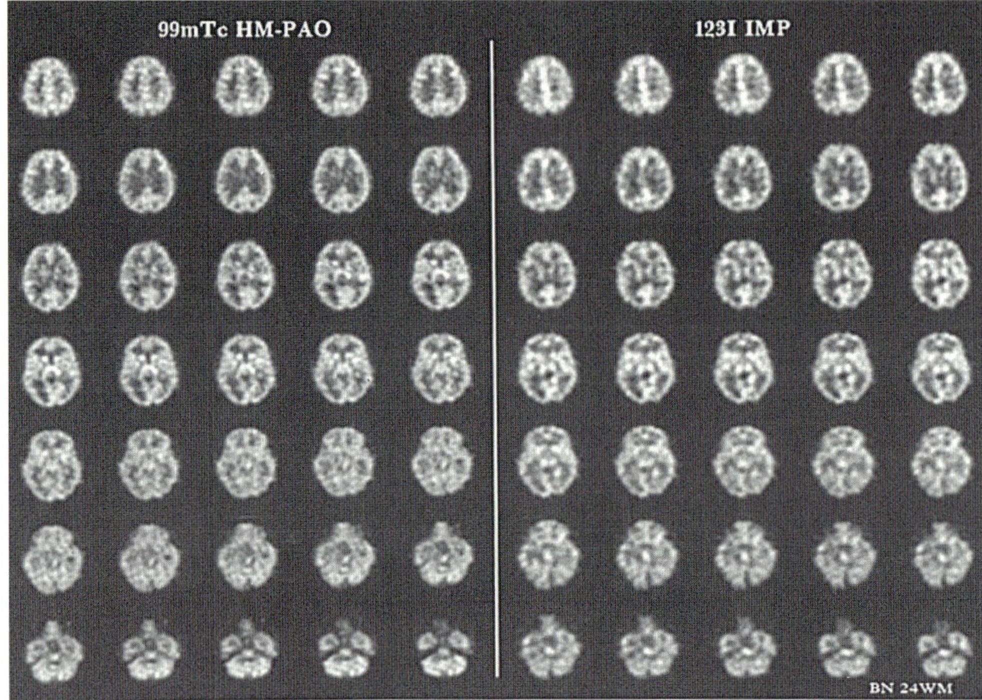

FIG. 1.7. Dual-isotope rCBF images in a normal volunteer demonstrating high-resolution images obtained with this technique for both ^{99m}Tc HMPAO and ^{123}I IMP.

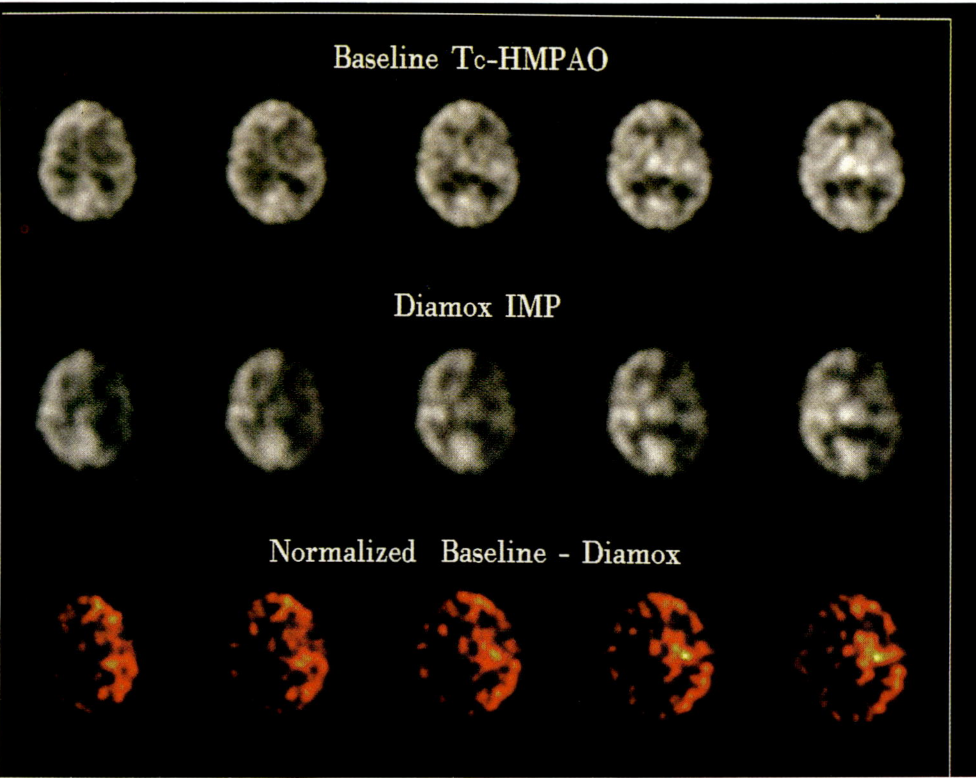

FIG. 1.8. Dual-isotope rCBF images in a patient with transient ischemic attacks (TIAs) demonstrating failed vasodilator reserve. Baseline study (^{99m}Tc HMPAO, **top row**) shows only mild left frontal hypoperfusion, while extensive reserve failure (^{123}I IMP, **middle row**) is seen after vasodilation with acetazolamide (Diamox). The distribution of failed reserve is seen in the subtraction images (**bottom row**), which are easily obtained since the dual-isotope technique produces image sets that are in perfect anatomic registration.

administered to a single subject. While we have documented the effectiveness of this technique in monitoring vasodilatory reserve (26), it should be possible to monitor any circumstance potentially producing a change in the perfusion state within 24 hr due to the *in vivo* stability of ^{99m}Tc HMPAO. Additional applications for dual-isotope imaging include ictal/interictal seizure imaging, monitoring acute therapeutic interventions, and single-session evaluations of cognitive or pharmaceutical challenge tests. Similarly, it would be possible to use this technique in receptor modeling studies by directly measuring rCBF (normally deduced by assumption) with a ^{99m}Tc-labeled flow tracer, while simultaneously using an ^{123}I-labeled receptor ligand.

Modern SPECT instruments have high resolution, reliable performance, and low cost. They function as full-volume imaging devices yielding multiple angle cross-sectional displays and true three-dimensional representations. Their computer systems provide potent image processing power and valuable flexibility. Some of these tomographs provide imaging opportunities (e.g., dual-isotope) not possible with PET systems. Consequently SPECT imaging can no longer be viewed as a poor man's PET, but as a mature technology.

RADIOPHARMACEUTICALS

Several ^{99m}Tc- and ^{123}I-labeled radiopharmaceuticals for the SPECT measurement of rCBF have been developed. It is also possible to measure regional cerebral blood volume (rCBV) using SPECT techniques. Receptor imaging with SPECT is still primarily a research tool, although at least one agent for D_2 receptor studies is commercially available in Europe (^{123}I IBZM). SPECT agents for D_1 dopaminergic, serotonergic, noradrenergic, cholinergic and gamma-aminobutyric acid (GABA)ergic receptor systems are in various stages of testing. At this moment there is no tracer for the measurement of cerebral metabolism by SPECT. However, two metabolism-related SPECT measurements can be made. The rCBF/rCBV ratio can be measured directly and is related to regional oxygen extraction. Also, several groups have recently tested a class of ^{99m}Tc- and ^{123}I-labeled agents that permit detection of hypoxic cerebral tissues.

Xenon 133

^{133}Xe, of course, is the original noninvasive brain blood flow marker (27–29). It has been in clinical use for several decades, and still has significant value (4,11). The cerebral transit of ^{133}Xe is very rapid, requiring complete tomographic scans every 10 sec to obtain accurate reconstructions (15). It undergoes no chemical interaction in the brain because it is an inert gas. The input function (i.e., the rate of arterial delivery to the brain), which must be known to measure rCBF quantitatively, can be easily measured by placing a scintillation probe over the lungs. SPECT studies of the transit of ^{133}Xe, when combined with a measure of the input function, can be fit to a mathematical model yielding quantitative estimates of brain blood flow (11,30–32). Unfortunately, the high sensitivity required for dynamic scanning has usually been obtained by sacrificing spatial resolution. Since ^{133}Xe has a short *biological* half-life, you can repeat examinations about every 15 min. For example, Fig. 1.9 shows ^{133}Xe rCBF scans in resting and

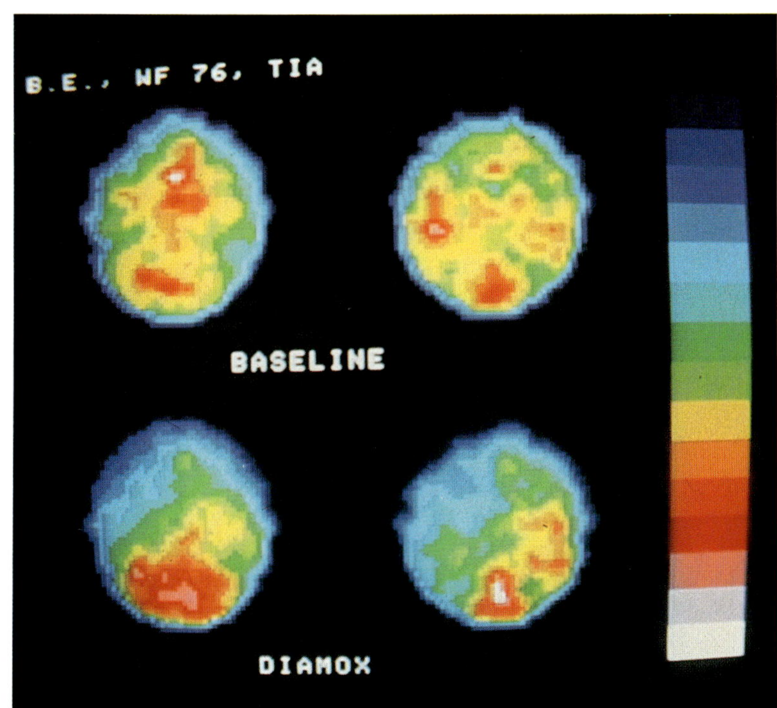

FIG. 1.9. Failed vasodilator reserve illustrated using ^{133}Xe SPECT and the Tomomatic 64 scanner in a 76-year-old woman suffering from TIAs. **Upper images** (2 and 6 cm above the CML) obtained in the resting state are nearly normal, while the **lower images,** obtained after vasodilation with Diamox, show middle and anterior cerebral artery reserve failure. Post-Diamox images were obtained 30 min after the resting study.

post-Diamox states from an elderly woman with transient ischemic attacks (TIAs). Images are relatively normal at baseline, but the scan obtained 15 min later after vasodilation with Diamox identifies an extensive area of failed vasodilatory reserve. Short imaging times and rapid isotope clearance greatly facilitate rest and stress brain imaging. In addition, the entire SPECT acquisition process is accomplished in 4 min, an important feature for difficult, uncooperative patients.

Static Tracers

All SPECT rCBF agents other than ^{133}Xe [e.g., IMP, HIPDM, HMPAO, and ethyl cysteinate dimer (ECD)]were designed for use with rotating gamma cameras, which have low sensitivity. Consequently, these agents must have a relatively stable *in vivo* distribution (at least 60 min). They are retained in brain (or at least diffusion from brain is hindered) by some trapping mechanism, such as metabolic degradation or conformational alteration. Such agents are commonly referred to as "chemical microspheres." Stable distribution permits prolonged imaging times (as long as the patient doesn't move) so that specialized collimators can be used to produce high-resolution images. While count ratios among brain regions correctly represent relative rCBF, most retention mechanisms do not lend themselves to simple mathematical models to provide absolute quantitation.

The original tracer microsphere model works reasonably well for IMP and HIPDM but not for ECD or HMPAO. More sophisticated models have been proposed, and one may ultimately prove to be effective. Unfortunately, these models depend on knowing the input function, which requires arterial blood sampling (not a routine practice in most nuclear medicine laboratories). If a simple method of measuring the input function is devised, then the microsphere-like compounds can be used to measure absolute rCBF as quantitatively as any other noninvasive modality (including PET).

Iodine 123 Regional Cerebral Blood Flow Tracers

The first rCBF agent for use on rotating gamma cameras was ^{123}I IMP, followed almost immediately by ^{123}I HIPDM. IMP (Spectamine) was developed by Winchell et al. (33) at MediPhysics, and HIPDM (Fig. 1.10) was developed by Kung et al. (34) at SUNY. Both are iodinated amines with fairly rapid brain uptake and good extraction. HIPDM has a 6 hour brain retention half-life. IMP has a much shorter brain retention half-life (on the order of 60–90 min). Both IMP (35–38) and HIPDM (39) follow higher cerebral blood flow levels more accurately than either HMPAO or ECD.

Some investigators have compared initial (early) with delayed IMP images (usually a 4-hr delay) to determine if changes in distribution over time relate to tissue status (3,6,7,40). This procedure is commonly referred to as redistribution imaging. Some reports suggest that filling in (redistribution) of lesions seen in early images is indicative of salvageable tissue. Current literature is contradictory, neither clearly supporting nor refuting the value of redistribution imaging with IMP.

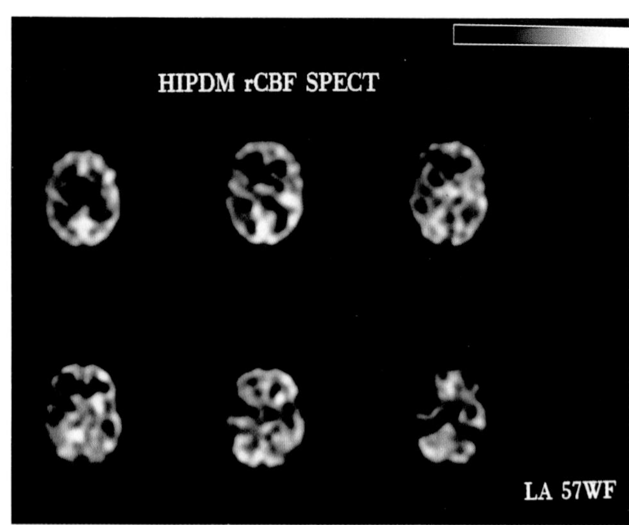

FIG. 1.10. SPECT rCBF images in a stroke patient obtained using ^{123}I HIPDM.

Technetium 99m Regional Cerebral Blood Flow Tracers

Investigators at Amersham (39,41) as well as Volkert et al. (42) at the University of Missouri developed the first of the technetium agents approved by the Food and Drug Administration (FDA) for use in humans, ^{99m}Tc HMPAO (Ceretec). ^{99m}Tc-ECD (Neurolite), of a class suggested by Kung et al. (43) and developed by DuPont (44,45) is under FDA review. Both agents have good brain uptake. The extraction of ECD is slightly lower, but the contrast (the gray-to-white matter ratio) is higher than for HMPAO. Both tracers image defects similarly, although there are suggestions that during luxury perfusion following stroke HMPAO will follow perfusion, while ECD will continue to show a defect at the site of injury. There is also a growing body of literature (mostly from Japan) that HMPAO and IMP mark somewhat different territories of damage in cerebrovascular disease (HMPAO underestimates IMP lesion size). Few data exist that compare ECD and IMP directly.

ECD may prove to be easier to use because HMPAO is unstable *in vitro* and requires freshly eluted $^{99m}TcO_4^-$. However, Amersham has a stabilized version of HMPAO (Fig. 1.11) under FDA review. ECD clears faster from the blood and from the body, consequently producing less radi-

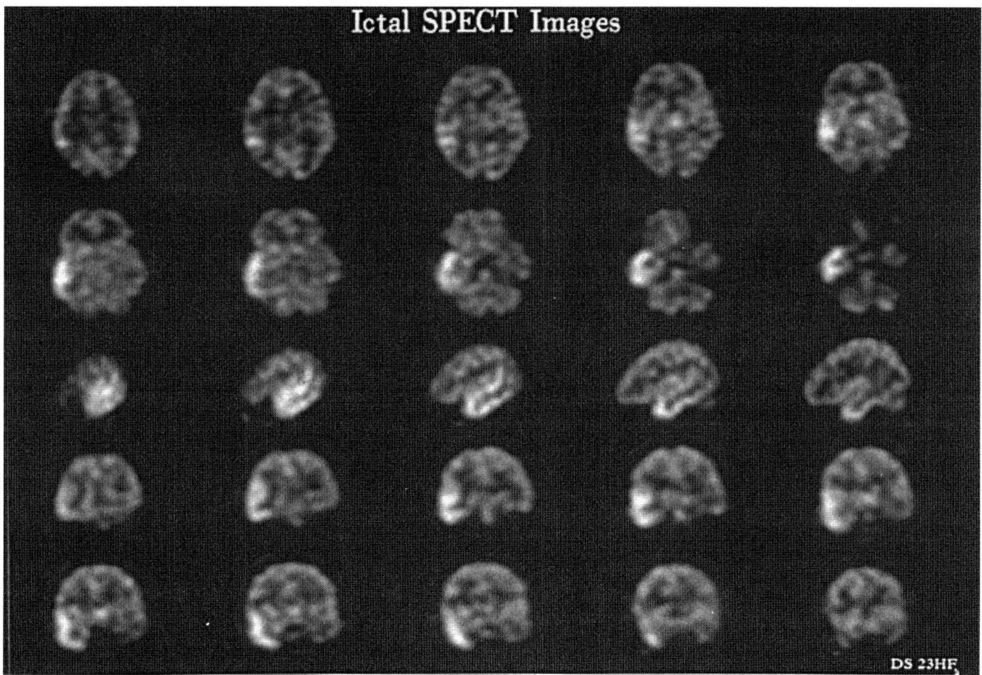

FIG. 1.11. Ictal rCBF SPECT images obtained in an epilepsy patient with complex partial seizures of temporal lobe origin using the stabilized form of ^{99m}Tc HMPAO.

ation exposure per mCi administered than HMPAO. In general, image contrast with ECD is superior to that with HMPAO, but recent studies with HMPAO obtained more than 90 min after injection demonstrate the potential for equivalent contrast (Fig. 1.5).

We have directly compared ^{99m}Tc ECD with ^{133}Xe SPECT in patients (46). On the left of Fig. 1.12 is a circumferential profile of uptake ratios (to whole brain) from regions of interest about 4 cm in size. The squares represent the ^{133}Xe data, and the ECD data are marked by asterisks. These were obtained with the same collimator at the same resolution without moving the subject between studies. In these data from 20 subjects the concordance of ECD and ^{133}Xe is quite striking. When the same data are displayed in a linear regression format (right side of Fig. 1.12), a strong linear relationship can be seen. ECD follows ^{133}Xe flow up to fairly high levels (80 ml/min/100 g). We recently obtained similar results in a comparison of ^{99m}Tc HMPAO to ^{133}Xe.

Regional Cerebral Blood Volume

Under most circumstances, cerebral blood flow is tightly coupled to tissue metabolism. However, rCBF is not the

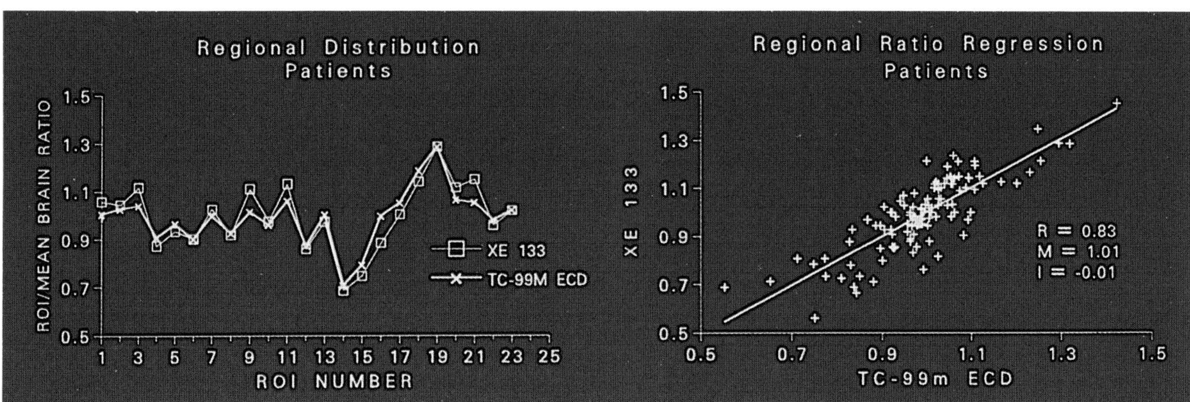

FIG. 1.12. A comparison of the distribution of rCBF measured with either ^{133}Xe or ^{99m}Tc ECD. ECD demonstrates a linear relation to true rCBF (^{133}Xe) up to flow levels of at least 80 ml/min/100 g.

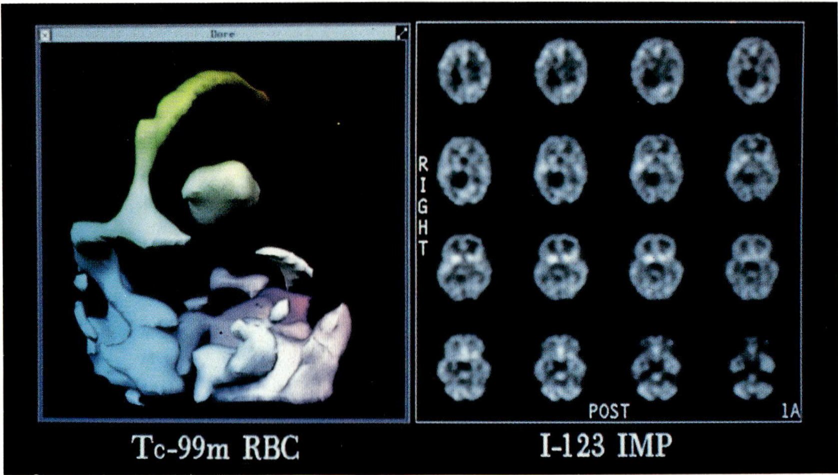

FIG. 1.13. Dual-isotope images of regional cerebral blood volume (rCBV) obtained with ^{99m}Tc-labeled red blood cells (**left image,** a three-dimensional right posterior oblique view) and rCBF obtained using ^{123}I IMP (**right image,** transverse cross sections) in a patient with an arteriovenous malformation (AVM). The AVM appears as a large mass just anterior to the descending sagittal sinus in the rCBV image, while it appears as a defect in the rCBF images since it does not retain the perfusion tracer.

only hemodynamic parameter that affects tissue metabolism. Regional cerebral blood volume and the extraction of oxygen can be important determinants of nutrient availability. Although direct measures of oxygen metabolism or extraction are not available by SPECT, the ratio of rCBF to rCBV is related to the regional oxygen extraction ratio (rOER). Thus an estimate of the rOER can be obtained from the rCBF/rCBV ratio (47). Regional cerebral blood volume imaging is conducted in a manner analogous to cardiac blood pool imaging: red cells are labeled with ^{99m}Tc, followed by static SPECT of the head. Quantitative values are obtained by SPECT imaging of a reference blood sample drawn from the subject at the time of rCBV imaging (48–51). The dual-isotope technique can be used to image rCBF and rCBV simultaneously (Fig. 1.13).

Receptor Imaging

Neuroreceptor imaging currently has no proven clinical role. However, early clinical trials and extensive PET experience suggest that SPECT imaging using specific receptor binding agents may soon find major clinical application. Radioligands are currently under study in human trials for quantitating dopaminergic (D_1 and D_2) (52), serotonergic (5-HT_2), benzodiazepine (53), and muscarinic cholinergic (54,55) systems. Most such agents rely on ^{123}I as the radiolabel. While these compounds differ structurally from their native analogs, their affinity for the specific receptor site often exceeds that of the native compound. In addition to their high affinity for the receptor site, many of these agents also have high total brain uptake (on the order of 10 percent). Such uptake is comparable to that seen with blood flow agents.

Potential clinical applications for receptor imaging would include the diagnosis of specific neurodegenerative diseases, quantitative assessment of therapeutic interventions designed to alter receptor function, and evaluation of interventions capable of producing prophylaxis. Such applications, in combination with or separate from perfusion imaging, may be particularly of interest in the study of psychiatric disorders, which are so commonly responsive to neurotransmitter-active pharmaceuticals. Areas for further investigation necessary to make receptor imaging a practical clinical tool include the establishment of correlations between the binding site concentration and the disease process, as well as the development of more accurate methods for absolute quantitation of the distribution of brain radioactivity. Fortunately, Innis et al. (56) have demonstrated that at least receptor affinity can be determined from data reflecting only relative count density. Advances in receptor imaging are also hampered by the fact that many neurotransmitters bind to a family of receptors. Unless more specific ligands are developed, receptor imaging may not reach its full potential. Combined use of receptor, perfusion, and structural imaging in a coregistration paradigm would also greatly enhance the quantitative data available.

Metabolism

Metabolic aspects of neuronal function can not be directly imaged with SPECT. We have no oxygen analog, even on the horizon. Glucose metabolism has been monitored by PET with ^{18}fluorodeoxyglucose (FDG) for years; it has been suggested that it might be possible to iodinate glucose analogs for SPECT that would behave like ^{18}FDG.

While there have been two promising preliminary reports, neither has come to fruition at this time.

In summary, SPECT measures of rCBF are well developed, perhaps more developed than for PET. Both dynamic and static techniques are effective. SPECT can also be used to image rCBV, although clinical application of this technique has been minimal. There is great potential for receptor imaging, which has now moved out of the basic science laboratory and into clinical research. Recent interest in ^{201}Tl as a SPECT brain agent has developed because it has been shown to be useful in imaging brain tumor viability after radiation therapy (57–59) and in staging brain tumors (60–62). Lastly, progress is being made with glucose metabolic imaging at the animal level.

FACTORS THAT AFFECT IMAGE APPEARANCE

Environmental Conditions

The conditions experienced by a subject during radiotracer administration play a significant role in determining the observed rCBF distribution. The coupling of rCBF to regional metabolism has been frequently demonstrated under not only resting conditions, but also during cognitive or motoric activation (63–69). Thus visual, auditory, and somatosensory stimuli can all be expected to impact the regional level of neuronal activity and thus rCBF (Fig. 1.14). Unfortunately, there are no clearly established standards describing the ideal conditions for any of these environmental parameters. Most investigators use an "eyes and ears open" imaging environment in which subjects are seated during radiotracer injection, since data from our group and from others have shown that quantitative flow or metabolism values are less variable under such conditions than in the eyes and ears closed setting (11,70). Room lights are often dimmed to provide a minimum and relatively standard visual stimulus. The degree to which surrounding personnel provide both auditory and visual stimuli should be (though seldom is) carefully controlled.

The duration of steady-state conditions necessary to ensure minimal variability induced by environmental conditions is also not well established. To some degree this is a radiotracer-dependent issue. For example, ^{99m}Tc HMPAO has very rapid first-pass extraction, while a component of ^{123}I IMP is retained by lung and likely affects brain tracer distribution for 5–10 min after injection. Xenon 133 is a dynamic tracer that must be imaged during administration. In each case, the requirements vary for how long environmental conditions must be constant both before and after tracer administration. As a general rule, we require steady-state environmental conditions for 10 min prior to and after tracer administration for injectables. No requirement after administration is needed for ^{133}Xe.

Subject Characteristics

Age, gender, handedness, anxiety, time of day (diurnal variations), blood pressure, arterial carbon dioxide levels, cognitive involvement (attention), and other factors are subject-specific determinants of rCBF. While it is clear that

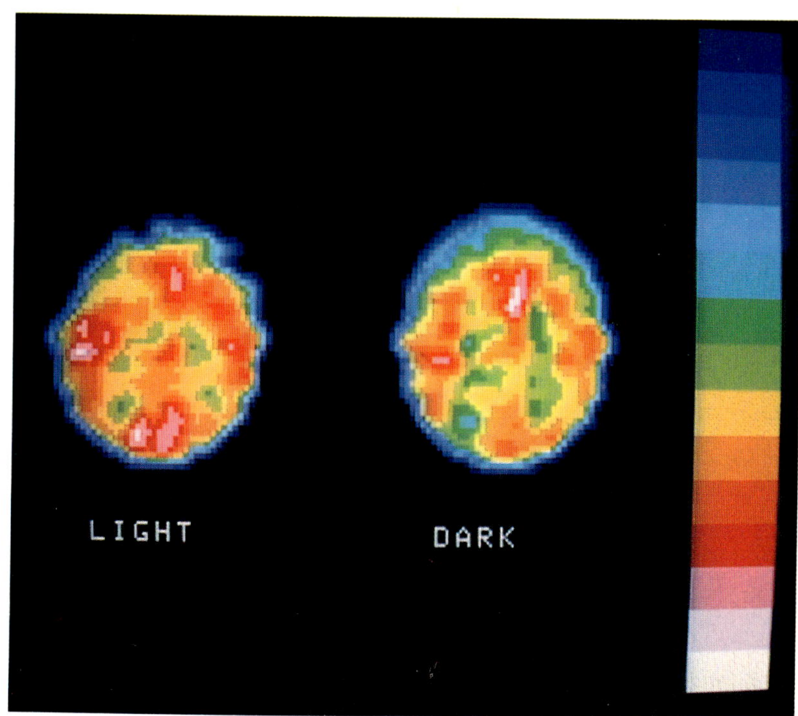

FIG. 1.14. The effect of visual stimulation on rCBF in a normal volunteer. Left image obtained in a dimly lit room in a subject with eyes and ears open. Right image obtained 20 min later in the same subject, now with eyes occluded and all room lights and machine lights turned off or covered. Note that perfusion decreases in the "dark" condition relative to the "light" condition not only in the primary visual cortex, but also in the associative cortices and in some remote areas as well.

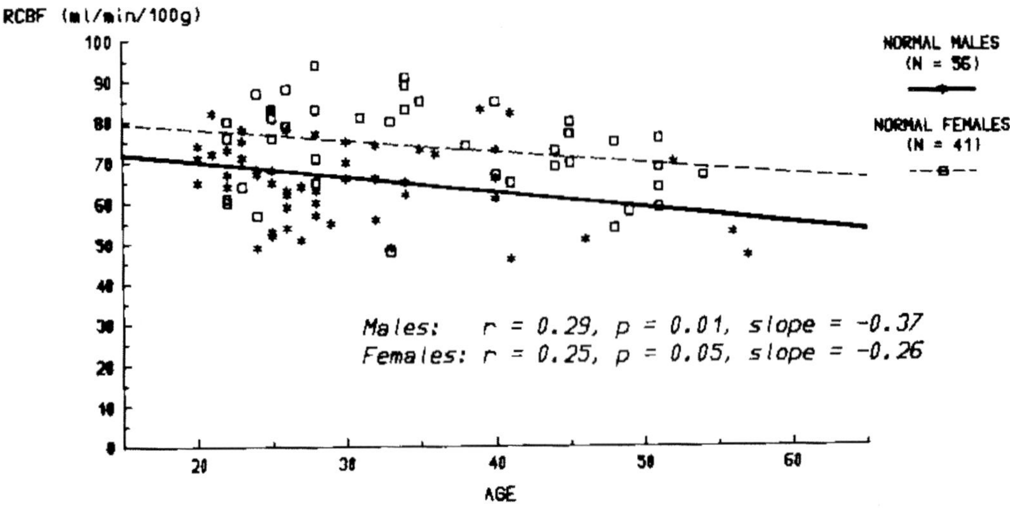

FIG. 1.15. Effect of age and gender on whole-brain rCBF as determined by ^{133}Xe SPECT. Note that rCBF declines with age for both genders, but is approximately 20 percent higher in females than in males across age.

there are both age (65,71–76) and gender (71,77–80) effects on whole brain blood flow (Fig. 1.15), regional effects are somewhat less well characterized (71,73,74,77, 78,80). Furthermore, recent studies suggest that these two factors affect rCBF in complex ways. For example, the decline in rCBF seen with age is not as marked in active elderly individuals as it is in age-matched inactive subjects (76). Also, gender effects seem dependent even on gender dominance within a particular gender (e.g., males with more feminine characteristics have higher flow than males with more masculine characteristics) (78).

Challenge Studies

Pharmacologic challenges induce alterations in rCBF that can provide both useful tools for the discrimination of disease and conundrums for image interpretation. For example, acetazolamide is a cerebral vasodilator commonly used in the determination of vasodilatory reserve (Figs. 1.8 and 1.9) (81–84). However, the consistency with which it alters or preserves regional patterns from a "resting" state is not well known. Caffeine, which may be present in subjects in various quantities, can lead to reductions in both global and regional CBF (85). The impact of other pharmacologic factors (e.g., antidepressants, antiepileptics, etc.) is only now being elucidated. It is advisable to eliminate all such complicating factors for as long as possible preceding a study. For caffeine, 24 hr may be effective. For antidepressants, drug clearance may not be complete for up to 14 days (86).

Cognitive challenges are also sources of valuable discrimination and unwanted variability. For example, mild visual stimulation (dimly lit room) seems to minimize variability among normals relative to deprivation of visual stimuli (11,70). However, specific visual stimuli can induce asymmetry (Fig. 1.16) and lead to activation not only of primary and associative visual cortices, but even of remote cortical and subcortical sites (67,87). Auditory stimuli must similarly be carefully controlled and evaluated (66,88). In general, consistency is the greatest asset, that is, study all subjects under as identical a set of conditions as possible.

Image Presentation

Recent advances in image processing instrumentation and SPECT tomographs have afforded the opportunity of presenting image data in a wide variety of formats. The degree to which conventional transverse cross-sectional images provide adequate information for image interpretation is being appropriately challenged. Sagittal, coronal, and other oblique angle reconstructions are readily produced by most computer systems. Experienced observers recognize that certain brain structures are more readily appreciated in nonconventional display orientations. For example, evaluation of the medial aspect of the orbital frontal cortex is more readily performed from sagittal cross sections than from transverse. Evaluation of mesial temporal lobe hypoperfusion in epilepsy is easiest in special oblique views designed to highlight the mesial temporal wall (Fig. 1.17)

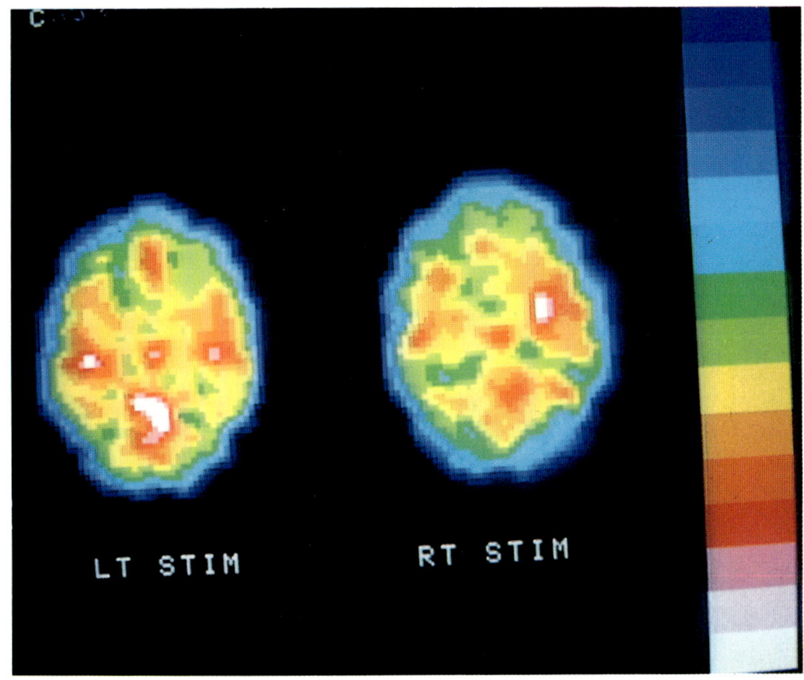

FIG. 1.16. Cognitive activation results in rCBF asymmetry. The "left" cognitive stimulus was a language task that actually resulted in bilateral activation of peri-sylvian sites, while the "right" task (facial discrimination) resulted in predominantly right-sided activation.

than in classic coronal, sagittal, or transverse views. It is wise to review studies in at least three orthogonal orientations.

Similarly, the modality employed for image review has a significant impact on interpretation. Conventional film-and-lightbox formats require the reviewer to consider all image data over a similar contrast range and often with a fixed degree of background subtraction. In contrast, direct viewing from a video display affords the opportunity for gray scale manipulation and dynamic background subtrac-

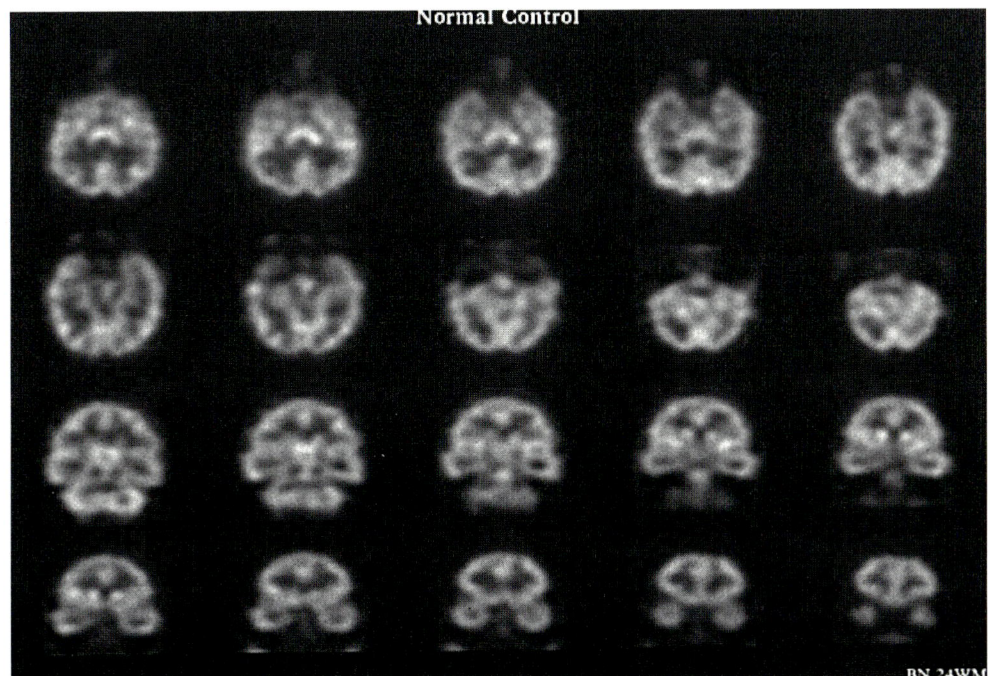

FIG. 1.17. Oblique cross-sectional views designed to facilitate visualization of the mesial temporal cortex. *Top two rows* are "transverse" sections cut parallel to the long axis of the temporal lobe; *bottom two rows* are "coronal" sections cut perpendicular to this same axis.

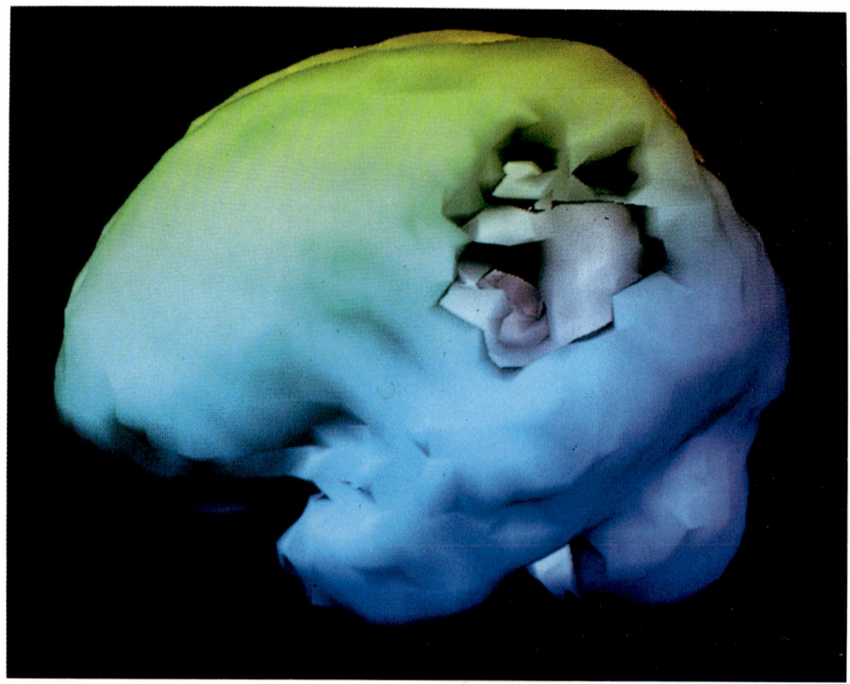

FIG. 1.18. Three-dimensional surface-rendered rCBF SPECT image in a patient with a left parietal stroke. Surface-rendered images are useful to assess the distribution (vascular territory) of cortical defects, but do not allow visualization of either defect magnitude (count density) or of subcortical abnormalities.

tion. Choosing between gray scale image displays and color image displays presents the viewer with yet another poorly defined dilemma. In general, most reviewers of high-resolution images prefer gray scales. The human visual system is better suited to gray scale discrimination across structural boundaries than it is to the same discrimination using a color-based scheme. However, with poorer resolution systems, or foreshortened image data sets (minimum pixel density), color scales can provide enhanced interpretation of abnormalities. Similarly, parametric displays in which color can be used to portray functional information may provide enhanced opportunities for lesion detection.

Recently, three-dimensional surface-rendered displays have become commonplace (Fig. 1.18), while more sophisticated three-dimensional displays of "see-through" or "smoked-glass" images are not as available (Fig. 1.19). The "dial-a-lesion" format of most surface-rendered images currently limits their routine applicability. Established standards for count-density threshold settings have not been published. Cinemagraphic displays of projection data also provide a certain three-dimensional quality. Their primary use is in monitoring patient motion as a source of image degradation.

Six conclusions can be drawn regarding image presentation.

1. SPECT rCBF studies should be presented in at least transverse, coronal, and sagittal cross sections.
2. The conditions under which subjects are studied should be established as a laboratory standard and maintained for all clinical and research studies. The most common standard is eyes and ears open in a dimly lit environment with minimal auditory "white noise."

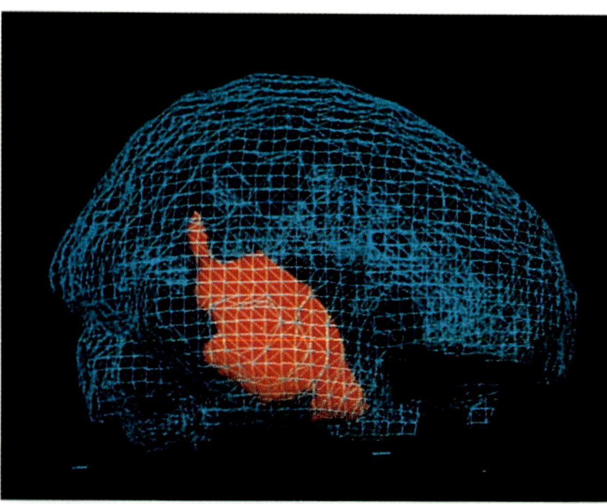

FIG. 1.19. Some "see-through" three-dimensional rCBF SPECT images combine multiple surfaces. In this case, a "wire-cage" surface is used to outline the brain, while a solid body is used to define the location of an area of high flow in an ictal study of rCBF in a seizure patient (same patient as shown in Fig. 1.11).

3. The normal distribution of rCBF in such a setting shows symmetric flow distribution between homologous regions.
4. Both age and gender effects can be noted. They are only well characterized for whole-brain blood flow, which is not readily measured by conventional SPECT techniques.
5. Among brain stress tests that could be employed to enhance discrimination of disease, the only well-established technique is the acetazolamide vasodilator test. Under most circumstances it reveals striking asymmetries in disease states of vascular origin. Its regional effects independent of global flow changes have not yet been established in normal controls.
6. Future research should focus on the establishment of normative databases and the effect of environmental variations on regional cerebral blood flow.

CONCLUSIONS

SPECT functional brain imaging is a powerful clinical and research tool. Several clinical applications have now been documented, a substantial number are under active investigation, and an even larger number are yet to be studied. Instrumentation continues to improve, although current SPECT tomographs yield excellent image quality. There is a rapidly expanding armamentarium of radiopharmaceuticals. Challenge tests, only well developed in cerebrovascular disease (the acetazolamide test for vasodilatory reserve), offer great promise in elucidating the extent and nature of disease, as well as predicting therapeutic responses. Some standards regarding patient imaging environment and image presentation are emerging. However, much is yet to be learned about the ideal circumstances for the performance and evaluation of SPECT functional brain imaging. Finally, we must keep in mind that SPECT will achieve its full potential as a clinical tool for the management of patients with cerebral pathology only through close cooperation between the nuclear medicine community and our colleagues in neurology, psychiatry, or neurosurgery.

ACKNOWLEDGMENTS

Many individuals have made important contributions to this chapter through their collaborative efforts. Chief among my clinical colleagues are Frederick J. Bonte, M.D., A. John Rush, M.D., and Robert F. Leroy, M.D. I would also like to acknowledge two extremely talented members of my staff: J. Kelly Payne, M.S., and James L. Lowe, M.S.

REFERENCES

1. Alavi A, Hirsch LJ. Studies of central nervous system disorders with single-photon emission computed tomography and positron emission tomography: evolution over the past 2 decades. *Semin Nucl Med* 1991;21:58–81.
2. Bonte FJ, Hom J, Tintner R, Weiner MF. Single-photon tomography in Alzheimer's disease and the dementias. *Semin Nucl Med* 1990; 20:342–352.
3. Brass LM, Rattner Z. Single photon emission computed tomography in cerebral vascular disease. In: Weber DA, Devous MD, Tikofsky RS, eds. *Workshop on brain SPECT perfusion imaging: optimizing imaging acquisition and processing.* DOE CONF-9110368; Washington, DC: Department of Energy; 1992: 77–88.
4. Devous MD Sr. Imaging brain function by single-photon emission computed tomography. In: Andreasen N, ed. *Brain imaging: applications in psychiatry.* Washington: American Psychiatric Press; 1988: 147–234.
5. Devous MD Sr, Leroy RF, Homan RW. Single photon emission computed tomography in epilepsy. *Semin Nucl Med* 1990; 20: 325–341.
6. Hellman RS, Tikofsky RS. An overview of the contributions of regional cerebral blood flow studies in cerebrovascular disease. Is there a role for single photon emission computed tomography? *Semin Nucl Med* 1990;20:303–324.
7. Holman BL, Devous MD Sr. Functional brain SPECT: the emergence of a powerful clinical method. *J Nucl Med* 1992;33:1888–1904.
8. Tikofsky RS, Hellman RS. Brain single photon emission computed tomography: new activation and intervention studies. *Semin Nucl Med* 1991;21:40–57.
9. VanHeertum RL, O'Connell RA. Functional brain imaging in the evaluation of psychiatric illness. *Semin Nucl Med* 1991;21:24–39.
10. Devous MD Sr. Image presentation and normal SPECT rCBF. In: Weber DA, Devous MD, Tikofsky RS, eds. *Workshop on brain SPECT perfusion imaging: optimizing image acquisition, processing, display and interpretation.* DOE CONF-9110368; Washington, DC: Department of Energy; 1992:56–62.
11. Devous MD Sr, Stokely EM, Bonte FJ. Quantitative imaging of regional cerebral blood flow in man by dynamic sngle-photon tomography. In: BL Holman, ed. *Radionuclide imaging of the brain.* New York: Churchill Livingstone; 1985:135–162.
12. Hoffer PB, Zubal G. A guide to SPECT equipment for brain imaging. In: Weber DA, Devous MD, Tikofsky RS, Woodhead AD, Vivirito KJ, eds. *Workshop on brain SPECT perfusion imaging: image acquisition, processing, display and interpretation.* DOE CONF-9110368; Washington, DC: Department of Energy; 1992:21–27.
13. Links JM. Optimization of acquisition parameters for brain SPECT. In: Weber DA, Devous MD, Tikofsky RS, Woodhead AD, Vivirito KJ, eds. *Workshop on brain SPECT perfusion imaging: image acquisition, processing, display, and interpretation.* DOE CONF-9110368; Washington, DC: Department of Energy; 1992:28–32.
14. Todd-Pokropek A. Image reconstruction in tomography: basics. In: Weber DA, Devous MD, Tikofsky RS, Woodhead AD, Vivirito KJ, eds. *Workshop on brain SPECT perfusion imaging: image acquisition, processing, display, and interpretation.* DOE CONF-9110368; Washington, DC: Department of Energy; 1992:33–41.
15. Stokely EM, Sveinsdottir E, Lassen NA, Rommer P. A single photon dynamic computer assisted tomograph (DCAT) for imaging brain function in multiple cross-sections. *J Comput Assist Tomogr* 1980; 4:230–240.
16. Kimura K, Hashikawa K, Etani H, et al. A new apparatus for brain imaging: four-head rotating gamma camera single-photon emission computed tomograph. *J Nucl Med* 1990;31:603–609.
17. Rogers WL, Clinthorne NH, Stamos J, et al. Performance evaluation of SPRINT, a single-photon ring tomograph for brain imaging. *J Nucl Med* 1984;25:1013–1018.
18. Kanno I, Uemura K, Miyura S, Miyura Y. HEADTOME: a hybrid emission tomograph for single-photon and positron emission imaging of the brain. *J Comput Assist Tomogr* 1981;5:216–226.
19. Logan KW, Holmes RA. Missouri University Multiplane Imager (MUMPI): a high-sensitivity rapid dynamic ECT brain imager. *J Nucl Med* 1984;25:PI05.
20. Smith AP, Genna S. Imaging characteristics of ASPECT, a single-crystal ring camera for dedicated brain SPECT. *J Nucl Med* 1989;30:796.
21. Stoddart HF, Stoddart HA. A new development in single-gamma transaxial tomography. Union Carbide focused collimator scanner. *IEEE Trans Nucl Sci* 1979;26:2710–2712.

22. Kirsch C-M, Moore SC, Zimmerman RE, English RJ, Holman BL. Characteristics of a scanning, multidetector, single-photon ECT body imager. *J Nucl Med* 1981;22:726–731.
23. Hill TC, Stoddart HF, Doherty MD, Alpert NM, Wolfe AP. Simultaneous SPECT acquisition of CBF and metabolism. *J Nucl Med* 1988;29:876.
24. Devous MD Sr, Bonte FJ. Initial evaluation of cerebral blood flow imaging with a high-resolution, high-sensitivity three-headed SPECT system (PRISM). *J Nucl Med* 1988;29:912.
25. Devous MD Sr, Lowe JL, Payne JK. Dual-isotope brain SPECT imaging with ^{99m}Tc and ^{123}I. Validation by phantom studies. *J Nucl Med* 1992;33:2030–2035.
26. Devous MD Sr, Payne JK, Lowe JL. Dual-isotope brain SPECT imaging with ^{99m}Tc and ^{123}I. Clinical validation using ^{133}Xe SPECT. *J Nucl Med* 1992;33:1919–1924.
27. Glass HI, Harper AM. Measurement of regional blood flow in cerebral cortex of man through intact skull. *Br Med J* 1963;2:1611.
28. Mallett BL, Veall N. The measurement of regional cerebral clearance rate in man using Xe^{133} inhalation and extracranial recording. *Clin Sci* 1965;29:179–191.
29. Obrist WD, Thompson HK, King CH, Wang HS: Determination of regional cerebral blood flow by inhalation of xenon-133. *Circ Res* 1967;20:124–135.
30. Kanno I, Lassen NA. Two methods for calculating regional cerebral blood flow from emission computed tomography of inert gas concentrations. *J Comput Assist Tomogr* 1979;3:71–76.
31. Celsis P, Goldman T, Henriksen L, Lassen NA. A method for calculating regional cerebral blood flow from emission computerized tomography of inert gas concentrations. *J Comput Assist Tomogr* 1981; 5:641–645.
32. Smith GT, Stokely EM, Lewis MH, Devous MD, Bonte FJ. An error analysis of the double-integral method for calculating brain blood perfusion from inert gas clearance data. *J Cereb Blood Flow Metab* 1984;4:61–67.
33. Winchell HS, Baldwin RM, Lin TH. Development of ^{123}I-labeled amines for brain studies: localization of ^{123}I iodophenylalkylamines in rat brain. *J Nucl Med* 1980;21:940–202.
34. Kung HF, Tramposh K, Blau M. A new brain imaging agent: (I^{123}) HIPDM: N,N,N′-trimethyl-N′-(2-hydroxy-3-methyl-5-iodobenzyl)-1,3-propanediamine. *J Nucl Med* 1983;24:66–72.
35. Lassen NA, Henriksen L, Holm S, et al. Cerebral blood-flow tomography: xenon-133 compared with isopropyl-amphetamine-iodine-123: concise communication. *J Nucl Med* 1983;24:17–21.
36. Kuhl DE, Barrio JR, Huang SC, et al. Quantifying local cerebral blood flow by N-isopropyl-p-[^{123}I]iodoamphetamine (IMP) tomography. *J Nucl Med* 1982;23:196–203.
37. Nishizawa S, Tanada S, Yonekura Y, et al. Regional dynamics of N-isopropyl-(^{123}I)p iodo-amphetamine in human brain. *J Nucl Med* 1989;30:150–156.
38. Nakano S, Kinoshita K, Jinnouchi S, Hiroaki H, Watanabe K. Comparative study of regional cerebral blood flow images by SPECT using xenon-133, iodine-123 IMP, and technetium-99m HM-PAO. *J Nucl Med* 1989;30:157–164.
39. Leonard J-P, Nowotnik DP, Neirinckx RD. Technetium-99m-d,l-HM-PAO: a new radiopharmaceutical for imaging regional brain perfusion using SPECT—a comparison with iodine-123 HIPDM. *J Nucl Med* 1986;27:1819–1823.
40. Defer G, Moretti JL, Cesaro P, Sergent A, Raynaud C, Degos JD. Early and delayed SPECT using N-isopropyl p-iodoamphetamine iodine 123 in cerebral ischemia. A prognostic index for clinical recovery. *Arch Neurol* 1987;44:715–718.
41. Neirinckx RD, Canning LR, Piper IM, et al. Technetium-99m d,l-HM-PAO: a new radiopharmaceutical for SPECT imaging of regional cerebral blood perfusion. *J Nucl Med* 1987;28:191–202.
42. Volkert WA, Hoffman TJ, Seger RM, Trounter DE, Holmes RA: Tc^{99m}-propylene amine oxime (Tc^{99m}-PnAO); a potential brain radiopharmaceutical. *Eur J Nucl Med* 1984;9:511–516.
43. Kung HF, Guo YH, Yu C-C, Billings J, Subramanyam V, Calabrese J. New brain perfusion imaging agents based on ^{99m}Tc-bis(aminoethanethiol) complexes: stereoisomers and biodistribution. *J Med Chem* 1989;32:437–444.
44. Walovitch RC, Hill TC, Garrity ST, et al. Characterization of technetium-99m-l,l-ECD for brain perfusion imaging, part 1: pharmacology of technetium-99m ECD in nonhuman primates. *J Nucl Med* 1989;30:1892–1901.
45. Leveille J, Demonceau G, De Roo M, et al. Characterization of technetium-99m-l,l-ECD for brain perfusion imaging, part 2: biodistribution and brain imaging in humans. *J Nucl Med* 1989;30:1902–1910.
46. Devous MD Sr, Payne JK, Lowe JL: Comparison of ^{99m}Tc-ECD to ^{133}Xe SPECT in normal controls and in patients with mild to moderate rCBF abnormalities. *J Nucl Med* 1993;34:754–761.
47. Gibbs JM, Wise RJS, Leendersbs, KL, Herold S, Frackowiak RS J, Jones T: Cerebral hemodynamics in occlusive carotid artery disease. *Lancet* 1985;1:933–934.
48. Kuhl DE, Reivich M, Alavi A, Nyary I, Staum M: Local cerebral blood volume determined by three dimensional reconstruction of radionuclide scan data. *Circ Res* 1975;36:610–619.
49. Buell U, Stirner H, Ferbert F: Cerebral blood flow-to-volume imaging by SPECT. *J Nucl Med* 1986;27:1938–1939.
50. Knapp WH, Kummer RV, Kubler W: Imaging of cerebral blood flow-to-volume distribution using SPECT. *J Nucl Med* 1986;27:465–470, 1986.
51. Toyama H, Takeshita G, Takeuchi A, et al. Cerebral hemodynamics in patients with chronic obstructive carotid disease by rCBF, rCBV, and rCBV/rCBF ratio using SPECT. *J Nucl Med* 1990;31:55–60.
52. Kung HF, Alavi A, Chang W, et al. In vivo SPECT imaging of CNS D-2 dopamine receptors: initial studies with iodine-123-IBZM in humans. *J Nucl Med* 1990;31:573–579.
53. Schubiger PA, Hasler PH, Beer-Wohlfahrt H, et al. Evaluation of multi-centre study with iomazenil: a benzodiazepine receptor ligand. *Nucl Med Commun* 1991;12:569–582.
54. Holman BL, Gibson RE, Hill TC, Eckelman WC, Albert M, Reba RC. Muscarinic acetylcholine receptors in Alzheimer's disease: in vivo imaging with iodine-123-labeled 3-quinuclidinyl-4-iodobenzilate and emission tomography. *JAMA* 1985;254:3063.
55. Weinberger DR, Gibson R, Coppola R, et al. The distribution of cerebral muscarinic acetylcholine receptors in vivo in patients with dementia. A controlled study with ^{123}IQNB and single photon emission computed tomography. *Arch Neurol* 1991;48:169–176.
56. Innis RB, Al-Tikriti MS, Zoghbi SS, et al. SPECT imaging of the benzodiazepine receptor, feasibility of in vivo potency measurements from stepwise displacement curves. *J Nucl Med* 1991;32:1754–1761.
57. Kim KT, Black KL, Marciano D, et al. Thallium SPECT imaging of brain tumors: methods and results. *J Nucl Med* 1990;31:965–969.
58. Mountz JM, Stafford-Schuck K, McKeever PE. Thallium-201 tumor/cardiac ratio estimation of residual astrocytoma. *J Neurosurg* 1988;68:705–709.
59. Schwartz RB, Carvalho PA, Alexander E III, Loeffler JS, Folkerth R, Holman BL. Radiation necrosis vs high-grade recurrent glioma: differentiation by using dual-isotope SPECT with ^{201}Tl and ^{99m}TC-HM-PAO. *AJNR* 1991;12:1187–1192.
60. Kaplan WD, Takvorian T, Morris JH, Rumbaugh CL, Connolly BT, Atkins HL. Thallium-201 brain tumor imaging: a comparative study with pathological correlation. *J Nucl Med* 1987;28:47–52.
61. Brismar T, Collins VP, Keeselberg M. Thallium-201 uptake relates to membrane potential and potassium permeability in human glioma cells. *Brain Res* 1989;500:30–36.
62. Black KL, Hawkins RA, Kim KT, Becker DP, Lerner C, Marciano D. Use of thallium-201 SPECT to quantitate malignancy grade of gliomas. *J Neurosurg* 1989;71:342–346.
63. Baron GC, Lebrun-Grandie P, Collard P, Crouzel C, Mestelan G, Bousser MG. Noninvasive measurement of blood flow, oxygen consumption and glucose utilization in the same brain regions in man by positron emission tomography. *J Nucl Med* 1982;23:391–399.
64. Ingvar DH, Risberg J. Increase of regional cerebral blood flow during mental effort in normals and in patients with focal brain disorders. *Exp Brain Res* 1967;3:195–211.
65. Kety SS, Schmidt CF. The nitrous oxide method for quantitative determination of cerebral blood flow in man: theory, procedure and normal values. *J Clin Invest* 1948;27:476–483.
66. Mazziotta JC, Phelps ME, Carson RE, Kuhl DE. Tomographic mapping of human cerebral metabolism: auditory stimulation. *Neurology* 1982;32:921–937.
67. Phelps ME, Kuhl DE, Mazziotta JC. Metabolic mapping of the brain's response to visual stimulation: studies in humans. *Science* 1981;211:1445–1448.

68. Raichle ME, Grubb RL, Gado MH, Eichling JO, Ter-Pogossian MM. Correlation between regional cerebral blood flow and oxidative metabolism. *Arch Neurol* 1976;33:523–526.
69. Roland PE, Eriksson L, Stone-Elander S, Widen L. Does mental activity change the oxidative metabolism of the brain? *J Neurosci* 1987;7:2373–2389.
70. Mazziotta JC, Phelps ME, Carson RE, Kuhl DE. Tomographic mapping of human cerebral metabolism: sensory deprivation. *Ann Neurol* 1982;12:435–444.
71. Devous MD Sr, Stokely EM, Chehabi HH, Bonte FJ. Normal distribution of regional cerebral blood flow measured by dynamic single-photon emission tomography. *J Cereb Blood Flow Metab* 1986; 6:95–104.
72. Gur RC, Gur RE, Obrist WD, Skolnick BE, Reivich M. Age and regional cerebral blood flow at rest and during cognitive activity. *Arch Gen Psychiatry* 1987;44:617–621.
73. Hagstadius S, Risburg J. Regional cerebral blood flow characteristics and variations with age in resting normal subjects. *Brain Cogn* 1989;10:28–43.
74. Kuhl DE, Metter EJ, Riege WH, Phelps ME. Effects of human aging on patterns of local cerebral glucose utilization determined by the ^{18}F fluorodeoxyglucose method. *J Cereb Blood Flow Metab* 1982; 2:163–171.
75. Mathew RJ, Wilson WH, Tant SR. Determinants of resting regional cerebral blood flow in normal subjects. *Biol Psychiatry* 1986; 21:907–914.
76. Rogers RL, Meyer JS, Mortel KF. After reaching retirement age physical activity sustains cerebral perfusion and cognition. *J Am Geriatr Soc* 1990;38:123–128.
77. Baxter LR, Mazziotta JC, Phelps ME, Selin CE, Guze BH, Fairbanks L. Cerebral glucose metabolic rates in normal human females vs. normal males. *Psychiatry Res* 1987;21:237–245.
78. Daniel DG, Mathew RJ, Wilson WH. Sex roles and regional cerebral blood flow. *Psychiatry Res* 1988;27:55–64.
79. Gur RC, Gur RE, Obrist WD, et al. Sex and handedness differences in cerebral blood flow during rest and cognitive activity. *Science* 1982;217:659–661.
80. Rodriguez G, Warkentin S, Risberg J, Rosadini G. Sex differences in regional cerebral blood flow. *J Cereb Blood Flow Metab* 1988; 8:783–789.
81. Bonte FJ, Devous MD Sr, Reisch JS. The effect of acetazolamide on regional cerebral blood flow in normal human subjects as measured by single photon emission computed tomography. *Invest Radiol* 1988;23:564–568.
82. Rogg J, Rutigliano M, Yonas H, Johnson DW, Pentheny S, Latchaw RE. The acetazolamide challenge: imaging techniques designed to evaluate cerebral blood flow reserve. *AJNR* 1989;10:803–810.
83. Sullivan HG, Kingsbury TB, Morgan ME, et al. The rCBF response to diamox in normal subjects and cerebrovascular disease patients. *J Neurosurg* 1987;67:525–534.
84. Vorstrup S, Brun B, Lassen NA. Evaluation of the cerebral vasodilatory capacity of the acetazolamide test before EC-IC bypass surgery in patients with occlusion of the internal carotid artery. *Stroke* 1986;17:1291–1298.
85. Mathew RJ, Barr DL, Weinman ML. Caffeine and cerebral blood flow. *Br J Psychiatry* 1983;143:604–608.
86. Rush AJ, Cain JW, Raese J, Stewart RS, Waller DA, Debus JR. The neurobiological bases for psychiatric disorders. In: RN Rosenberg, ed. *Comprehensive neurology.* New York: Raven Press; 1991: 555–603.
87. Fox PT, Mintun MA, Raichle ME, Miezen FM, Allman JM, Van Essen DC. Mapping human visual cortex with positron emission tomography. *Nature* 1986;323:806–809.
88. Petersen SE, Fox PT, Posner MI, Mintun M, Raichle ME. Positron emission tomographic studies of the cortical anatomy of single-word processing. *Nature* 1988;331:585–589.

Cerebral SPECT Imaging, Second Edition,
edited by R.L. Van Heertum and R.S. Tikofsky.
Raven Press, Ltd., New York © 1995.

CHAPTER 2

Technique and Pitfalls

Ronald L. Van Heertum and Ronald S. Tikofsky

SPECT imaging systems, ranging from single-head to multidetector systems, have proliferated rapidly. Dedicated brain imaging devices using ring detectors have also been developed. Although the manufacturers of these systems provide basic guidelines for use, adjustments in protocols routinely have to be made by each laboratory. There are no generally accepted protocols for image acquisition and processing for the equipment that is currently available. Therefore, we suggest that each nuclear medicine laboratory establish suitable acquisition and processing protocols in conjunction with the manufacturer of the system being used.

RADIOPHARMACEUTICAL QUALITY CONTROL

Iodine 123 *N*-isopropyl-*p*-iodoamphetamine (IMP), described in the first edition of this text, is no longer commercially available. This radiopharmaceutical did not require any reconstitution prior to injection. The quality control procedures are described in Van Heertum and Tikofsky (1) and the package insert (2).

The only presently available radiopharmaceutical for SPECT brain imaging is ^{99m}Tc Exametazime [hexamethylpropyleneamine-oxime (HMPAO); Ceretec, Amersham Corporation]. Procedures for kit preparation and quality control are described in the package insert. A short method of kit preparation is described by Hung et al. (3). Whichever kit preparation technique is used, it is strongly recommended that the radiotracer be injected as soon as possible after reconstitution of the radiopharmaceutical. A stabilized version of ^{99m}Tc HMPAO is currently before the Food and Drug Administration (FDA). This version will allow for a greater (up to 6 hr) interval between kit preparation and injection.

Another technetium-based radiopharmaceutical, ^{99m}Tc Bicisate (Neurolite, Du Pont Pharma), is currently under consideration by the FDA. It also comes in kit form and requires reconstitution prior to injection. Procedures for preparation are described by Tikofsky et al. (4).

TECHNIQUE

Patient Preparation

Some of the interview time should be devoted to explaining the procedure and allaying patient concerns. It is also advisable to obtain a brief history, including information concerning handedness. This type of information is particularly useful when evaluating patients with cerebrovascular disease.

If the study is to be done with IMP, particularly when dealing with dementia patients, this sort of communication will be best accomplished with other members of the patient's family. Although advance time with the patient is important with any type of nuclear medicine study, this approach is absolutely essential to ensure a successful cerebral SPECT study.

Following the orientation, the patient should be given three drops of a saturated potassium iodide solution in orange juice or a similar beverage. This preparation is necessary to minimize thyroid gland irradiation from uptake of the radioactive ^{123}I. Prior to the injection, the patient should be requested to void (5).

After completing the orientation and preparation procedures, the patient is comfortably positioned on the imaging couch with arms resting at the sides. In some systems, the imaging couches have removable wing armrests that can be used to allow greater ease of positioning and patient comfort during injection of the radiopharmaceutical. The imaging room environment should be carefully controlled,

R. L. Van Heertum: Department of Radiology, Columbia University College of Physicians and Surgeons, and Department of Nuclear Medicine, Columbia Presbyterian Medical Center, New York, New York 10032.

R. S. Tikofsky: Department of Radiology, Section of Nuclear Medicine, Medical College of Wisconsin, Milwaukee, Wisconsin 53226.

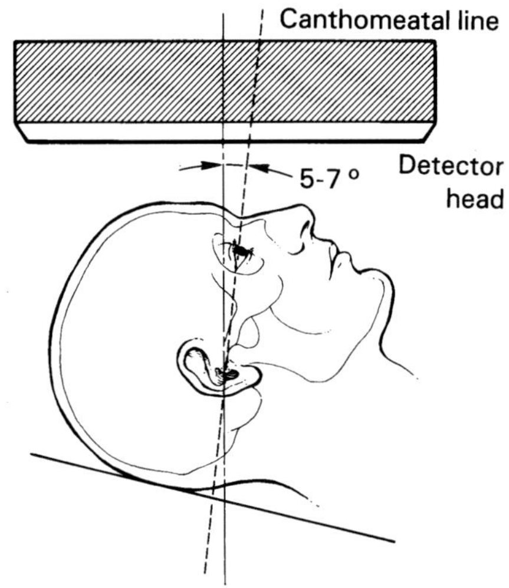

FIG. 2.1. Detector head in relation to canthomeatal line.

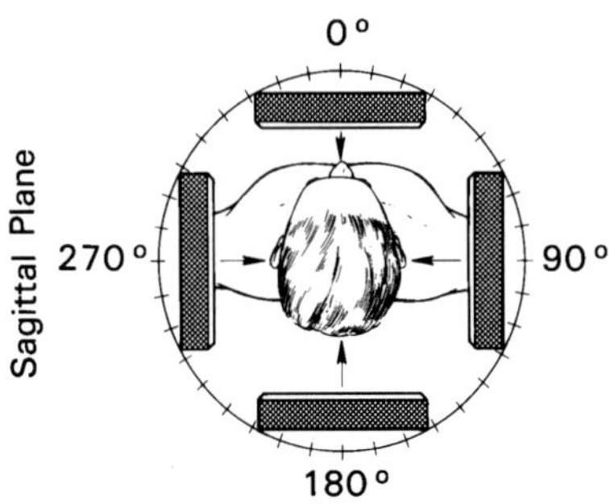

FIG. 2.2. Relation of detector to patient's head at 0°, 90°, 180°, and 270°.

with low noise, low light, and minimal traffic. The patient should be instructed, whenever possible, to keep eyes open during the injection and the ensuing equilibration period (15 to 20 mins after the injection). A dose of 3 to 5 mCi (111 to 185 mBq) ^{123}I-labeled IMP or 10 to 20 mCi (370 to 740 mBq) ^{99m}Tc-labeled HMPAO is administered intravenously. Following the radiopharmaceutical injection, the patient should remain in a quiet, comfortable, motionless position for the next 20 mins. During this time, the technologist begins the actual set-up and positioning of the detector system so that the image acquisition can begin immediately thereafter.

When imaging with ^{99m}Tc HMPAO, the patient should be brought into an injection area that is free of noise, but with the lights on. An intravenous line is then put in place. The patient is then asked to remain quiet (no talking) for approximately 5 mins, at which point the ^{99m}Tc HMPAO is injected, and continue in this environment for an additional 5-10 mins post-injection. Following an interval of 30 mins to 2 hrs, the patient can return for imaging. If sedation is necessary, it should be administered after injection, and just prior to imaging.

Acquisition Technique

Specific acquisition techniques will vary depending on the equipment used, but a number of considerations apply to all cerebral SPECT studies. In all instances, the patient should be comfortably positioned on the imaging couch with the head "immobilized" in a radiolucent head holder. The patient's head is fixed so that a line perpendicular to the detector head runs 5°to 7°cephalad to the canthomeatal line (Fig. 2.1). Furthermore, the patient and detector should be positioned in such a manner that the imaging device remains parallel to the coronal plane at the 0°and 180°detector positions and parallel to the sagittal orthogonal plane at the 90°and 270°positions (Fig. 2.2). It is also essential that the patient be centered so that the brain remains within the field of view on all of the individually acquired projection images. In addition, the detector should be positioned as close to the patient's brain as possible, preferably with a radius of rotation of 14 cm or less from the surface of the collimator to the center of the patient's brain. This tight radius of rotation can be achieved by using a variety of approaches, including a cut-off detector head, long-bore fan beam collimation, and frontal tomography (6–8) (Fig. 2.3). The cut-off or "shaved" detector is specifically designed so that the detector will clear the patient's shoulders. When a cut-off detector is not available, alternative approaches include either long-bore fan beam collima-

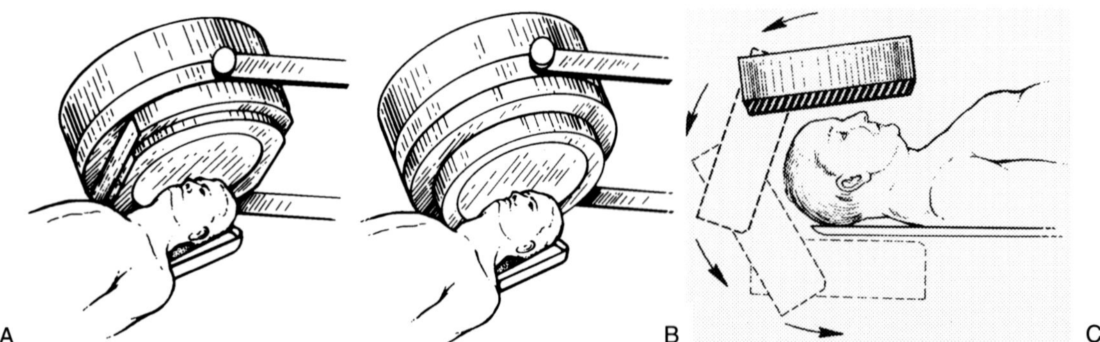

FIG. 2.3. A: Cut-off head configuration. B: Long-bore collimator. C: Frontal tomography.

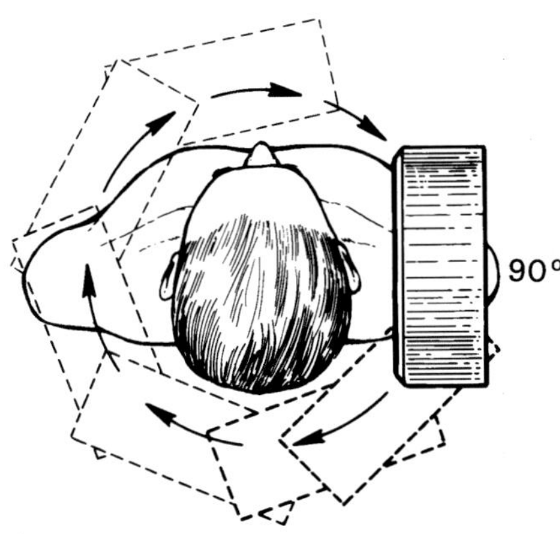

FIG. 2.4. Clockwise rotation of detector head starting on patient's right side.

tion or frontal tomography, both of which have been shown to be useful for cerebral SPECT imaging studies.

Following proper positioning of the patient and detector, the actual acquisition procedure can begin. In general, 64 to 128 projection images are acquired, for a total imaging time of 30 to 45 mins on single detector and 10 to 20 mins on multi-detector systems. It is recommended that acquisition begin with the detector positioned to the side of the patient's head, in a clockwise fashion (Fig. 2.4).

This image acquisition technique is particularly useful with anxious, agitated, or claustrophobic patients, since the detector first rotates posteriorly and thus allows the patient to become acclimated to the procedure before the detector moves anteriorly over the face at the end of the procedure. A 360°rotation orbit should be used whenever possible. In compromise situations—as with difficult or agitated patients—a reduced imaging time for each projection image on multiple rapid acquisition systems (RAS) with a multidetector device will usually prove to be a viable solution.

The type of collimation for the procedure will vary depending on the equipment used. To ensure that a proper study has been obtained, the projection images should be evaluated before the patient leaves the department. A useful method for performing this assessment is to display the acquired projection images in a closed-loop cine display. An alternative is to use a horizontal profile region of interest (ROI) analysis of the acquired data to generate a sinogram display (9). (These approaches are discussed in detail in the Pitfalls section.)

Processing Technique

After the study has been acquired and assessed for adequacy, the preprocessing and reconstruction procedures are performed. The images should be routinely uniformity corrected and reconstructed with attenuation correction. Spe-

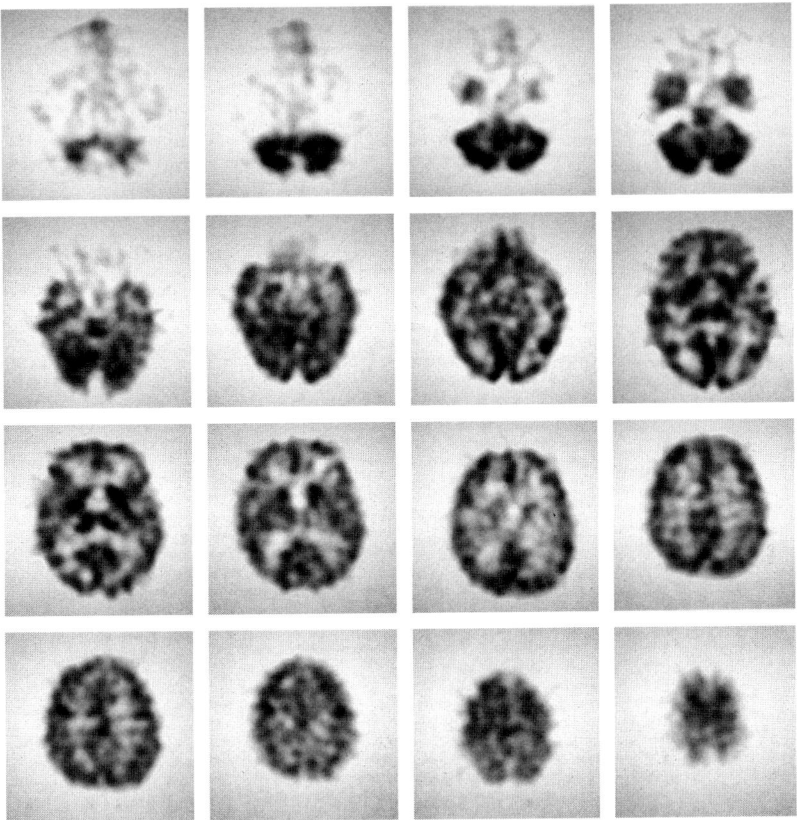

FIG. 2.5. Normal cerebral SPECT images. Transaxial plane (inferior to superior).

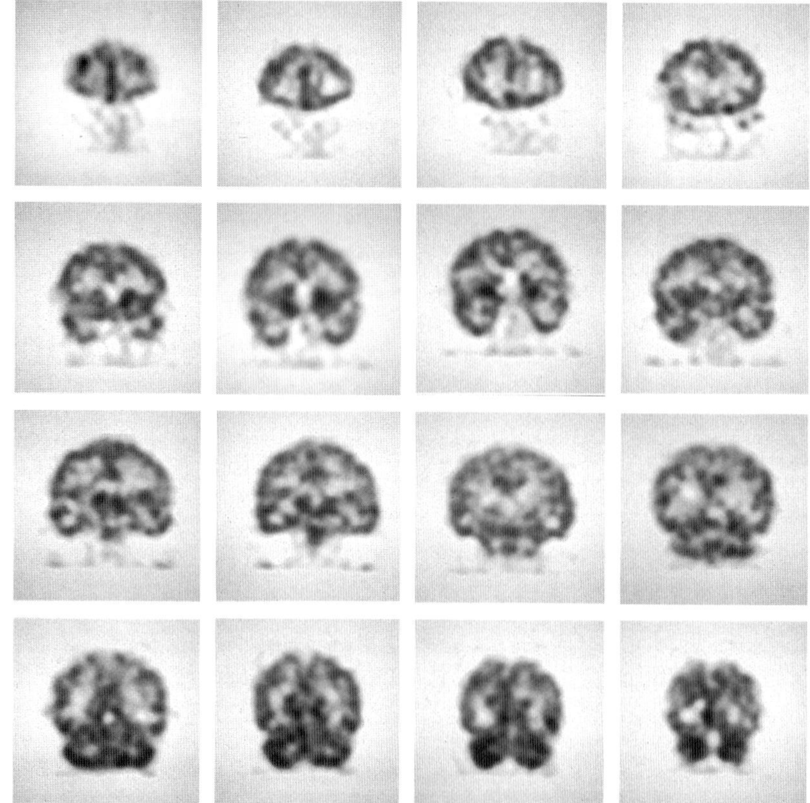

FIG. 2.6. Normal cerebral SPECT images. Coronal plane (anterior to posterior).

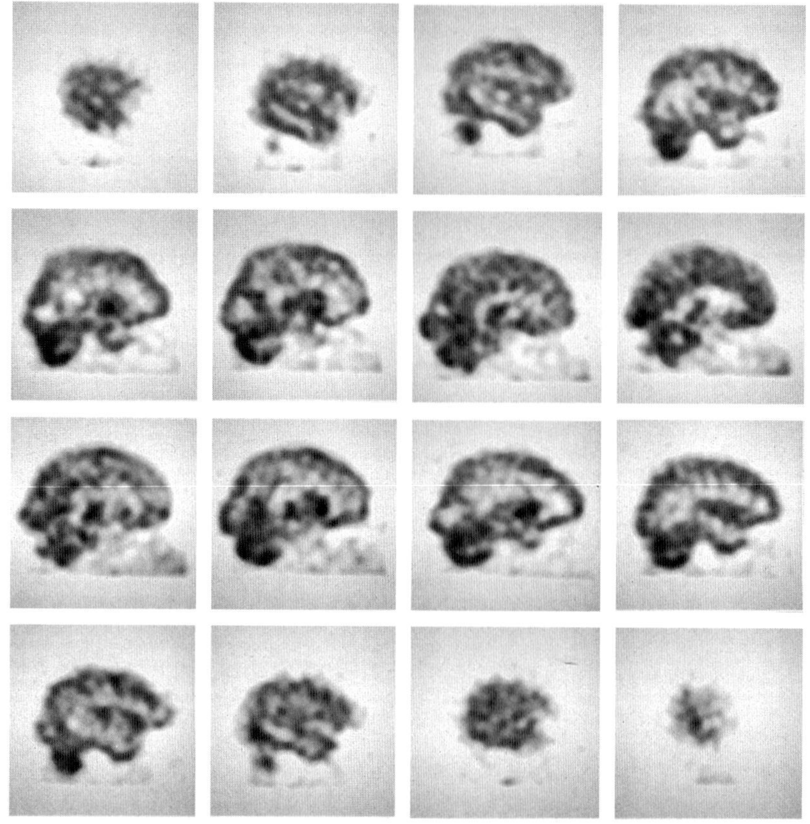

FIG. 2.7. Normal cerebral SPECT images. Sagittal plane (right to left).

cific processing protocols will vary from system to system. In general, the images are either spatially filtered before (preprocessed) or after (postprocessed) the reconstruction process, using a filtered back-projection technique. The reconstructed transaxial sections are then reoriented and displayed in the coronal and sagittal planes.

Display Technique

All three orthogonal imaging planes should be displayed. The transaxial images are generally displayed in the same format as transmission computed tomography (CT) or magnetic resonance imaging (MRI) scans. The sections begin inferiorly and continue superiorly in a contiguous manner (Fig. 2.5). The coronal and sagittal planes are displayed in the same manner as MRI studies (Figs. 2.6 and 2.7). (These presentations are reviewed in greater detail by Noback et al. in Chapter 3, this volume.)

Although the images are generally displayed and archived on transparency film, direct viewing of the images on the monitor screen can be very helpful, since additional information can be obtained from such observations. The three-dimensional surface display is an alternative technique that may become more useful.

PITFALLS

A wide variety of potential pitfalls may be encountered when performing cerebral SPECT imaging studies. The most common pitfalls fall into one of three major categories: patient, pharmaceutical and technical, and interpretive.

Patient Factors

The major patient factors are patient size; patient motion; patient position; head holder; and low count rates.

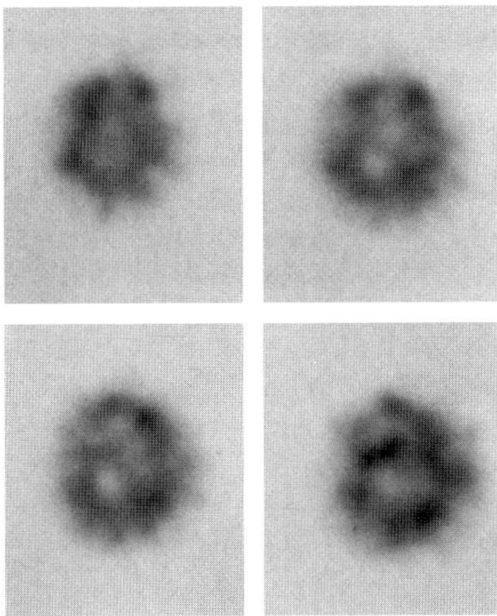

FIG. 2.8. Increased radius of rotation resulting in loss of spatial resolution in a very obese patient.

Patient Size

In cerebral SPECT imaging, there may be difficulty in the proper positioning of the patient in the gantry system and also maintaining the detector head as close to the patient's head as possible. Getting the detector close to the patient's head is of particular concern with obese patients, for whom even a cut-off configuration detector may not be able to clear the shoulders and allow adequately short radius of rotation. The result is a longer than desirable radius of rotation (>14 cm), which gives rise to a loss of spatial resolution (Fig. 2.8).

Patient Motion

Movement of the patient's head during the SPECT acquisition will also degrade image quality. Proper quality control during the acquisition procedure will usually detect this abnormality and should be performed on a routine basis (Fig. 2.9). The technologist should make every effort to keep the patient's head movement to a minimum. When the radiotracer being used is technetium based, it is possible to use sedation to control patient movement. Sedation is not given at the time of injection but is administered prior to imaging. The type and amount of sedation is determined by the referring physician. This approach to controlling patient movement, particularly in demented and psychiatric patients has proved to be quite useful.

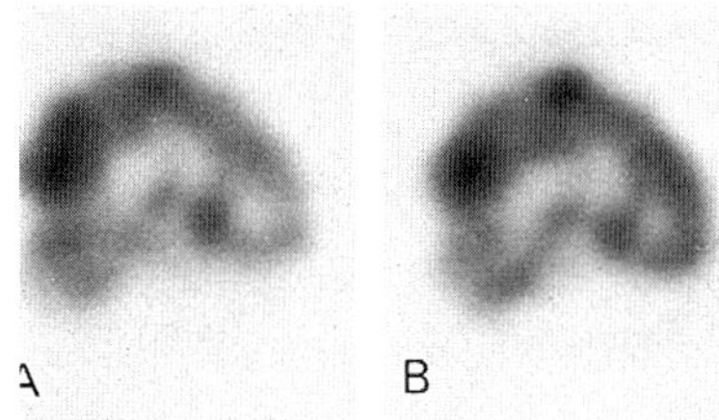

FIG. 2.9. A: Sagittal plane study with motion. **B:** Sagittal plane study with motion correction and improved spatial resolution.

Patient Position

Improper positioning of the detector in relation to the patient's canthomeatal line can give rise to images that may easily be improperly interpreted (Fig. 2.10). This type

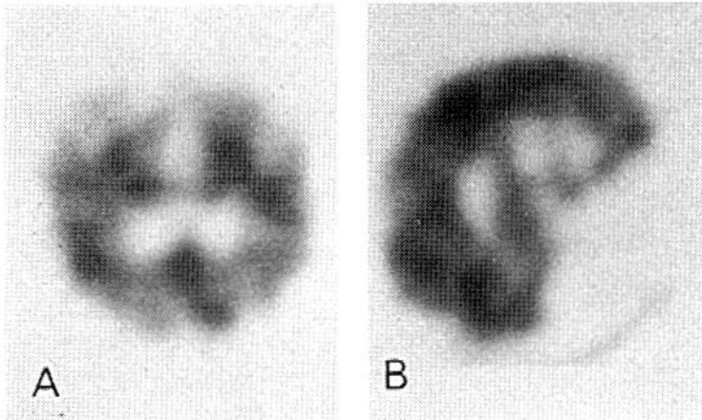

FIG. 2.10. Transaxial plane **(A)** and sagittal plane **(B)** images with patient in extended neck position causing inadequate delineation of the temporal lobes on the transaxial plane.

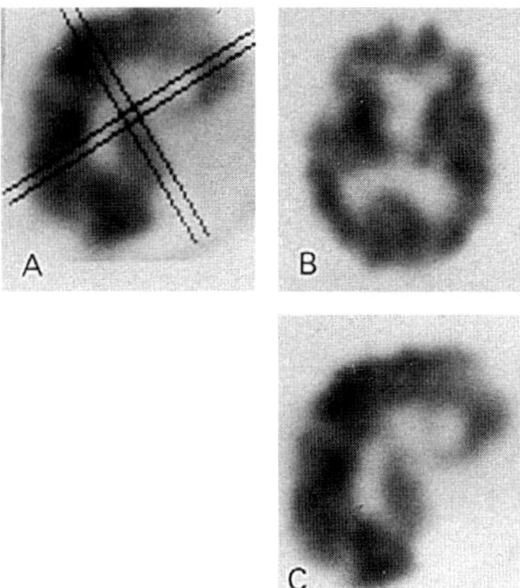

FIG. 2.11. Oblique angle reorientation of images resulting in better delineation of the temporal and frontal lobes. **A:** Cursor position for oblique angle technique. **B:** Corrected transaxial plane. **C:** Corrected sagittal plane.

of malpositioning can be corrected using an oblique angle image reorientation algorithm similar to that currently available from a number of commercial vendors for myocardial SPECT imaging procedures (Fig. 2.11). Although other types of tilting of the patient's head can be corrected with this approach (Fig. 2.12), not all malalignments can be resolved without doing the study a second time.

One patient positioning problem that cannot easily be corrected is yaw (malalignment in the coronal plane). Some of the newer software now available for brain scanning does provide such correction. However, it is a tedious and iterative procedure.

Head Holders

There is great variation among the head holders used in SPECT imaging systems. Some allow great flexibility, but those used with multidetector systems tend to have fewer options for adjustment. Their ability to cradle the patient's head also varies greatly. These factors can lead to patient motion and can create problems in securing images that will include the total brain and cerebellum. When repeat studies are required for either clinical or research purposes, a thermoplastic mask may be fitted to the patient's face to reduce motion and slippage and to enhance reproducibility.

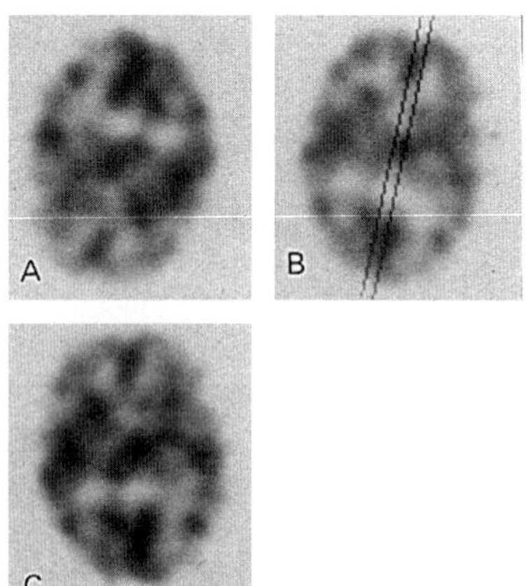

FIG. 2.12. A: Transaxial plane image rotated to patient's left side. **B:** Cursor placement for oblique angle correction technique. **C:** Corrected transaxial plane image.

Low Count Rates

The most frequent cause of a low count rate examination is infiltration of a portion of the injected intravenous dose. The result is usually a noisy reconstruction that may be difficult to interpret. The use of a butterfly intravenous injection set-up with a 25-gauge needle taped in place before the start of the procedure will reduce the likelihood of an infiltration.

Technical Factors

Pitfalls related to technical factors can be categorized into one of four major groups corresponding to the main technical aspects of the imaging procedure: pharmaceutical preparation (4), acquisition, processing, and display factors (10).

Pharmaceutical Preparation

Attention and care must be given to the proper preparation of the radiopharmaceutical and the timing of the injection. Specific procedures for preparation of the radiopharmaceuticals suitable for cerebral SPECT studies are described by Tikofsky et al. (4). The availability of stabilized preparations is likely to reduce problems related to the timing of injections following kit preparation. However, time of injection relative to time of onset of symptoms should be recorded since this may be a variable in interpretation for pathologic states such as an acute stroke, transient ischemic attacks, seizures, and the appearance of luxury perfusion.

Acquisition Factors

Two of the most important instrumentation problems that can cause significant image artifacts during the acquisition procedure are detector nonuniformity and center-of-rotation errors. Detector nonuniformity can give rise to troublesome ring image artifacts that may inadvertently be interpreted as disease (Fig. 2.13). This type of artifact is avoided by proper calibration of the detector photomultiplier tubes and uniformity correction using high count density correction maps. Detector head center-of-rotation errors are another source of artifacts. This type of image distortion be-

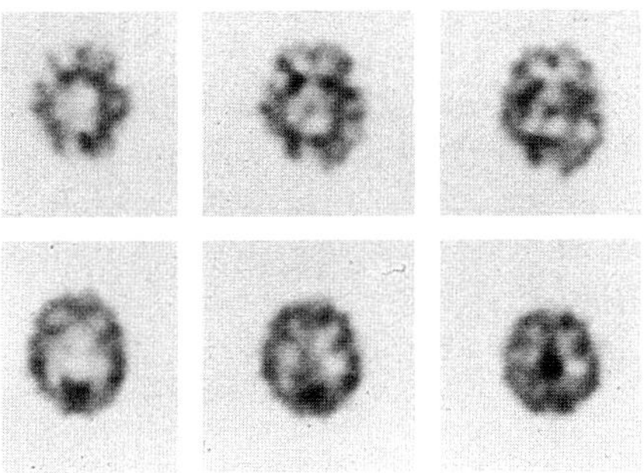

FIG. 2.13. Ring artifact secondary to detector nonuniformity.

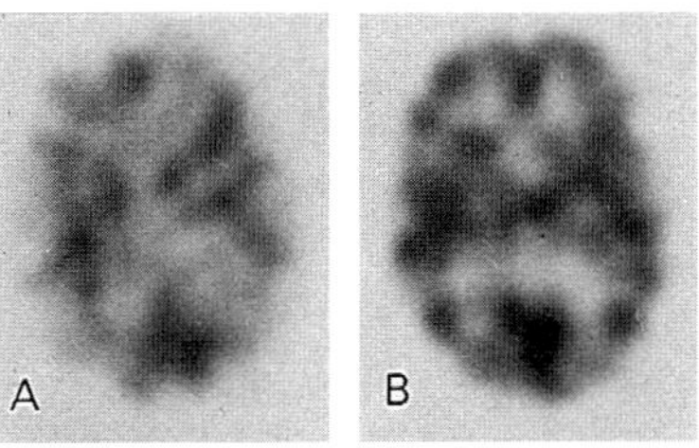

FIG. 2.14. A: Image distortion secondary to center of rotation error. **B:** Proper center of rotation.

comes increasingly apparent as the size of the center-of-rotation error increases (Fig. 2.14). This particular problem can be readily identified by routinely performing a center-of-rotation quality control check as, discussed in the Quality Control section of the Appendix. Other acquisition problems that can give rise to potential pitfalls include incomplete acquisition protocols (Fig. 2.15) as well as inadequate angular sampling (Fig. 2.16) and spatial sampling.

The problems described above are compounded when multidetector imaging systems are used for cerebral SPECT imaging because it is necessary to account for two or three detectors. Each detector must have similar peaking, uniformity, sensitivity, and linearity. Establishing the center-of-rotation for multidetector imaging systems when the detectors are not fixed is more elaborate and requires more care than that for a single detector system.

Patient motion also influences image acquisition. A technique to reduce the effect of patient motion during acquisition is to perform serial short acquisitions with the camera going back and forth, and then eliminating all images with significant patient motion. The transverse reconstructed slices that do not show patient motion are then added together.

Processing Factors

Processing problems that can cause significant image degradation usually arise from abusive filtering techniques and patient slippage in the head holder. Excess filtration of the images will, for example, result in an image that is "oversmoothed" (Fig. 2.17). Oversmoothed images generally have poor spatial resolution (Fig. 2.18). On the other hand, inadequate filtration will result in an excessive image noise, which can likewise make image interpretation very difficult (Fig. 2.19). Pixel sizing represents another potential pitfall. Pixel size of the transaxial sections is an area of real concern when reconstructing the reoriented coronal and sagittal planes. The transaxial sections used for reconstruction of the coronal and sagittal planes should be 1 pixel thick (3 to 4 mm); otherwise, significant image distortion may result (Fig. 2.20).

Patient motion may also effect processing. Patients tend to slide down from the head holder, representing longitudinal displacement. Postacquisition processing can be done to align the brain activity at the vertex from all projections. Although patient motion does degrade image quality, the larger effects of longitudinal displacement can be ameliorated by this technique. A shift greater than 1 cm constitutes a large effect. Some commercial software to deal with this problem is available.

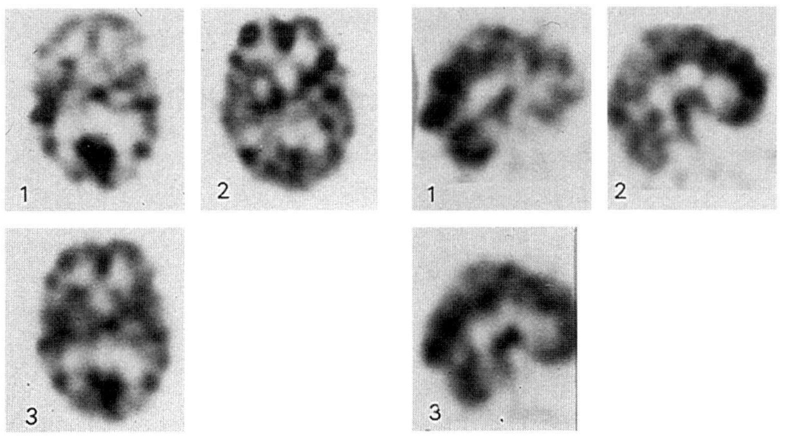

FIG. 2.15. A: Transaxial plane—180° vs. 360°acquisition. *1,* 180°posterior; *2,* 180°anterior; *3,* 360°acquisition.

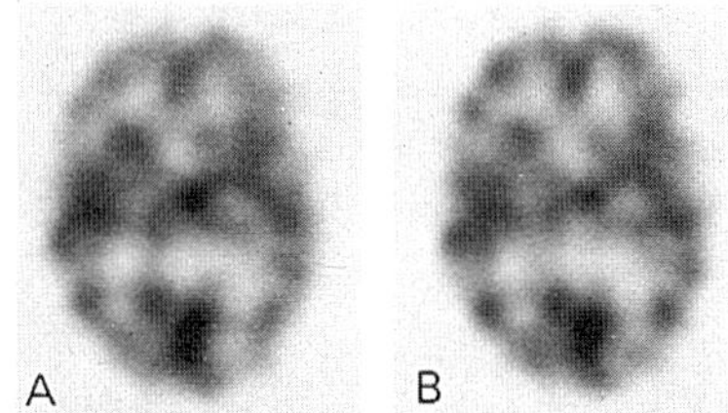

FIG. 2.16. Angular sampling. **A:** 32 frame. **B:** 128 frame.

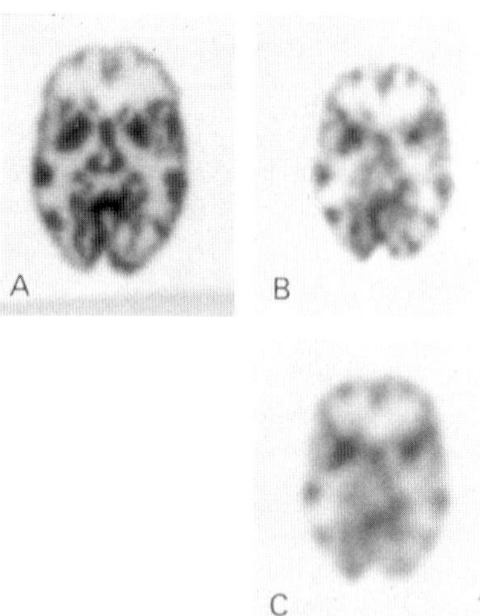

FIG. 2.17. A: High-resolution planar image of Hoffman brain phantom. **B:** Properly filtered transaxial plane SPECT image. **C:** Overfiltered transaxial plane SPECT image with loss of spatial resolution.

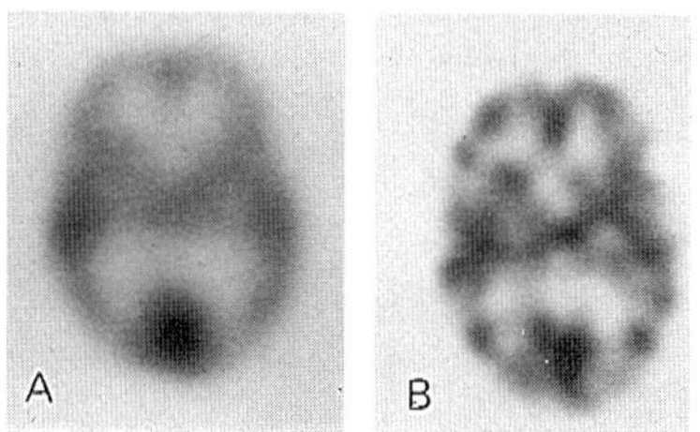

FIG. 2.18. A: Overfiltered transaxial plane SPECT image of a patient. **B:** Properly filtered image of same patient with improved spatial resolution.

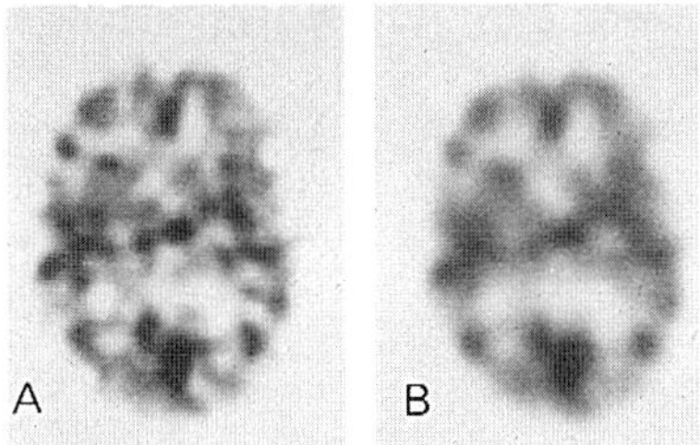

FIG. 2.19. A: Underfiltered transaxial plane SPECT image of a patient resulting in an excessively noisy image. **B:** Properly filtered image of same patient with improved spatial resolution.

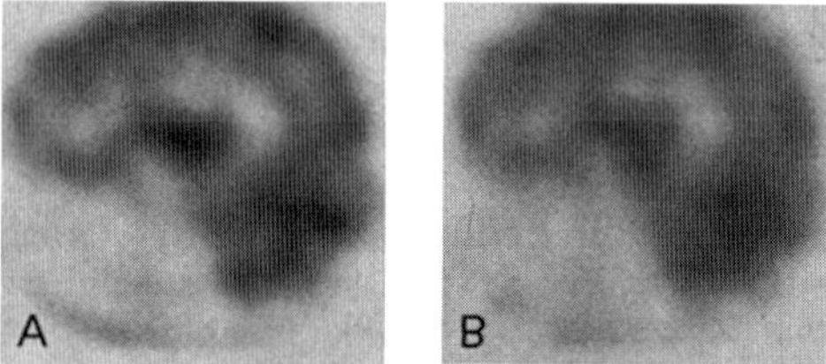

FIG. 2.20. Pixel sizing. **A:** Distorted sagittal plane secondary to reconstruction from 3-pixel-width transaxial plane study. **B:** Improved image resolution in sagittal plane study reconstructed from 1-pixel-width transaxial plane study.

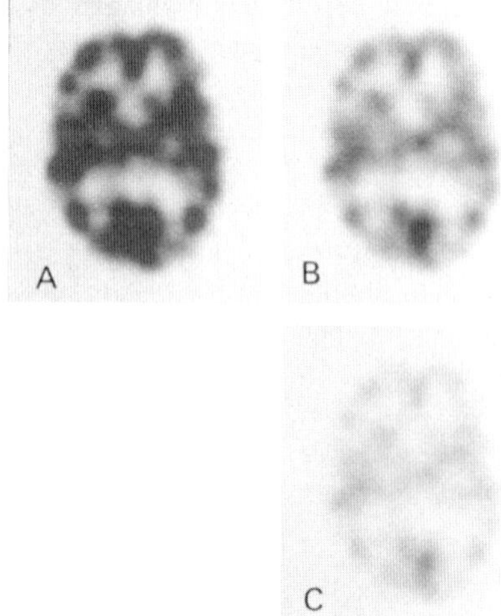

FIG. 2.21. Image display intensity. **A:** Excessively dark image. **B:** Proper intensity. **C:** Excessively light image.

Display Factors

Slice thickness and pixel size should be at least twice that of the expected resolution. For example, if slices are 8 mm thick, then changes <16 mm in size ($2 \times 8 = 16$) cannot be detected.

Great care should be given to the proper choice of transparence film used to archive the cerebral SPECT imaging study. Consideration must also be given to the type of black-and-white and color maps used to display the data on the computer monitor and the type of map utilized for the image formatter display. Scales favoring midrange enhancement may be advantageous for qualitative image evaluation. Low display level can also aid in qualitative image analysis (lower thresholding). However, whatever approach to display is taken, it should be minimally operator dependent and be used in a consistent fashion. These variables should be properly established when first initiating cerebral SPECT imaging studies and then checked on an ongoing basis. Once these factors are carefully controlled and the film formatters are properly maintained, the most frequent cause for display problems relates to the use of an improper display intensity. Image displays that are either too light or too dark may result in the loss of important data that may be pertinent to the study (Fig. 2.21).

Interpretive Factors

Most of the pitfalls described above can produce images with artifacts that either simulate pathology or make image interpretation very difficult or impossible. Proper quality control and standardization of the imaging technique should significantly reduce interpretive errors. A knowledge of the previously discussed pitfalls, should they occur, will also result in a further reduction in the number of misinterpretations of cerebral SPECT studies. In addition, it is essential that the physician interpreting the cerebral SPECT images have a fundamental understanding of the cross-sectional anatomy of the brain in all three orthogonal planes, plus a firm understanding of the major normal variants in anatomic structures.

REFERENCES

1. Van Heertum RL, Tikofsky RS. *Advances in cerebral SPECT imaging.* New York: Tirvirum; 1989.
2. SPECTamine package insert. Schaumberg, IL: IMP Incorporated; April, 1991.
3. Hung JC, Corlija M, Volkert WA, Volkert WA, Holmes RA. Kinetic analysis of technetium-99m d,l-HM-PAO decomposition in aqueous media. *J Nucl Med* 1988;29:1568–1576.
4. Tikofsky RS, Trembath LA, Voslar MA. Radiopharmaceuticals for brain imaging: the technologist's perspective. *J Nucl Med Technol* 1993;21:57–60.
5. Hellman RS, Tikofsky RS, Collier BD, Joestgen TM. *A new era in functional brain imaging in the evaluation of stroke: a monograph.* New York: Medi-Physics; 1988.
6. Hellman RS, Collier BD. Single photon emission computed tomography: a clinical experience. In: Freeman LM, Weissmann HS, eds. *Nuclear medicine annual 1987.* New York: Raven Press; 1987;51–101.
7. Polak JF, English RJ, Holman BL. Performance of collimators used for tomographic imaging of I-123 contaminated with I-124. *J Nucl Med* 1983;24:1065–1069.
8. Larson SA, Bergstrand G, Berstedt H, et al. A special cut-off gamma camera for high resolution SPECT of the head. *J Nucl Med* 1984;25:1023–1030.
9. Woronowicz EM, Eisner RL, Gullberg DJ et al. Factors affecting single photon emission computed tomography image quality and recommended QC procedures. In: *General Electric medical systems operations.* Milwaukee: General Electric Company; 1982.
10. Weber DA, Devous, Sr. MD, Tikofsky RS. *Brain SPECT perfusion imaging: image acquisition, processing, display and interpretation.* DOE CONF-9110368; Washington, DC: US Department of Energy; 1992.

Cerebral SPECT Imaging, Second Edition,
edited by R.L. Van Heertum and R.S. Tikofsky.
Raven Press, Ltd., New York © 1995.

CHAPTER 3

Normal and Correlative Anatomy

Charles R. Noback, David L. Daniels, Leighton P. Mark, and Robert S. Hellman

The frontal, temporal, parietal, and occipital lobes are seen on the lateral view of the brain (Fig. 3.1). The central sulcus (fissure of Rolando) separates the frontal from parietal lobes. The Sylvian fissure divides the frontal from temporal and parietal lobes. There is no clear demarcation dividing the parietal from the occipital lobe. Functionally, the anterior portions of the frontal lobes are concerned with memory and emotional control, while the posterior portions are involved with the initiation and voluntary control of motor activity. The temporal lobe is involved with auditory function, and on the left side language comprehension. The parietal lobe is involved with the appreciation and interpretation of sensory input relating to form, shape, and weight. The occipital lobe is involved with primary visual function. The cerebellum is primarily involved with overall coordination of movement, including gait and balance. It is important to note that the two cerebral hemispheres do not have perfectly symmetric gross and microscopic anatomy, nor do they provide equivalent cognitive functions.

SAGITTAL VIEW OF THE BRAIN

The two hemispheres are interconnected by a large band of nerve fibers, the corpus callosum. The limbic (fifth) lobe, consisting of the cortex and associated structures superior to the corpus callosum, is involved in emotions, drives, and behavioral expression (Fig. 3.2).

The brain stem is involved in the control of respiration and cardiovascular activity. In addition, the major sensorimotor pathways pass through the brain stem to and from the cortex. The cerebellum, as noted above, is involved with motor coordination, gait, and balance.

C. R. Noback: Department of Anatomy, Columbia University College of Physicians and Surgeons, New York, New York 10032.

D. L. Daniels, L. P. Mark, and R. S. Hellman: Department of Radiology, Medical College of Wisconsin, Milwaukee, Wisconsin 53226.

THE VENTRICULAR SYSTEM

The ventricular system (Fig. 3.3) and subarachnoid space surrounding the brain are filled with cerebrospinal fluid (CSF). The fluid is formed by the choroid plexus in each ventricle. The CSF flows from the lateral ventricles through the interventricular foramen of Monro to the third ventricle, and then through the cerebral aqueduct and the fourth ventricle to the subarachnoid space. The system provides a fluid cushion upon which the brain "floats," protected from physical injury.

VASCULAR DISTRIBUTION

The arterial blood supply to the brain is derived from two major sources, i.e., the paired internal carotid (ICAs) and vertebral arteries (Fig. 3.4). The vertebral arteries join to form the basilar artery, which in turn usually terminates by dividing into the posterior cerebral arteries (PCAs). Branches of the PCAs supply blood to the brain stem, cerebellum, occipital lobes, and inferior portion of the temporal lobes. The ICAs usually terminate by dividing into anterior cerebral arteries (ACAs) and middle cerebral arteries (MCAs). The anterior and posterior circulations connect via the circle of Willis, an arterial ring found at the base of the brain.

As seen in the lateral view, the MCA extends laterally from the sylvian fissure to supply regions of the frontal, temporal, parietal, and occipital lobes (Fig. 3.5). However, the ACA provides the major arterial supply to the medial surface of the brain, in particular the superior surface of the corpus callosum with branches reaching to the frontal and parietal lobes (Fig. 3.6). The PCA extends posteriorly and supplies the medial and posterior aspects of the temporal and occipital lobes.

On the coronal view, the MCAs are seen to extend between the temporal and parietal lobes (Fig. 3.7). Their deep branches—striate arteries—supply the corpus striatum of the basal ganglia and the internal capsules.

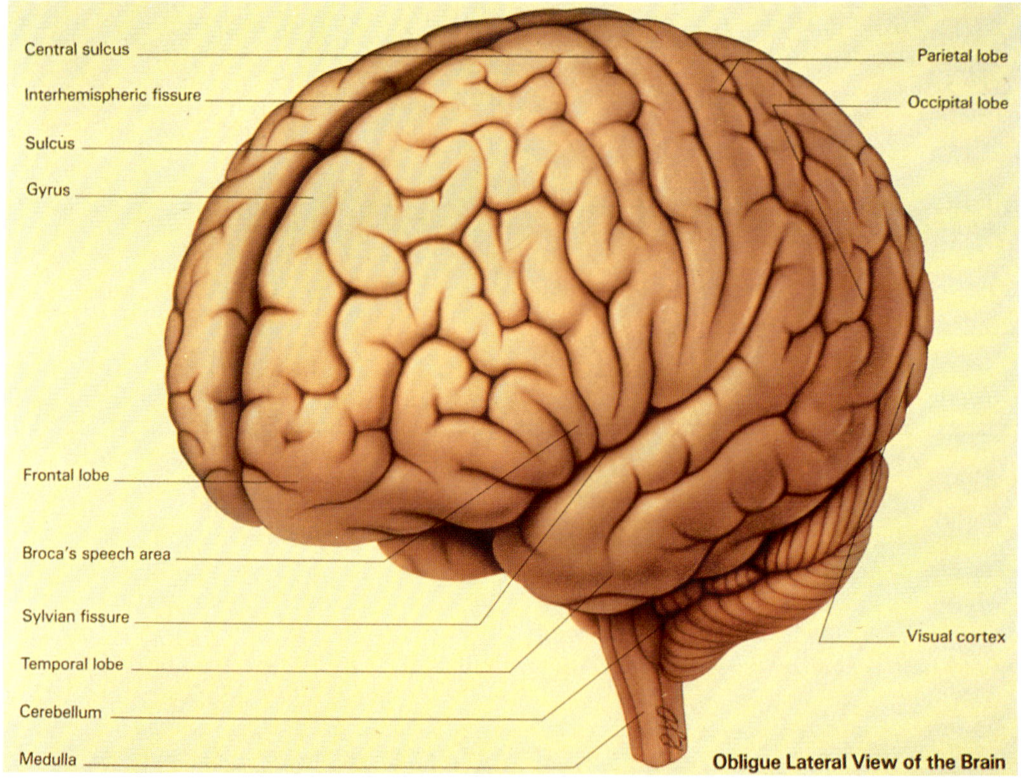

FIG. 3.1. Oblique lateral view of the brain.

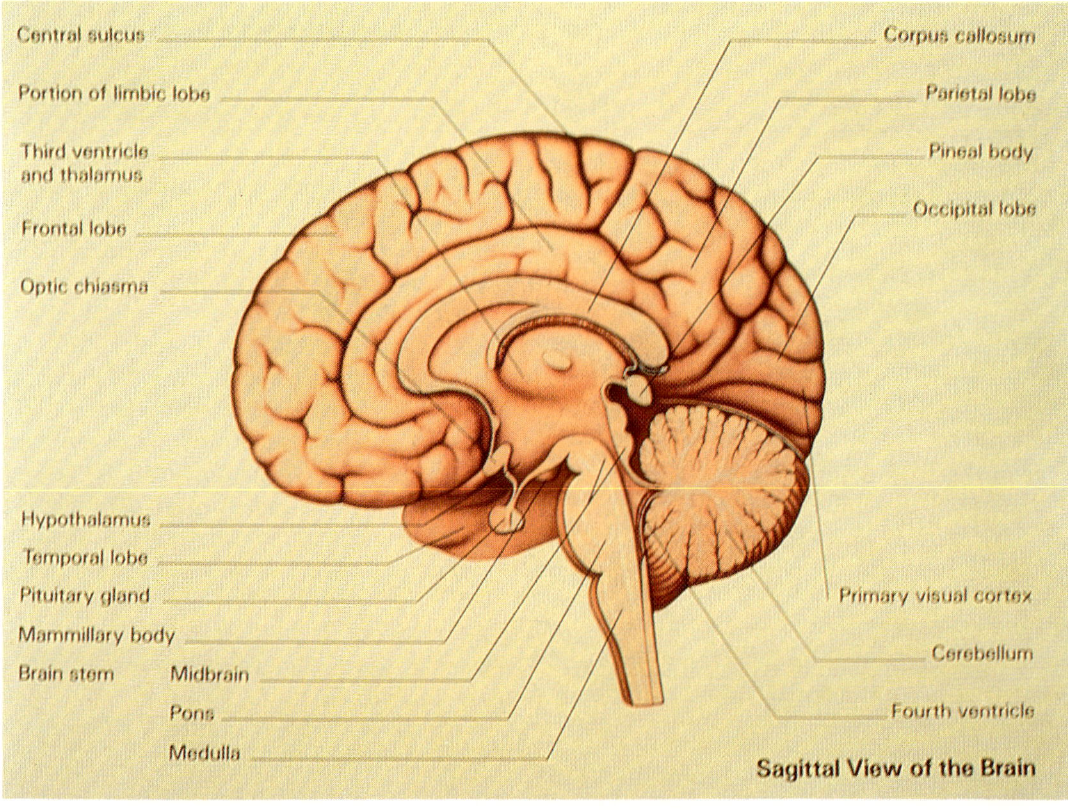

FIG. 3.2. Sagittal view of the brain.

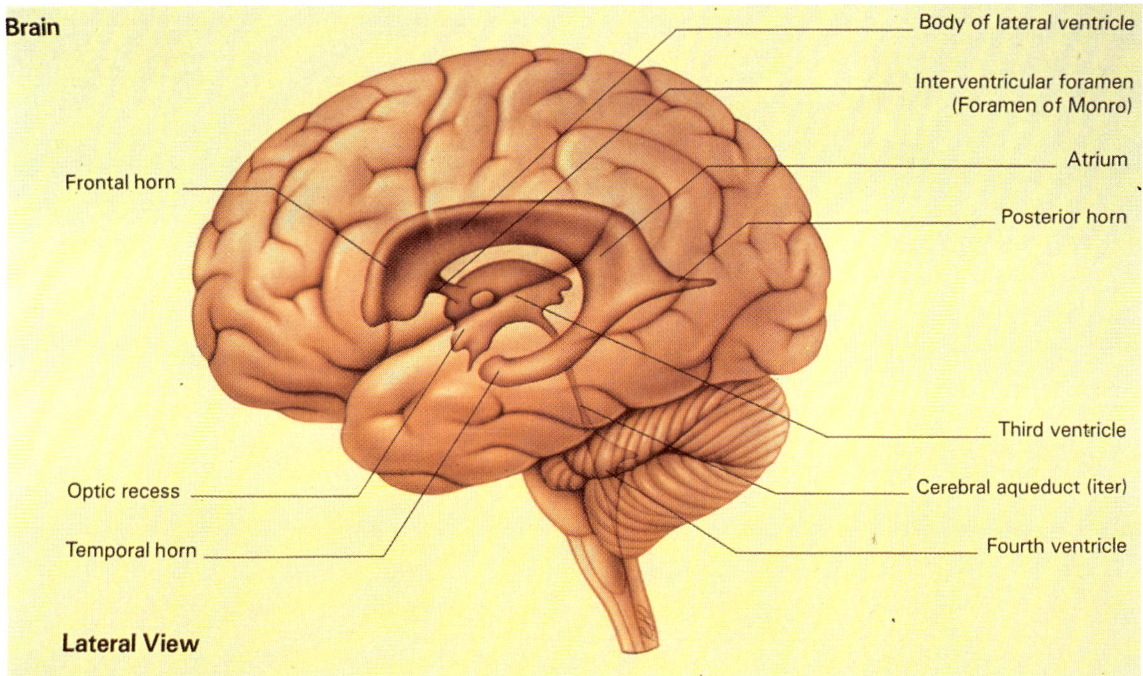

A

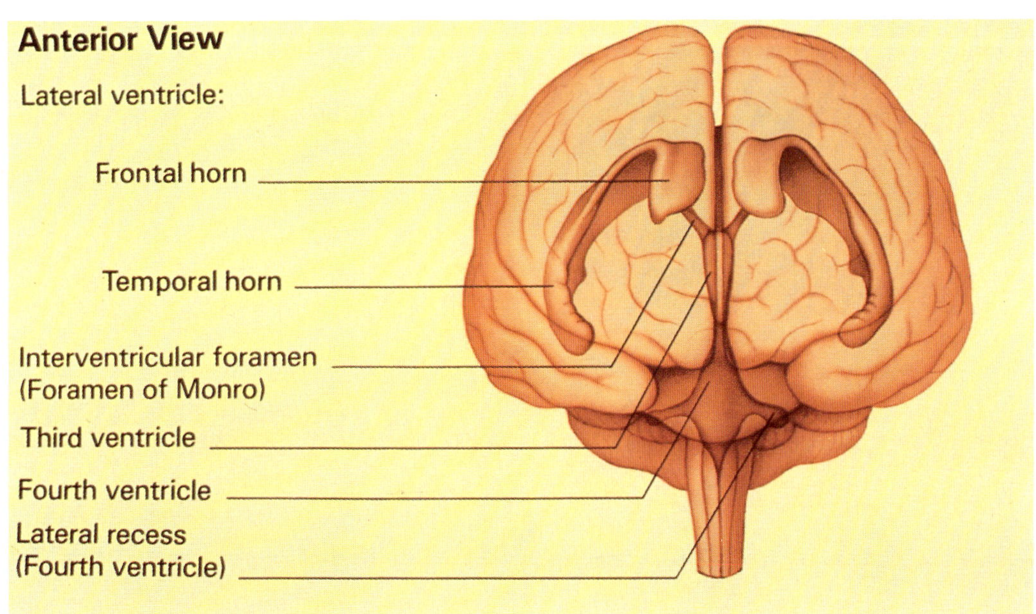

B

FIG. 3.3. Lateral **(A)** and anterior **(B)** views of the ventricles.

TRANSAXIAL VIEW OF THE BRAIN

The anterior and posterior limbs of the internal capsule are involved in motor activity. The caudate and putamen, structures making up part of the basal ganglia are involved in fine motor coordination. The thalamus is a major structure for the perception of many types of sensory stimuli. It sends projections to the primary sensory/motor areas of the cerebral hemispheres (Fig. 3.8).

CORRELATIVE ANATOMY

Cerebral SPECT studies are displayed in transaxial, coronal, and sagittal planes (Fig. 3.9) adjacent to the corresponding MR images.

The major structures of the cerebrum such as the frontal, temporal, parietal, and occipital lobes are identified. The cerebellar hemispheres and basal ganglia are also shown. However, the spatial resolution of SPECT images is less

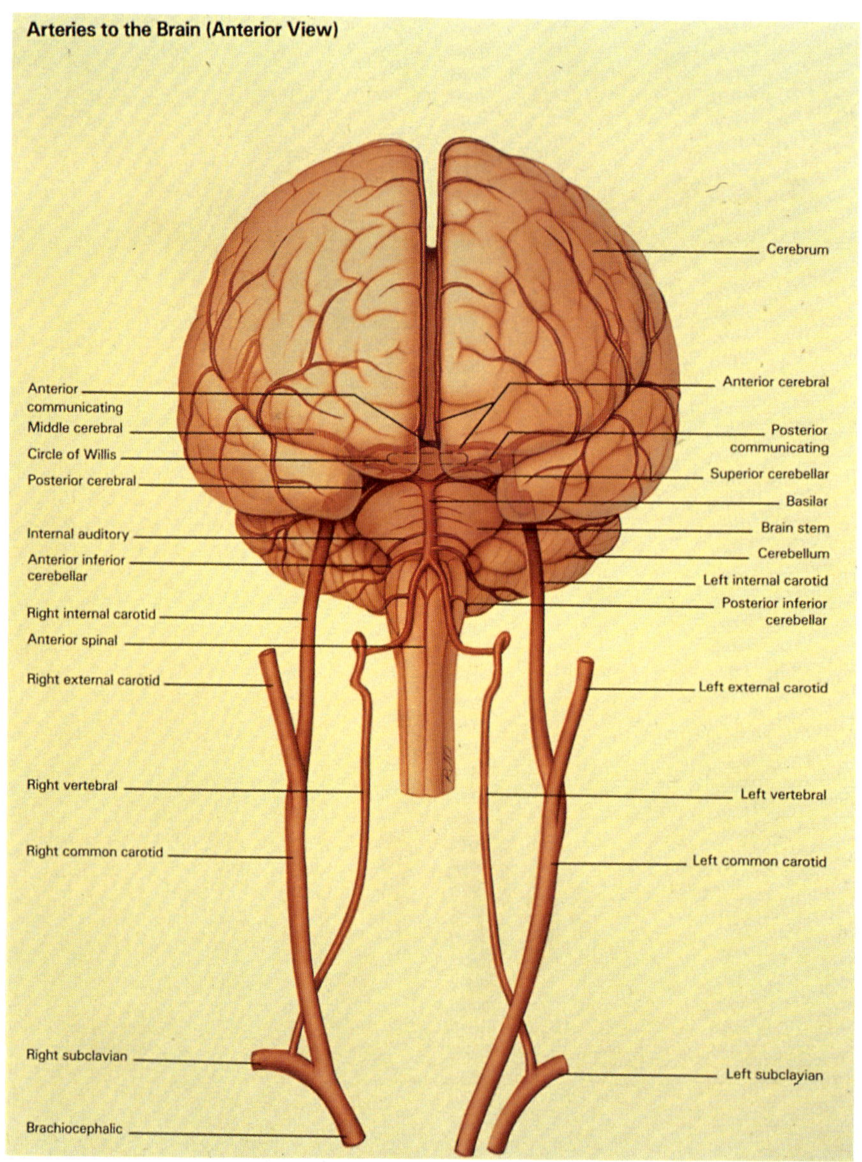

FIG. 3.4. Anterior view of the cerebral arteries.

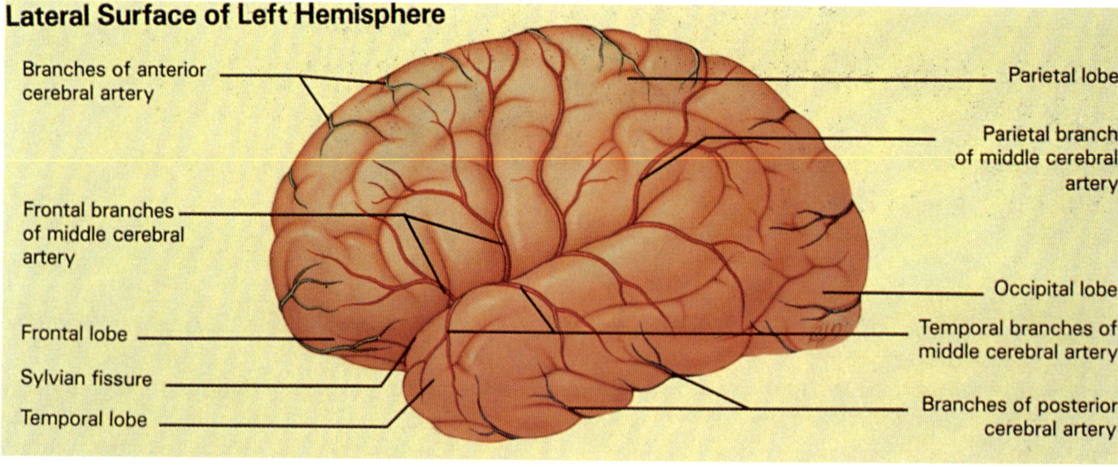

FIG. 3.5. Lateral surface of the left hemisphere.

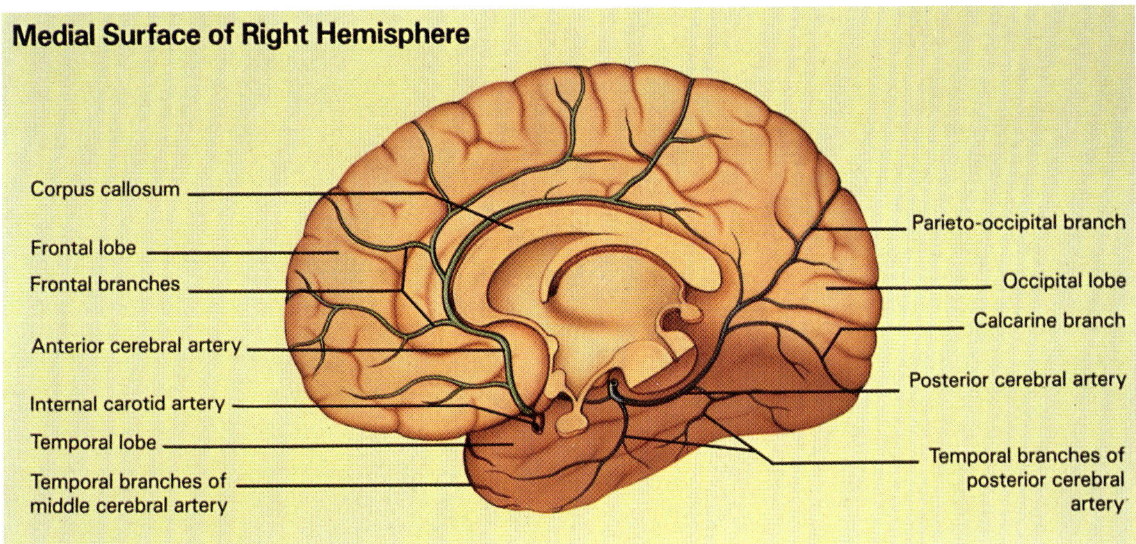

FIG. 3.6. Medial surface of the right hemisphere.

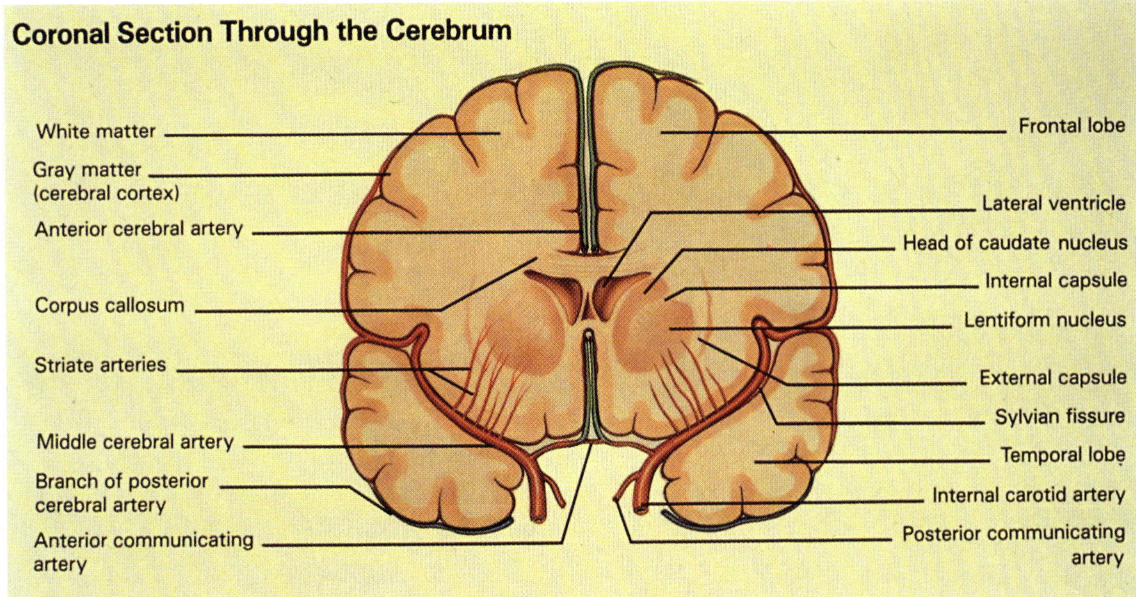

FIG. 3.7. Coronal section through the cerebrum.

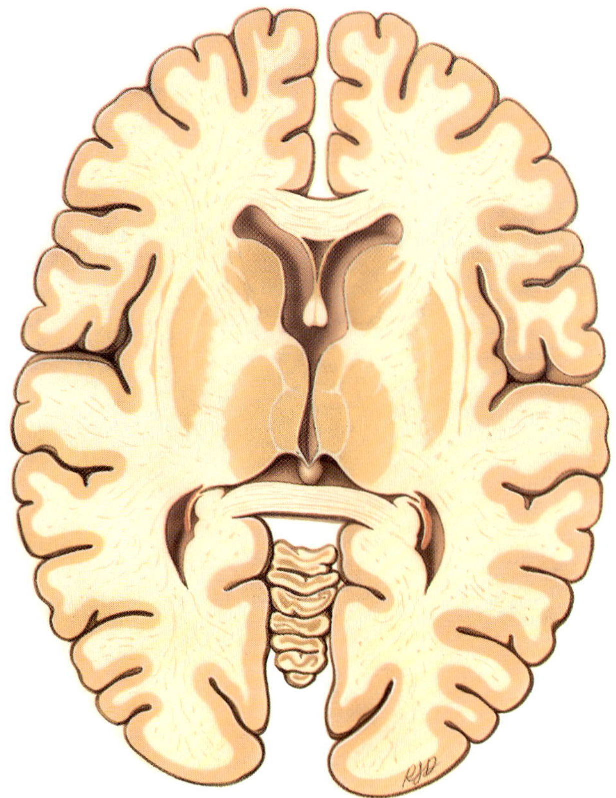

FIG. 3.8. Transaxial view of the brain.

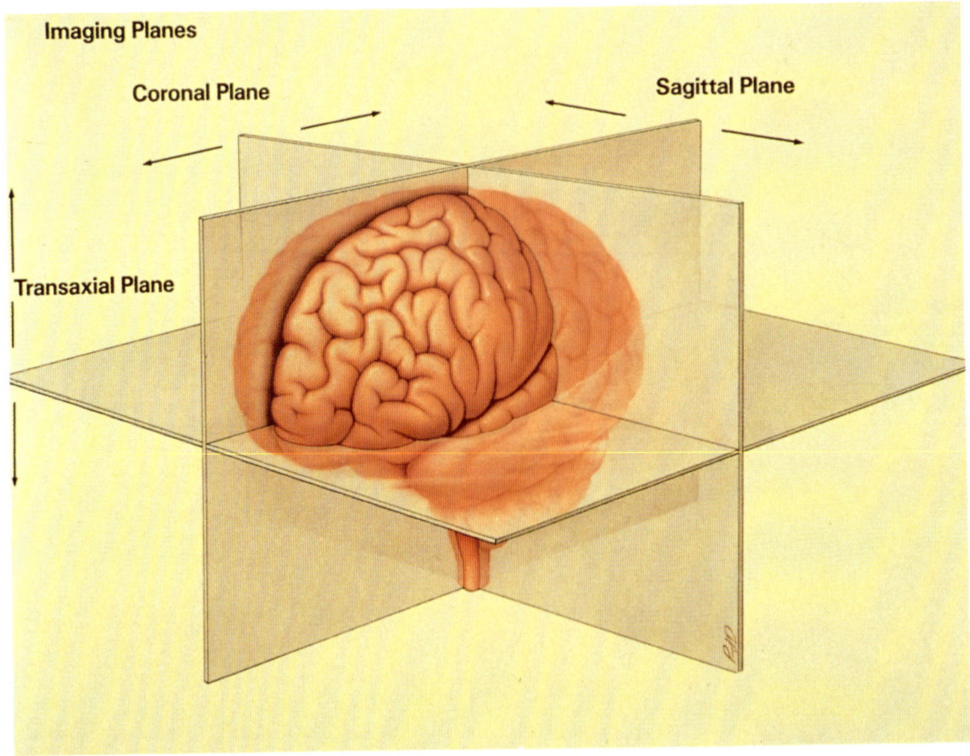

FIG. 3.9. Imaging planes.

than that of MRI. Thus, SPECT images do not demonstrate the different structures of basal ganglia, brain stem, and the edge between white matter and the ventricles.

SPECT images should not be used to show detailed anatomy although they demonstrate the major anatomic landmarks. SPECT imaging—when correlated with anatomic studies such as MRI and CT—may be useful in delineating some pathologic processes using multiple planes. More importantly, in some disease states, changes in blood flow and metabolism may only be appreciated with SPECT imaging, but not with CT or MRI. Figures 3.10, 3.11, and 3.12 illustrate representative SPECT images for single head (IMP), triple head (HMPAU), adjacent to corresponding MRI images.

TRANSAXIAL PLANE

The transaxial cerebral SPECT sections are displayed in the same format as the MRI images. The sections begin inferiorly in the cerebellum and continue superiorly through the entire cerebrum (Fig. 3.10).

CORONAL PLANE

The coronal cerebral SPECT sections are displayed in the same format as the MRI images. The sections begin anteriorly in the frontal lobes and continue posteriorly through the entire brain (Fig. 3.11).

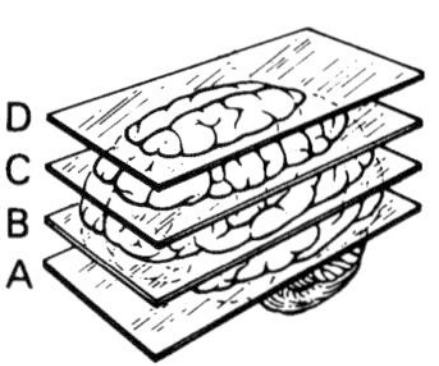

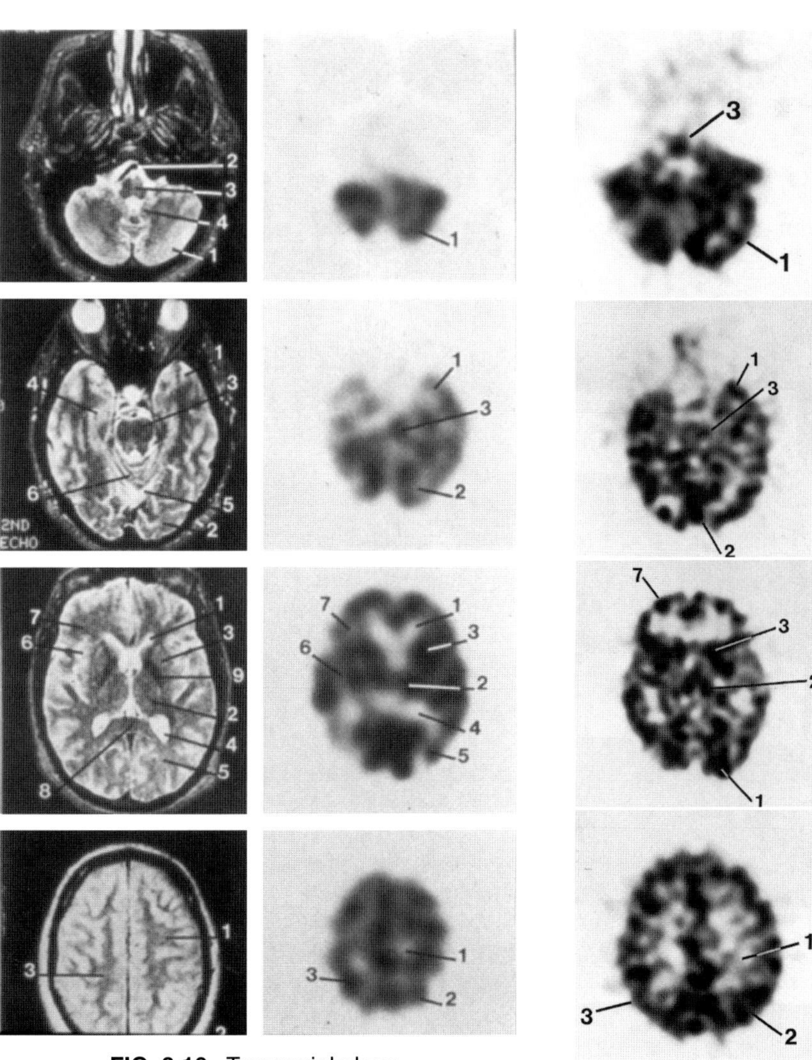

A. 1. Cerebellar hemisphere
2. Vertebral artery
3. Medulla oblongata
4. Cerebellar tonsil

B. 1. Temporal lobe
2. Occipital lobe
3. Upper brain stem
4. Temporal horn
5. Tentorial notch
6. Cerebellar vermis

C. 1. Frontal horn
2. Thalamus
3. Basal ganglia—lentiform nucleus
4. Occipital horn
5. Occipital lobe
6. White matter
7. Frontal lobe
8. Splenium of corpus callosum
9. Internal capsule

D. 1. White matter
2. Gray matter
3. Parietal lobe

FIG. 3.10. Transaxial plane.

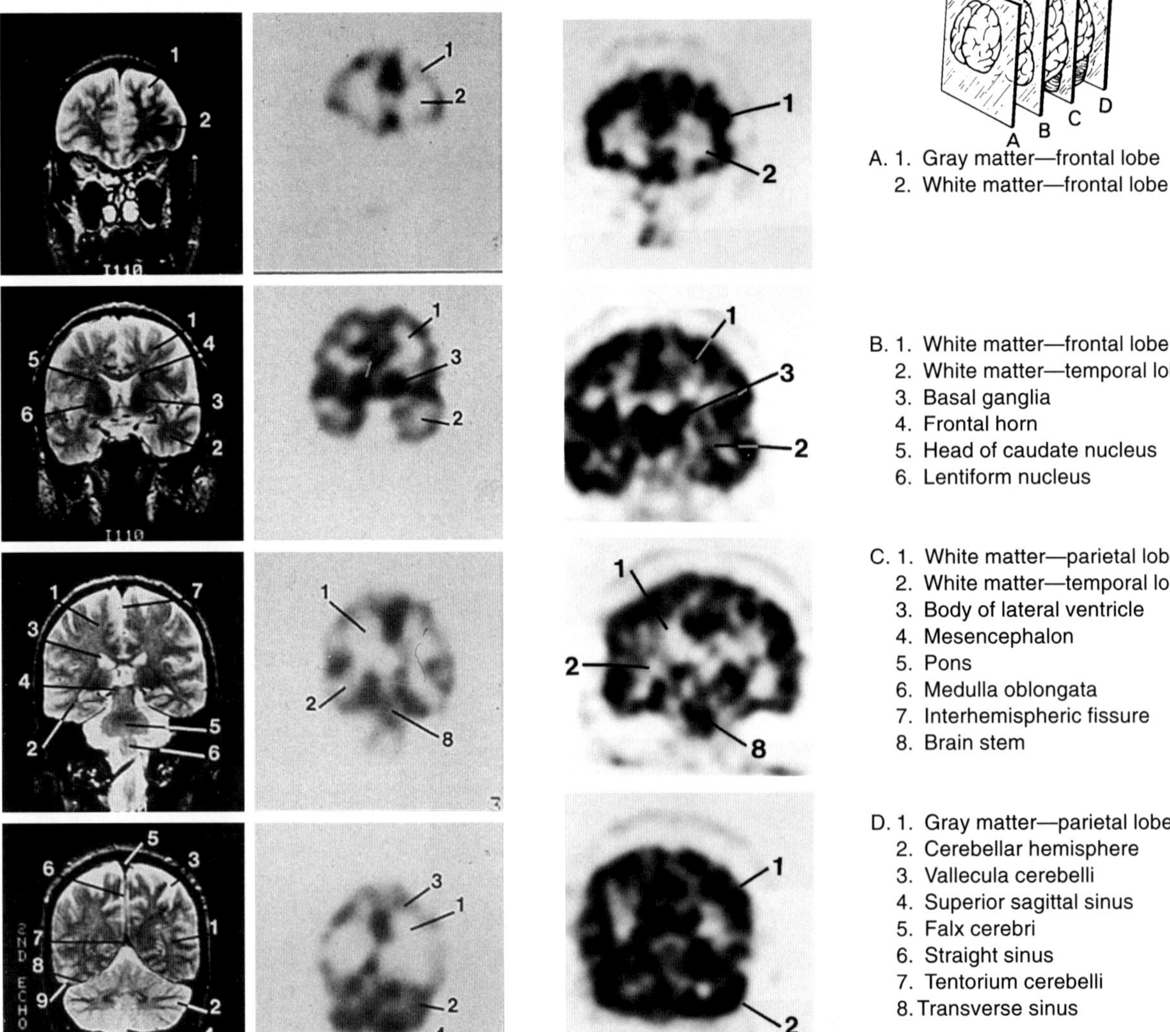

FIG. 3.11. Coronal plane.

SAGITTAL PLANE

The sagittal cerebral SPECT sections are displayed in the same format as the MRI images. The images extend from the right side of the brain to the midline (Fig. 3.12).

HELPFUL HINTS

The examples that follow are designed to provide an overview of the general characteristics observed in normal and pathological regional cerebral blood flow/SPECT brain images. They serve as a general point of reference for comparison with the case presentations in the chapters that follow.

Normal Tracer Uptake

Typically, there is symmetric distribution of tracer uptake in both hemispheres. The basal ganglia, occipital cortex, and cerebellum will often appear darker than other regions. Ventricles will not be as sharply defined as with CT or MRI because the tracer is not taken up by the ventricles or white matter surrounding the ventricles. When imaging is performed with multidetector systems it is possible to distinguish the heads of the caudate nuclei, the body of the caudate, and other lenticular structures. In addition, the thalamus can also be visualized in the transaxial images (Fig. 3.13).

Absent Tracer Uptake

Absent tracer uptake implies that tracer uptake is not present in a zone extending from deep within the brain through the cortical rim. These regions of absent uptake often have the appearance of a bite or wedge taken out of the brain. This type of finding is associated with a region of infarction seen on CT or MRI (Fig. 3.14). Areas of absent tracer uptake may also be observed in case of trauma and surgical resection.

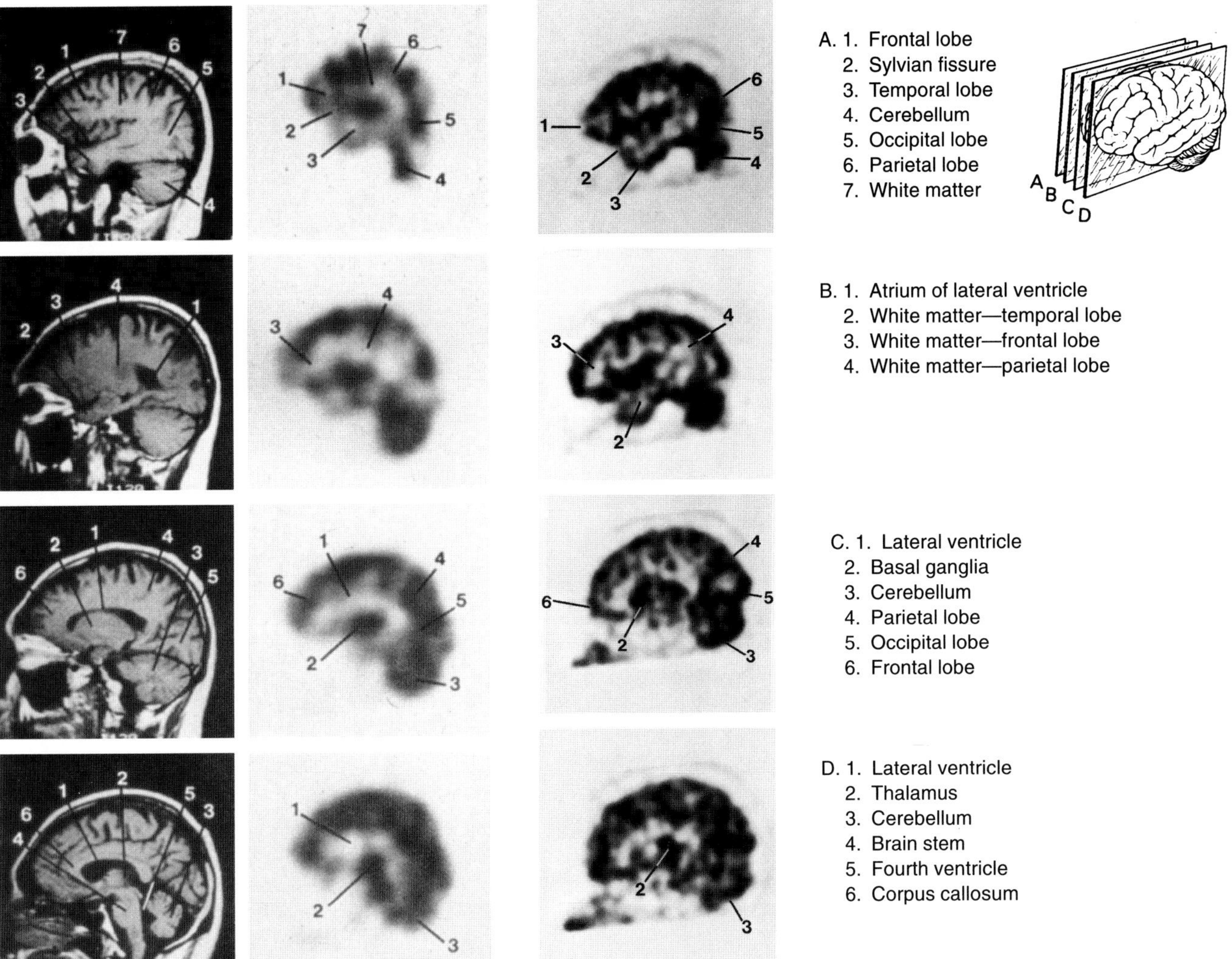

FIG. 3.12. Sagittal plane.

Reduced but not Absent Tracer Uptake

Regions of reduced but not absent tracer uptake usually appear "less intense" than do the surrounding cortical regions and corresponding regions of the contralateral hemisphere. They also will appear "thin" or "less intense" in comparison to equivalent regions seen in normal studies. It is also useful to compare regions thought to show reduced but not absent tracer uptake with the basal ganglia, occipital cortex, and cerebellum. This finding is typically associated with the presence of ischemia and is not necessarily evident on CT or MRI images. It is a common finding in the dementias and may be seen in depressed patients (Fig. 3.15).

Increased Tracer Uptake

Regions of increased tracer uptake usually appear to have "greater intensity" than do the surrounding cortical regions and corresponding regions of the contralateral hemisphere. They will also appear "thicker" and "darker" than the equivalent regions seen in normal studies. Findings of increased tracer uptake have been associated with one of two conditions: regions of hypermetabolism such as seizure activity (Fig. 3.16) or luxury perfusion (Fig. 3.17 A, B).

Findings of increased tracer uptake have been associated with one of two conditions: regions of hypermetabolism such as seizure activity (Fig. 11), or luxury perfusion (Fig. 3.17 A, B).

Distortion of the Cortical Surface

Regions of "misshapen" or "distorted" cortical rim are often seen when there is an accumulation of extra axial fluid or blood following trauma, and when there is an extra axial mass. The extent of distortion is related to the amount of fluid accumulation and the size of the mass (Fig. 3.18).

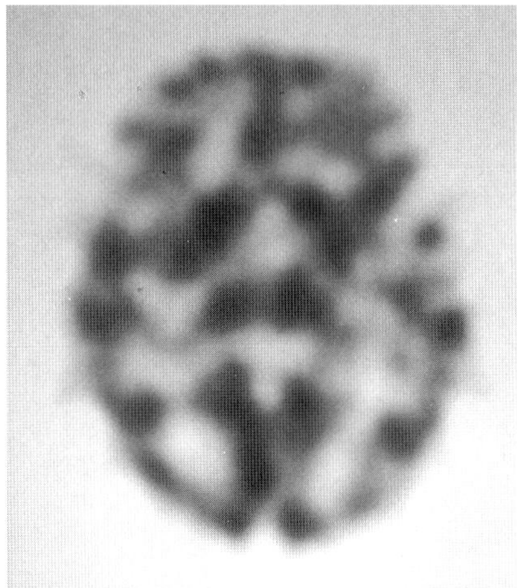

FIG. 3.13. Normal distribution.

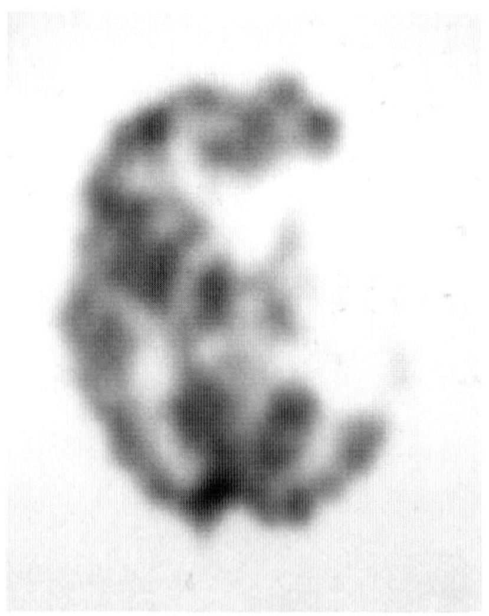

FIG. 3.15. Reduced tracer uptake.

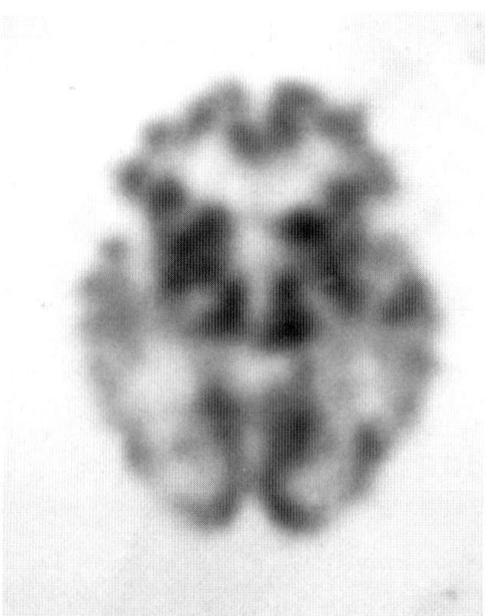

FIG. 3.14. Absent tracer uptake.

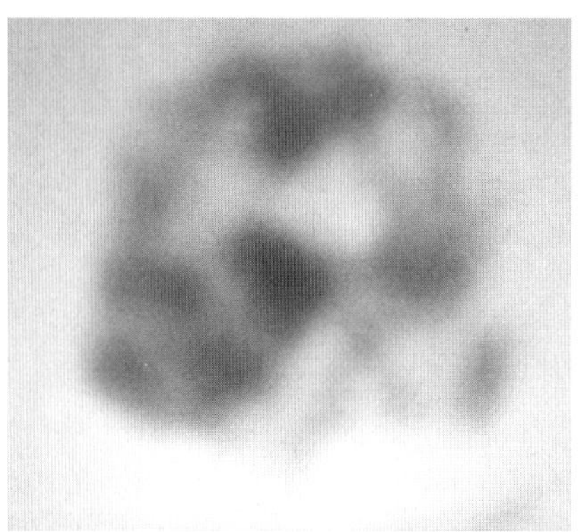

FIG. 3.16. Increased tracer uptake.

A

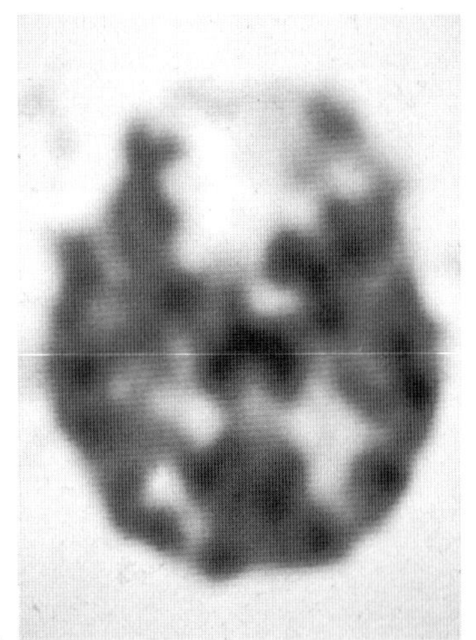

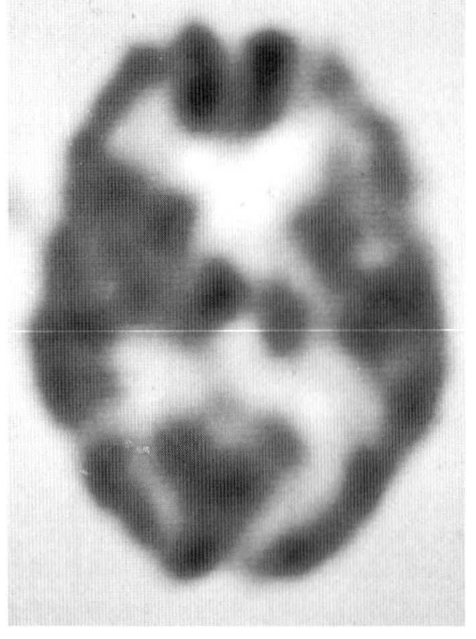

B

FIG. 3.17. Absent tracer uptake before luxury perfusion **(A)** and after the onset of luxury perfusion **(B)**.

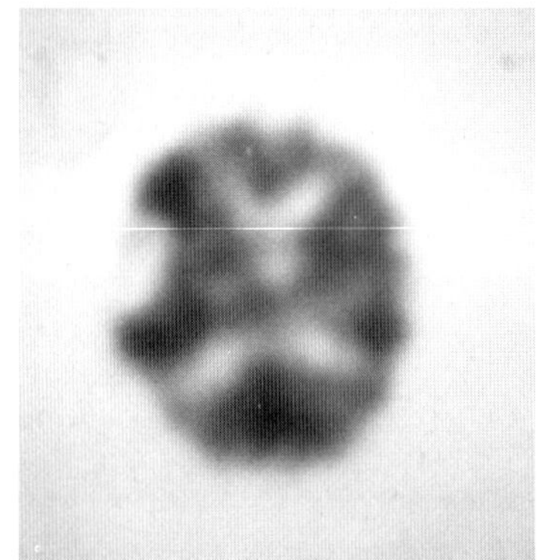

FIG. 3.18. Compressed cortex.

Cerebral SPECT Imaging, Second Edition,
edited by R.L. Van Heertum and R.S. Tikofsky.
Raven Press, Ltd., New York © 1995.

CHAPTER 4

Functional Anatomy and SPECT Imaging

H. Branch Coslett

Interest in the anatomic underpinnings of behavior has a venerable history, dating at least to the ancient Greeks. In the fifth century BC, for example, Hippocrates of Croton argued that the brain was the organ of intellect whereas the heart was the organ of the senses. In the second century, Galen was the first to claim that cognition resided in the substance of the brain rather than the ventricles.

Perhaps the first modern attempt to localize behaviors to specific brain structures is found in the work of the phrenologist Franz Joseph Gall, who in the late nineteenth and early twentieth centuries espoused the theory that mental faculties were localized in "centers" in the brain; unfortunately, Gall is primarily remembered at this point not for his belief that definable brain regions were implicated in specific behaviors but for his additional incorrect assertion that, because the brain's form shapes the overlying skull, the status of an individual's cognitive and behavioral capacities could be inferred by measuring the external contours of the skull.

Although ultimately discredited, the teachings of the phrenologists are clearly relevant to contemporary accounts of brain-behavior relationships in that these teachings exerted a significant influence on the French and German physicians of the mid-nineteenth century such as Paul Broca and Carl Wernicke, whose seminal contributions constitute the beginnings of the contemporary doctrine of the localization of cerebral functions. After hearing Aubertin, a student of Gall, describe the significance of the frontal lobes in speech, Broca (1) investigated a series of patients with "aphemia" (only later designated *aphasia*) and subsequently determined that the left frontal lobe is critical for speech. Additional observations by Hughlings Jackson (2), Bastian (3), and Wernicke (4) supporting the consistent association between sites of brain injury and specific behavioral disorders quickly followed. Indeed, the exploration of brain-behavior relationships, to which SPECT brain imaging has made important contributions in recent years, continues to be a major subject of research in modern cognitive neuroscience.

In this chapter, we will provide a brief overview of insights on the functional anatomy of the human brain afforded by investigations conducted over the last 130 years. The *ablation paradigm,* that is, the investigation of the behavioral consequences of focal brain injury such as stroke or intracerebral hemorrhage, has been the richest source of information regarding the functional anatomy of the cerebral cortex. It should be noted, however, that a number of other lines of investigation including brain stimulation in humans and animals, electrophysiological recordings in animals, manipulation of neurochemical systems in animals and, more recently, "activation" studies using SPECT positron emission tomography (PET), and magnetic resonance imaging (MRI) scans have also contributed substantially to this body of knowledge.

Prior to a consideration of the behavioral disorders associated with dysfunction of different brain regions, it is important to note that the likelihood that brain dysfunction will result in the "classical" pattern of behavioral disturbance is influenced by a number of factors. The *age* at which the pathologic process is initiated, for example, may be critical to the outcome; thus, while the association between language dysfunction and left hemisphere perisylvian dysfunction in right-handers has been repeatedly demonstrated since the time of Broca, a number of investigators have demonstrated that left hemisphere insult—even including left hemispherectomy (5)—may cause minimal language dysfunction when the insult occurs prior to the age of 6. Similarly, the *nature* of the underlying pathologic process may play an important role in modulating the behavioral consequences of brain dysfunction; behavioral disturbances associated with right (nondominant) parietal lobe dysfunction may appear quite different in patients with brain tumors, for example, compared with stroke. Additional factors that may substantially influence the behavioral consequences of brain dysfunction include the time

H. B. Coslett: Department of Neurology, Temple University School of Medicine, Philadelphia, Pennsylvania 19140.

since insult, the rate of evolution of the pathologic process, depth and surface area of the lesion, and, of course, premorbid factors such as handedness and presence of previous neurologic or psychiatric disorders.

As the present volume provides an excellent account of the utility of SPECT brain imaging in defining the functional anatomy of behavioral disorders, we have elected to describe the functional anatomy of the cerebral cortex with respect to specific brain regions (e.g., the temporal lobe) rather than, for example, describing the localization of specific behavioral disorders such as amnesia or aphasia. We have opted to present what we believe to be the most "typical" or consistent pattern of localization of function; in light of the complexity of the psychological processes underlying human behavior, we wish to make clear that many clinical syndromes may be associated with lesions in different brain regions.

FRONTAL LOBES

Describing the scope and characteristics of human cognition, the eminent Russian neuropsychologist A. Luria (6) wrote:

> Man not only reacts passively to incoming information, but creates *intentions,* forms *plans* and *programs* of his actions, inspects their performance, and *regulates* his behavior so that it conforms to these plans and programs; finally, he *verifies* his conscious activity, comparing the effects of his actions with the original intentions and correcting many mistakes he has made (pp. 78–79).

In fact, as we shall see below, it is the frontal lobe that provides the substrate for much of what Luria believed to be the essence of creative, synthetic, and goal-directed human behavior.

Perhaps the most striking evolutionary alteration in human brain structure has been the dramatic enlargement of the frontal lobe; the human frontal lobe comprises approximately 50 percent of brain volume and is characterized by both anatomical and functional diversity. The anatomical diversity is illustrated, for example, by the fact that the influential human neuroanatomist Brodmann identified 11 distinct cytoarchitectonic regions in the frontal lobe (Fig. 4.1).

In light of the size and complexity of this portion of the brain, it is perhaps not surprising that many different patterns of impairment may be observed as a consequence of frontal lobe lesions. Thus, despite the fact that clinicians frequently refer to a "frontal lobe syndrome," there is no single constellation of symptoms and signs that characterize frontal lobe lesions. Rather, the specific behavioral disturbance associated with frontal lobe pathology is to a large extent a function of the site of damage within the frontal lobe. Thus, although a seemingly bewildering array of behavioral deficits have been observed in association with frontal lobe dysfunction, a number of clinicoanatomical correlations have been established. For present pur-

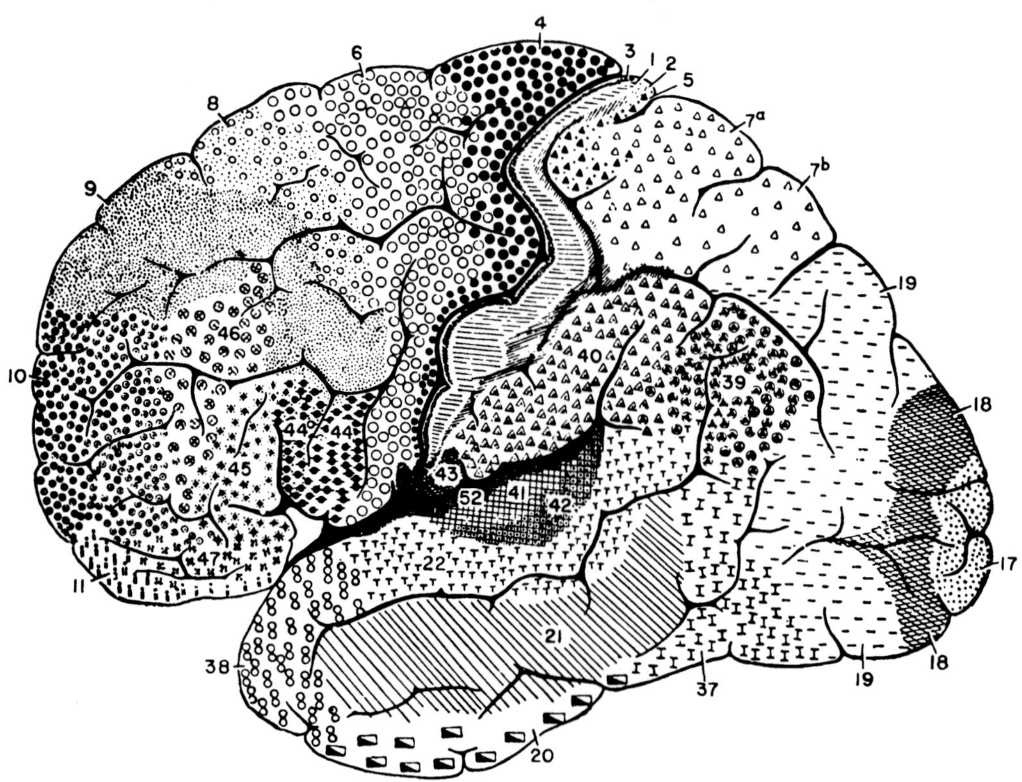

FIG. 4.1. Brodmann map—lateral view.

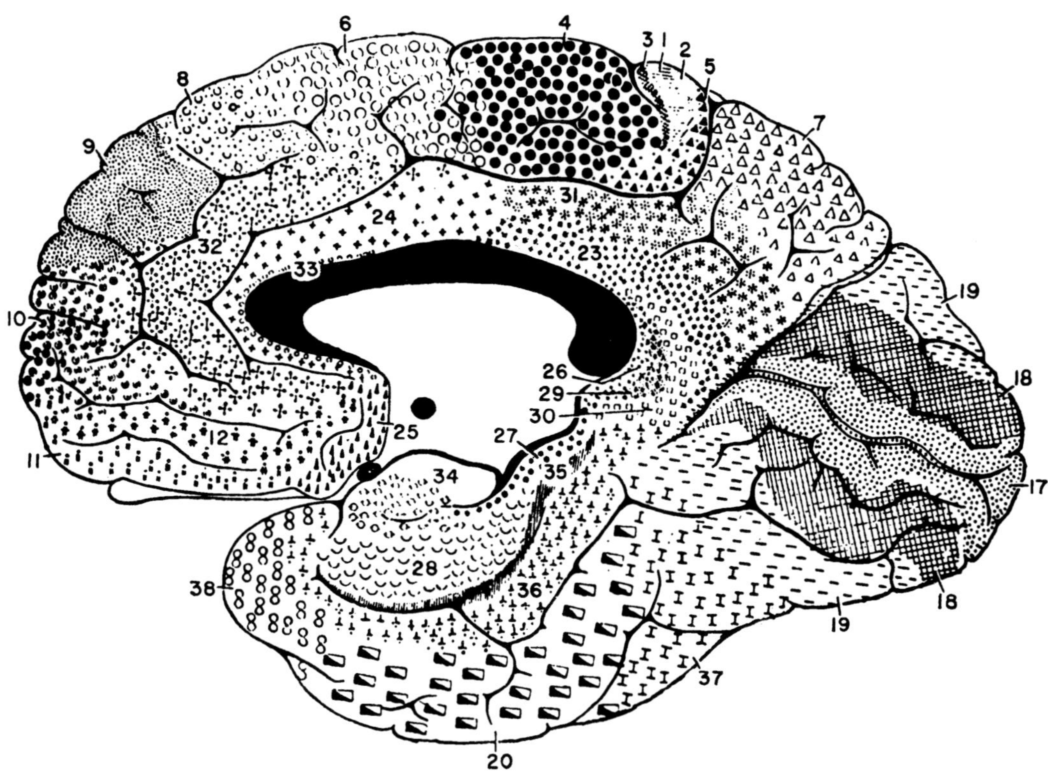

FIG. 4.2. Brodmann map—medial view.

poses, one may distinguish four distinct functional regions of the frontal lobe, damage to which typically is associated with different patterns of behavioral deficits.

The first of the functional regions, the *motor cortex,* extends from the sylvian fissure laterally to the medial surface of the frontal lobes and encompasses the precentral gyrus or "primary" motor cortex (Brodmann area 4) as well as the "premotor" cortex, comprised of the posterior portions of the three horizontally aligned frontal gyri (Brodmann area 6). These cortical regions are, of course, critical for fine motor activity; the majority of the axons comprising the corticospinal tract arise from neurons in these regions. As the primary behavioral consequences of damage to the motor cortex—that is, motor deficits ranging from clumsiness with mild weakness to hemiparesis—are well known, these regions will not be considered further.

The balance of the frontal cortices, often designated the "prefrontal" cortex, includes three regions that are, at least in part, functionally distinct. These include the *orbitofrontal* cortex on the undersurface of the frontal lobe, the *dorsolateral* frontal cortices on the lateral surface of the frontal lobes (including at least portions of Brodmann areas 8, 9, 10, 44, 45, 46, and 47), and the *medial* cortex of the frontal lobe (including parts of Brodmann areas 8, 9, 10, and 24). These three regions are discussed separately below.

Orbitofrontal Cortex

Dysfunction of the orbitofrontal cortex is typically associated with profound changes in personality characterized by emotional instability and unpredictability; damage to these structures is thought to be, at least in large part, responsible for symptoms and signs such as a "pseudobulbar affect," which is characterized by inappropriate expressions of emotion, and the closely related phenomenon of "Witzelsucht." Interestingly, "intelligence," at least as assessed by standard tests of cognitive ability, may be normal.

The consequences of bilateral orbitofrontal lesions may be illustrated by the following accounts of two patients with damage to the orbitofrontal cortex.

Patient E.V.R.

Eslinger and Damasio (7) described a patient, E.V.R., who exhibited dramatic changes in behavior after resection of an orbitofrontal meningioma as well as substantial portions of the bilateral orbitofrontal cortex. By age 32, E.V.R. was married and had two children; he was a church elder and the comptroller of an accounting firm. Shortly thereafter, however, he began to exhibit changes in personality, marital difficulties, and an inability to discharge his professional responsibilities. These difficulties worsened over the course of the next several years, leading to his suspension from his job. At age 35, a large orbitofrontal meningioma, which was compressing the anterior frontal lobes, was resected.

After the resection, E.V.R.'s problems apparently continued unabated. When able to resume work, he returned to accounting for a short time before going into business with a man of dubious moral character. Against the advice of friends and family, he invested his entire savings in a venture that failed, forcing him to declare bankruptcy. He subsequently took and lost a number of jobs ranging from accountant to warehouse laborer. Within 2 years of his operation, his wife left him and filed for divorce. E.V.R. remarried within a month of his divorce and divorced again 2 years later. Interestingly, an extensive inpatient psychiatric evaluation revealed him to be of above normal intelligence with "no evidence of organic brain syndrome or frontal dysfunction" (7).

Subsequent evaluation at the University of Iowa several years later demonstrated that E.V.R. performed well on many conventional measures of intelligence and memory. For example, he obtained a verbal IQ of 129 (97th percentile) and a performance IQ of 135 (99th percentile) as well as a Weschler Memory Scale Score of 143 (well above average).

Patient C.C.

We recently investigated a patient, C.C., whose behavior also illustrates the consequences of dysfunction of the orbitofrontal cortex. C.C. was a seemingly happy and well-adjusted young girl until the age of approximately 15, when she was noted by family and teachers to become increasingly "difficult" and unpredictable. Attributed initially to an adolescent adjustment reaction, over the course of several years her behavior deteriorated to the point at which she displayed "sociopathic" and on occasion violent behavior, ultimately leading to her suspension from school. At the age of 17 she complained of increasingly severe generalized headaches; medical evaluation at that point revealed a large (8 × 8 cm) meningioma arising from the right sphenoid wing and extending superiorly into the posterior portion of the orbitofrontal cortex and basal forebrain; the tumor and surrounding edema distorted most of the orbitofrontal cortex bilaterally as well as portions of the mesial frontal lobes.

Following resection of the tumor and small amounts of surrounding basal forebrain, a dramatic change in C.C.'s behavior was observed. Her irritability, aggressiveness, and unpredictability disappeared, and the previous observed warm and affectionate relationships with family and friends resurfaced. Thus, according to her mother, C.C.'s personality reverted to that she had exhibited as a child.

C.C. did not, however, return to her premorbid state in all respects; she continues to exhibit a prominent and disabling deficit often associated with lesions of the posterior portions of the orbitofrontal cortex and basal forebrain, amnesia (see below).

These two cases, as well as those of previously reported patients (8), attest to the role of the orbitofrontal cortex in the mediation of complex social behavior as well as memory.

Medial Frontal Cortex

The mesial frontal cortex receives projections from the limbic system and has extensive reciprocal projections with the polymodal sensory association cortex as well as cortical regions mediating motor planning. Thus, as emphasized by Mesulam (9), the medial frontal cortex (and cingulate gyri in particular) may play an important role in the integration of limbic information that pertains to motivational significance and emotional valence; such information combines with sensory input and other data about past experience and current needs to generate plans of action. In other words, the medial frontal cortex may be critical for generating and initiating behavior that serves to modulate current and anticipated needs and goals.

This hypothesis is consistent with observations regarding the effects of brain lesions in humans. For example, bilateral lesions of the medial frontal lobes produce the syndrome of akinetic mutism; patients with this disorder may be awake and apparently alert yet they fail to interact with the examiner or with their environment more generally; when spoken to, these patients may not respond and when asked to execute a movement they typically produce no response. Observation of the patients often reveals the movements made by a normal resting individual (e.g., eye-blinking, grooming movements) to be markedly reduced.

Patients with medial frontal lesions typically adopt a quite passive attitude toward their environment, exhibiting little initiative. Laplane et al. (10), for example, reported a patient with destruction of portions of the bilateral medial frontal cortex who, despite a lack of food for 24 hr, never complained of hunger or initiated any action to obtain food. When finally provided a meal tray, she expressed no surprise or relief but ate in her usual fashion. Interestingly, when provided a second meal a short while later, she expressed no consternation but consumed the meal just as she had the first.

Finally, a striking flatness of affect or emotional expression is a frequent consequence of medial frontal damage. These patients typically appear neither happy nor sad but are seemingly indifferent to the emotional valence and content of social interactions.

Unilateral lesions of the mesial frontal cortex typically produce similar but far less dramatic deficits. Damage to the left medial frontal region is associated with an akinesia of speech, that is, "transcortical motor aphasia," which is characterized by a marked reduction in the length and frequency of utterances but a relative preservation of the ability to repeat.

Patient M.S.

The behavioral deficits associated with lesions of the medial frontal cortex are illustrated by the following account. Patient M.S. was a high-ranking executive until the age of 60, when he was noted by business colleagues to be less "energetic" and motivated. Although the quality of his work remained exemplary, he failed to complete his usual tasks despite working the same schedule. At approximately the same time, his wife noted him to become less affectionate; he exhibited less and less interest in his friends and hobbies and spent increasing amounts of leisure time "just sitting." During the ensuing 2 years, the symptoms became more pronounced. After being encouraged to take early retirement, he finally sought medical attention.

Neurological examination revealed M.S. to be alert and oriented, with excellent mathematical and analytical skills. Memory appeared normal. Two striking abnormalities were observed, however. First, although cooperative and responsive, M.S. virtually never initiated interactions with his wife or the examiner. He sat passively in a wheelchair, exhibiting little affect and rare spontaneous movements. He exhibited normal strength and only mild rigidity; when asked to walk, however, he stood but appeared to be rooted to the floor; when sufficient force was exerted to displace his center gravity, he recovered his balance and, seemingly without effort, walked a few steps; while sitting, he was able to demonstrate the stepping movements with both legs.

Second, M.S. manifested a dramatic delay in responding. When greeted, for example, he invariably provided an appropriate (if bland) salutation but required up to 30 secs to respond. Similar delays were noted in response to commands to execute movements. He required as much as a minute to generate a (usually correct) response to a simple problem. Although spontaneous speech was markedly diminished, he exhibited no impairment in accuracy of naming, reading, writing, or comprehension. M.S. was frequently incontinent of urine; he stated that he sensed when his bladder was full and could inhibit evacuation but was indifferent to the incontinence.

SPECT scan exhibited a substantial reduction in blood flow in the medial frontal cortex and anterior temporal lobes bilaterally.

Dorsolateral Frontal Lobes

Although recent investigations in nonhuman primates (11) have demonstrated the dorsolateral frontal cortex (cortex surrounding the arcuate and principal sulci) to be implicated in a variety of motor, sensory, and even visual functions, investigations of patients with lesions of the dorsolateral frontal lobes suggest that the primary consequence of dysfunction in this region is an impairment in planning, problem solving, abstract reasoning, and high-level cognitive abilities more generally.

Patients with bilateral dorsolateral frontal lesions frequently exhibit a lack of flexibility in their thinking and planning and appear rigid and perseverative. Many, but not all patients with these lesions exhibit deficits on standard intelligence tests (e.g., Weschler Adult Intelligence Scale—Revised or Raven's Progressive Matrices); other patients, often with less extensive lesions, may appear to family and friends to be less insightful, innovative, or analytical in their thinking but do not demonstrate clear-cut cognitive abnormalities.

As noted above with respect to other frontal lobe regions, unilateral lesions of the dorsolateral frontal cortex often produce substantially less prominent symptoms and signs of cognitive dysfunction. Lesions of the left (that is, dominant) dorsolateral frontal cortex, for example, are typically associated with language deficits, whereas lesions of the right dorsolateral frontal lobe are often associated with an impairment in the expression of emotion in conjunction with a relatively preserved ability to apprehend the emotional significance of affect expressed in speech or facial expressions (12).

The severity of the language deficit associated with left dorsolateral frontal lobe damage varies widely. Extensive lesions that disrupt the posterior portion of the left dorsolateral frontal lobe (e.g., Brodmann areas 44 and 45, or Broca's area) as well as portions of the motor cortex and insular cortex typically produce the syndrome of Broca aphasia, characterized by nonfluent, halting, "telegraphic" speech. In contrast, lesions *restricted* to the dorsolateral frontal lobe are typically not associated with a severe aphasia but manifest as an impairment in verbal fluency and sometimes subtle impairment in the ability to adequately express oneself (13). Thus, Mohr et al. (14) have demonstrated that lesions restricted to Broca's area, for example, are not associated with Broca's aphasia.

PARIETAL LOBES

For the sake of convenience, the parietal lobes may be divided into three distinct regions, the *primary sensory cortices* (Brodmann areas 1, 2, and 3), the *inferior parietal lobule* (Brodmann areas 39 and 40), and the *superior parietal lobule* (Brodmann areas 5 and 7).

Lesions restricted to the primary sensory cortex of the post-central gyrus are infrequent. These lesions may be asymptomatic or may be associated with relatively minor and restricted primary sensory deficits such as a reduction or alteration in the perception of light touch. In light of their rarity and relatively straightforward nature of the associated deficits, these impairments will not be discussed further.

Inferior Parietal Lobule

Lesions of the inferior parietal lobule, in contrast, are commonly observed in infarctions in the territory of the middle cerebral artery (MCA), in association with damage to either the frontal and/or parietal lobes, or, in the case of an embolus, the posterior portion of the superior division of the MCA.

The behavioral deficits associated with unilateral lesions of the inferior parietal lobules differ markedly as a function of the side of the lesion. Dysfunction of the left inferior parietal lobule is typically associated with a deficit in speech comprehension, often in the presence of preserved repetition (that is, transcortical sensory aphasia). Additionally, at least since Dejerine's (15) classical description over 100 years ago of alexia with agraphia, damage to the dominant inferior parietal lobule has been associated with impairments in reading and writing.

Other cognitive deficits typically associated with damage to the left inferior parietal lobule include an impairment in the ability to perform calculations and right/left confusion. When encountered in conjunction with finger agnosia and agraphia (an impairment in writing), acalculia and right/left orientation are designated Gerstmann's syndrome, a constellation of deficits claimed by many investigators to be associated with dysfunction of the dominant angular gyrus.

Lesions of the right inferior parietal lobule are frequently associated with two behavior deficits. The first is the neglect syndrome, a striking and disabling disorder characterized by a failure to report, orient to, or respond to salient stimuli presented in the side opposite a brain lesion that is not attributable to a primary sensory deficit (e.g., hemianopia) or weakness (16). Although observed in conjunction with lesions in a number of cortical (e.g., dorsolateral frontal, dominant inferior parietal lobule) and subcortical (e.g., thalamus) structures, the neglect syndrome is most frequently encountered in association with dysfunction of the nondominant inferior parietal lobule.

Patients with neglect may fail to groom or dress the neglected side of their body; for some patients with this syndrome, the neglect of their extremities is so severe that they fail to recognize their arms as their own; thus patients who have felt their neglected extremity with their "good" arm may complain that another person has climbed into their bed. Interestingly, the sensory and motor performance of patients with neglect may be influenced by factors such as the location with respect to their bodies in which testing occurs; these patients may, for example, exhibit greater "strength" when power is assessed with the hand placed on the *ipsilesional* compared with the contralesional side of the body.

The second deficit frequently associated with nondominant inferior parietal lobule lesions is an impairment in the ability to understand affect, whether expressed in speech or by means of facial expressions. At least in part as a consequence of this deficit, these patients are often judged by family members and friends to be emotionally flat and indifferent.

Focal structural lesions of the bilateral inferior parietal lobules are relatively rare but are associated with dramatic behavioral deficits such as simultanagnosia, a condition in which patients "see" only one object at a time despite the fact that they have normal visual acuity and visual fields. We have recently reported a patient with this striking disorder (17).

Patient B.P.

B.P., a 67-year-old woman, had suffered a small infarct of the left inferior parietal lobe as well as a larger right inferior parietal infarct. The patient's major complaint was that her environment appeared fragmented; although she saw individual items clearly, they appeared to be isolated, and she could not discern any meaningful relationship among them. She stated, for example, that she could find her way in her home (in which she had lived for 25 years) with her eyes closed, but she became confused with her eyes open. On one occasion, for example, she attempted to find her way to her bedroom by using a large lamp as a landmark; while walking toward the lamp, she fell over her dining room table. Although she enjoyed listening to the radio, television programs bewildered her because she could only "see" one person or object at a time and therefore could not determine who was speaking or being spoken to; she reported watching a movie in which, after hearing a heated argument, she noted to her surprise and consternation that the character she had been watching was suddenly sent reeling across the room, apparently as a consequence of a punch thrown by a character she had never seen. Although she was able to read single words effortlessly, she stopped reading because the "competing words" confused her. She was unable to write as she was able to see only a single letter; thus, when creating a letter she saw only the tip of the pencil and the letter under construction and "lost" the previously constructed letters.

Neurologic examination at that time revealed her to be alert and oriented. Cranial nerve examination revealed normal visual fields to confrontation and normal ocular movements; strength, reflexes, sensation, and coordination were normal. Examination of higher nervous system functions revealed no general intellectual impairment. The patient performed well on tests of abstract reasoning. She demonstrated no impairment in the production or recognition of gesture. No hemisensory neglect or extinction of auditory, tactile, or visual stimuli was noted. She exhibited a profound dressing impairment; B.P. was unable to put on a single item of clothing without assistance.

The most frequent clinical setting in which bilateral inferior parietal dysfunction is encountered is in the context of dementing illnesses such as Alzheimer's disease. Although the full spectrum of behavioral disorders observed in these patients varies widely, presumably as a function of the extent of dysfunction in other brain regions such as the temporal and frontal lobes, some patients with dementing illness appear to present with dysfunction at least relatively restricted to the inferior parietal lobules. The behavioral deficits exhibited by these patients are similar in many crucial respects to those demonstrated by patients with structural abnormalities in the same regions. The following case report illustrates the pattern of deficits typically encountered in these patients.

Patient R.C.

R.C. is a 60 year-old right-handed man who at age 55 first noted difficulty locating tools on his cluttered workbench. At approximately the same time he also noted difficulties in reading text, which he attributed to "getting lost" on the page. Over the ensuing 5 years, his difficulties in reading and locating objects embedded in an array slowly progressed. At the time of the evaluation reported here, for example, he stated that he could not visually locate items in the refrigerator but identified them by palpation. Over the course of the last 2 years, he began to notice difficulties recognizing some objects, particularly large ones. He experienced less trouble with small objects and, for example, routinely assisted his wife by threading her needles.

He denied tripping over or bumping into stationary objects and drove a car without incident until shortly before the time of the present evaluation. He had only recently become forgetful; he has not noted problems with names, language, or simple calculations.

Neurologic examination revealed that he was able to reach to visualized targets accurately with either hand but performed poorly, especially with the left hand, when asked to point to a target after closing his eyes.

Visual acuity was 20/25 ou with correction, and ocular movements were normal except for a modest reduction in upgaze. Visual field examination to confrontation revealed that he detected finger movements in both visual fields quickly and accurately.

Magnetic resonance imaging (MRI) scan revealed mild generalized atrophy; SPECT scan demonstrated markedly diminished perfusion of the inferior parietal and lateral occipital regions with normal perfusion of primary visual cortex. Consistent with the asymmetric visual field deficit, the perfusion defect was worse in the right hemisphere.

Superior Parietal Lobules

The association cortex of the superior parietal lobules (Brodmann areas 5 and 7) appears to be critical for integration of multiple sensory and motor inputs for the body and external space. The posterior superior parietal lobule receives dense projections from the visual association cortex; experiments in monkeys suggest that this cortical region is critical for the "where" component of the visual system, that is, the representation of peri- and extrapersonal space. This contention is supported by Gordon Holmes's (18) elegant investigations of the behavioral consequences of penetrating missile injuries of the superior parietal lobules. Holmes described patients with bilateral superior parietal damage who, although able to identify and describe visually presented objects normally, were unable to reach to grasp the visualized object, a phenomenon termed "optic ataxia." Similarly, these patients were able to identify their cot, for example, but were utterly unable to walk to it; while attempting to reach the cot, the patients walked into chairs and even walls.

The anterior portion of the superior parietal lobule (Brodmann area 5) appears, in contrast, to represent high-level, multimodal sensory information including a representation of the body in three-dimensional space. We have observed patients with ischemic infarction restricted to Brodmann area 5 on the left who, in spite of apparently normal sensory thresholds to pin, temperature, and light touch, were unable to name from touch objects placed in the right hand. The same objects were accurately named when placed in the left hand, demonstrating that the impaired performance with the right hand was not attributable to a language deficit.

The clinical deficits associated with dysfunction of the superior parietal lobule are illustrated by the following case history.

Patient G.W.

G.W., a 63-year-old right-handed woman, was in good health until approximately 6 years prior to our evaluation when she began to have difficulty driving. She was involved in five accidents over the course of approximately 1 year, all of which she attributed to an inability to determine the spatial relationships between her car and other cars or objects. Over the ensuing years she experienced increasing difficulty in navigating through familiar areas such as her town and even her house; despite having clearly seen and identified objects around her, she tended to bump into things on either side of her. She also began to have difficulty sitting down in chairs and positioning herself to lie in bed. Early in the course of her illness, for example, she attempted to take her seat in a restaurant only to miss the chair and find herself sprawled on the floor.

A second problem of which G.W. was aware was an inability to localize sounds. While crossing a street, for example, she was unable to determine if the sound of a horn honking emanated from a car to her left or right. Similarly, it was noted that she often turned in the wrong direction when greeted by someone who was out of her line of vision.

G.W. experienced no difficulties recognizing people or objects. She also denied problems with language or memory and stated that she continued to enjoy reading although she admitted to losing her place on the page when reading text. She experienced no difficulties in tasks such as locating a magazine on a crowded desk or eating from a tray. Despite her problems, the patient was able to continue working until approximately 18 months prior to the time of testing.

Neurologic examination performed 6 years after the onset of symptoms revealed mild rigidity of all extremities that was more pronounced on the left. No spasticity or weakness was noted, but the left arm was often held in an awkward manner, with adduction of the upper arm and flexion of the elbow, causing her left hand to rest on or below her chin. Occasional myoclonic jerks were observed, the vast majority of which involved the left arm. With eyes open, she accurately touched the examiner's finger with either hand; when instructed to touch the examiner's finger after closing her eyes, however, she appeared to grope aimlessly while stating that the finger had "disappeared." Similarly, she was unable, with eyes closed, to touch her free hand to her stationary, extended hand. She was slower with the left hand on both tasks. With eyes open or closed she was able to point to named proximal body parts such as her elbow, chest, or knee.

Perhaps the most striking abnormality on the neurologic examination was the patient's inability to position herself in space. When instructed to lie down on her bed with her head on the pillow, she sat on the edge of the bed and over the course of approximately 10 minutes made many futile attempts (some of which caused her to almost fall off the bed) to orient her body in the desired fashion. During this time, she was consistently able to articulate her objective, point to the pillow, and provide a description of the action that would permit her to achieve that end.

Unlike R.C., G.W. was not simultanagnosic. She was able to interpret complex scenes when shown a series of line drawings and pictures. She quickly and accurately identified the contents of the scenes but made occasional errors in identifying the spatial relationships between the objects or individuals in the scenes.

Magnetic resonance imaging (MRI) scan revealed focal atrophy in the superior parietal lobules bilaterally.

TEMPORAL LOBES

Four major functional systems may be identified in the temporal lobe. The superior temporal gyrus contains the primary (Brodmann areas 41 and 42) as well as secondary (Brodmann area 22) auditory cortex, which is critical for the conscious perception and interpretation of sound. Although unilateral lesions restricted to these structures appear to produce little functional deficit, bilateral disruption of these structures may be associated with syndromes ranging from cortical deafness, a quite rare disorder characterized by the loss or substantial reduction in the ability to detect sound, to auditory agnosia and pure word deafness. Auditory agnosia is characterized by the preserved ability to detect and discriminate sounds but an impaired ability to recognize sounds; patients with this disorder may, for example, "hear" a telephone ringing but cannot name or indicate the meaning of the sound. Patients with pure word deafness, in contrast, recognize nonverbal sounds but are unable to understand speech. For example, we reported a patient with this disorder who after identifying a series of nonverbal sounds correctly, responded to a verbal request by saying "I know you are talking to me, but I can't understand a word you are saying." Pure word deafness is differentiated from aphasia by the preservation of all language skills (such as naming, reading, writing, and speech production) that are not dependent on auditory input.

The second functional system mediated at least in part by the temporal lobe is language. The posterior portion of the superior temporal gyrus, or Wernicke's area, appears to be critical for the comprehension of speech. Dysfunction in this region causes a receptive or Wernicke's aphasia characterized by an inability to understand speech and the fluent production of semantically impoverished speech that typically contains distorted or contextually inappropriate words ("paraphasic errors"). It should be noted that severe Wernicke's aphasia is typically associated with lesions that extend into the inferior parietal lobule or inferiorly into the middle temporal gyrus (Brodmann area 21).

The third distinct functional system supported by the temporal lobe is memory. Since the landmark investigations by Milner and colleagues (19) of the patient H.M. in the 1950s, it has been clear that the limbic structures of the mesiobasal temporal lobe, in particular the hippocampi and surrounding cortex, are critical for memory. Since undergoing bilateral anterior temporal lobe (including amygdala and hippocampus) ablations for the treatment of intractable epilepsy, H.M. has exhibited a profound and utterly disabling inability to acquire new information (that is, H.M. exhibits an "anterograde amnesia"). Although able to recall information about events prior to the operations, H.M. has failed to learn such basic information as the name of present-day politicians, athletes, and celebrities; when asked the ages of his children, he provides ages appropriate to the time of the operation.

We recently evaluated a patient (R.H.) with bilateral infarctions of the mesiobasal temporal lobes whose behavior is quite similar to that of H.M. Although he possesses an IQ of 129 and performs normally on a variety of tests of facial recognition, he fails to recognize people whom he has met on approximately 40 occasions. Similarly, he cannot find his way from the front door of the building to our laboratory, although he has visited over 50 times. A self-described football fan, R.H. names Johnny Unitas (who retired in 1974) as his favorite active player and cannot name a single current player.

The fourth functional system supported by the temporal lobes is the "what" component of the visual system, for which the inferior temporal cortex is critical. In contrast to the "where" processing stream supported by the superior parietal lobule, the "what" system appears to be critical for object identification. Bilateral inferior temporal lobe (and, occasionally, unilateral left) lesions may produce the clinical syndrome of "visual object agnosia," characterized by an inability to recognize visually presented objects that is not attributable to low-level visual deficits. Although there is substantial variability in this poorly defined clinical syndrome, at least some patients with this disorder may be unable to name or match to sample visually presented objects or pictures despite normal visual fields and acuity. The preserved ability to name the same objects from palpation demonstrates that the impairment is not simply attributable to language or general cognitive deficits.

More recent investigations suggest that the inferior temporal cortex may be important not only for the visual aspects of object identification but also for supporting the general body of knowledge about objects and concepts that constitute the semantic system. A number of patients with lesions of the inferior temporal cortex have been described who exhibit selective impairment in knowledge of specific categories of knowledge; patients have been reported who had a relatively selective impairment in the recognition and knowledge of animals but who had preserved information on a variety of other domains such as nonliving things. Once again, we recently evaluated a patient whose performance is relevant in this context.

Patient D.M.

D.M. is a 56-year-old right-handed professional who presented for evaluation of slowly progressive forgetfulness and difficulty reading. Although able to work full time for several years after the onset of symptoms, he frequently complained that he was "overwhelmed" by his professional responsibilities and simply could not keep up with his work.

The patient's wife and colleagues also noted a deterioration in his performance. One of the striking observations made by his wife was that he appeared to have lost knowledge about a variety of subjects; one subject about which he became increasingly confused, for example, was animals. When asked by his wife to name a squirrel running across his lawn, for example, he stated that it was "a deer, but awfully small"; additionally, when questioned about the attributes of common animals with which he had been familiar, he frequently responded incorrectly. It should be noted that in spite of his gradual loss of information (or "semantic knowledge"), D.M.'s personality and behavior remained largely unchanged. He was aware of his cognitive deficits and pursued a vigorous course of remediation to no avail.

When examined in our laboratory, the neurologic examination was normal except for a mild dementia. D.M.'s IQ was 86, a score that certainly represents a decline from his premorbid level of function. Memory was mildly impaired. Extensive testing of visual processing demonstrated normal visual acuity and visual fields. He did, however, exhibit an impairment in the recognition of at least some types of objects. For example, D.M. was able to name line drawings of tools and furniture substantially better than he was able to name drawings of animals and kitchen utensils.

His knowledge of the world was tested in a variety of ways. On the "Pyramids and Palm Trees" test, on which the subject is shown a picture (e.g., a pyramid) and must select which one of two other pictures (e.g., palm tree or pine tree) is most closely related or associated, D.M. performed significantly worse than controls, indicating a loss of stored information.

One of the most striking aspects of his performance was a preservation of information pertaining to "abstract" compared with "concrete" words. In this context, the abstract/concrete dimension refers to the extent to which the referent of a word can be experienced by the senses; thus concrete words include apple, table, and bunion, whereas abstract words include destiny, thought, and passion. Unlike normal controls and the vast majority of patients with brain lesions, D.M. performed *better* on a variety of tasks with abstract compared with concrete words.

SPECT scan demonstrated decreased blood flow to the anterior portions of the inferior temporal and occipitotemproal gyri that was greater on the left than on the right.

OCCIPITAL LOBES

The occipital lobes, which include the primary and secondary visual cortex, are critical for the conscious processing of visual stimuli. Lesions of the occipital lobe typically cause a homonymous visual field deficit that may range in severity from a mild deficit (e.g., color desaturation) to a complete loss of vision in the affected portion of the visual field contralateral to the affected hemisphere. Large, bilateral lesions of the occipital lobes may cause the syndrome of "cortical blindness," in which patients fail to detect visual stimuli. Occasionally, patients with acquired blindness secondary to cortical pathology or dysfunction elsewhere in the visual system explicitly deny their visual loss; this condition is termed Anton's syndrome.

Although investigations in human brains have delineated only a relatively small number of visual areas defined on the basis of cytoarchitectonic grounds (e.g., Brodmann areas 17, 18, and 19), recent investigations in monkeys have identified at least 20 distinct cortical regions differing in function. Evidence consistent with such a differentiation in visual cortex in humans comes from observations of the effects of brain lesions in humans. Achromatopsia, or the acquired inability to discriminate color, for example, has been consistently observed in association with lesions of the inferior surface of the occipital lobe, in particular the lingual and fusiform gyri. Unilateral inferior occipital lesions may produce achromatopsia only in the contralateral visual field, whereas bilateral lesions produce a complete loss of ability to discriminate color. Similarly, recent PET studies have defined a lateral temporo-occipital lesion that may be important for the appreciation of motion which may be analogous to are MT in monkeys which mediates, at least in part, the perception of movement.

As illustrated by the previous brief discussions of the behavioral consequences of brain dysfunction, progress in understanding brain-behavior relationships has been substantial. The tentative nature of the previous discussion and the presence of obvious gaps in the current knowledge base demonstrate compellingly, however, that a great deal remains to be learned. In light of the achievements of the last decade and the accelerating rate of technological advancement, we believe that functional brain imaging techniques such as SPECT will continue to provide critical insights into the functional anatomy of complex human behaviors.

REFERENCES

1. Broca P. Sur la faculté du langage articule. *Bull Soc Anthr Paris* 1865;6:337–393.
2. Jackson H. On the affections of speech from disease of the brain. *Brain* 1878;1:304–330.
3. Bastian HC. On the various forms of loss of speech in cerebral disease. *Br Foreign Medico-Surg Rev* 1869;43:470–492.
4. Wernicke C. *Des aphasische Symptomenkomplex.* Breslau: Cohn and Weigart; 1874.
5. Dennis M, Whitaker HA. Language acquisition following hemidecortication: linguistic superiority of the left over the right hemisphere. *Brain Lang* 1976;3:404–433.
6. Luria A. *The working brain.* London: Allan Lane, Penguin Press; 1973.
7. Eslinger PJ, Damasio AR. Severe disturbance of higher cognition after bilateral frontal lobe ablation: patient EVR. *Neurology* 1985;35:1731–1741.
8. Brickner RM. *The intellectual functions of the frontal lobes: study based upon observation of a man after partial bilateral frontal lobectomy.* New York: Macmillan; 1936.
9. Mesulam M-M. A cortical network for directed attention and unilateral neglect. *Ann Neurol* 1980;10:309–325.
10. Laplane D, Degos JD, Baulac M, Gray F. Bilateral infarction of the anterior cingulate gyri and of the fornices. *J Neurol Sci* 1981;51:289–300.
11. Goldman-Rakic PS. Topography of cognition: parallel distributed networks in primate association cortex. *Annu Rev Neurosci* 1988;11:137–156.
12. Ross E. The aprosodias. *Arch Neurol* 1981;38:561–569.
13. Coslett HB, Bowers D, Verfaellie M, Heilman KM. Phonological amnesia. *Arch Neurol* 1991;48:949–955.
14. Mohr JP, Pessin MS, Finkelstein S, Funkenstein HH, Duncan GW, Davis KR. Broca aphasia: pathologic and clinical. *Neurology* 1978;28:311–324.
15. Dejerine J. Sur un cas de cecite verbale avec agraphie, suivi d'autopsie. *Mem Soc Biol* 1891;3:197–201.
16. Heilman KM, Watson RT, Valenstein E. Neglect and related disorders. In: Heilman KM, Valenstein E, eds. *Clinical neuropsychology.* New York: Oxford University Press; 1985.
17. Coslett HB, Saffran EM. Simultanagnosia: to see but not two see. *Brain* 1991;114:1082–1107.
18. Holmes G. Disturbances of vision by cerebral lesions. *Bri J Ophthal* 1918;2:353–384.
19. Milner B. Amnesia following operation on the temporal lobes. In: Whitty CWM, Zangwill OL, eds. *Amnesia.* London: Butterworth; 1966

SECTION II

Clinical Disease States

Cerebral SPECT Imaging, Second Edition,
edited by R.L. Van Heertum and R.S. Tikofsky.
Raven Press, Ltd., New York © 1995.

CHAPTER 5

Cerebrovascular Disease

Alan B. Rubens and H. Branch Coslett

Cerebral infarctions can be divided into two major groups, hemorrhagic infarctions, which comprise about 15 percent of all infarctions, and ischemic or "bland" infarctions, which constitute approximately 85 percent of infarcts. Ischemic infarcts may, in turn, be divided into two major groups on the basis of the presumed pathophysiologic mechanism; embolic infarctions are thought to be caused by substances in the arterial circulation lodging in the lumen of the carotid, vertebral, or intracranial arteries and thereby disrupting the blood flow to structures irrigated by that vessel. Most emboli originate from intraarterial atheromatous plaque, often from the bifurcation of the internal and external carotid arteries. Alternatively, emboli may originate in the heart, typically from mural thrombi or heart valve vegetations; recent investigations have also emphasized that emboli may arise in the systemic circulation and reach the brain by means of a right-to-left shunt in the heart ("paradoxical" emboli). Thrombotic infarctions, in contrast, are attributable to a reduction or obliteration of the arterial lumen caused by the accumulation of atheromatous plaque or fibris containing debris.

Although it is frequently difficult or even impossible to distinguish between ischemic and embolic infarctions on the basis of clinical considerations alone, most neurologists believe that the sudden onset of maximal deficit in the absence of prodromal symptoms is suggestive of an embolus.

Intracerebral hemorrhages are usually, but certainly not invariably, encountered in patients with hypertension. "Hypertensive" hemorrhages tend to occur deep in the brain, arising in the thalamus, basal ganglia, or internal capsule. The clinical deficit associated with intracerebral hemorrhage usually differs from that of ischemic stroke in that, following an abrupt onset of symptoms, the patient's signs and general level of consciousness often worsen substantially over the course of hours.

A. B. Rubens: Department of Neurology, University of Arizona College of Medicine, Tucson, Arizona 85724.
H. B. Coslett: Department of Neurology, Temple University School of Medicine, Philadelphia, Pennsylvania 19140.

PATHOPHYSIOLOGY OF STROKE

In all instances of cerebrovascular disease (CVD) there is interference with the normal flow of blood to the brain. Brain activity is dependent for its metabolic activity on an adequate supply of oxygenated blood. It is known that in normals there is a close linkage between blood flow and metabolism. Autoregulation and vasodilatory reserve permit minor modifications of flow to be matched to metabolic demand. However, if there is significant alteration of blood flow to the brain, as in the case of a cerebrovascular accident, then there is an onset of neurological deficit due to the reduction or interruption of the blood supply to vessels subserving the regions of the brain producing the deficit. Thus, the deficit occurs because the blood flow to the brain has dropped to a point at which increasing oxygen extraction can no longer sustain normal metabolic activity.

When blood flow exceeds the metabolic demand of the tissue involved, as in the case of cerebral infarction, "luxury perfusion" will often occur. This phenomenon can occur in the acute phase, 3 to 7 days after onset, when normal cerebrovascular autoregulation fails, or in the period 14 to 21 days after onset, when it is the result of capillary hyperplasia. Therefore, when imaging with hexamethylpropyleneamine-oxime (HMPAO), which will show luxury perfusion, it is necessary to be aware of the time the SPECT study is performed relative to onset of symptoms (1). This phenomenon will not be seen on scans obtained with IMP or ECD (2).

SPECT is of considerable clinical value in stroke because it provides a three-dimensional representation of perfusion that is neither invasive nor expensive. It requires low doses of radiation, it is widely available, and it uses conventional nuclear medicine equipment. In CVD, SPECT is useful in a spectrum of conditions ranging from transient ischemic attacks (TIAs) (3) to completed stroke (4–6).

In acute cerebral infarction, SPECT imaging demonstrates hypoperfusion in the early hours after onset, a period when computed tomography (CT) scans are usually still normal. In the acute period, used in conjunction with CT scans, SPECT is helpful in distinguishing between frank infarction and reversible ischemia (7,8). In patients with chronic symptoms and signs of CVD but a negative CT, a positive SPECT study implicates cerebral ischemia and suggests the presence of hemodynamically significant arterial stenosis or occlusion (9). SPECT also has a clinical application in monitoring ischemia associated with vasospasm following subarachnoid hemorrhage (10,11). This is of great importance in planning surgical management. SPECT imaging therefore complements the information available from CT, magnetic resonance imaging (MRI), and cerebral angiography. By showing both brain perfusion and brain metabolism (on delayed scans), the technique holds great promise in delineating the physiological evolution of acute infarction and in identifying areas of viable but ischemic brain tissue surrounding chronic infarcts (12). However, the development of this aspect of SPECT brain imaging has been severely limited because *N*-isopropyl-*p*-iodoamphetamine (IMP) is not commercially available at present in the United States. More recently, SPECT's role in planning of therapy and predicting short-term prognosis in acute stroke has become more clearly defined (13,14). In addition, its role in determining prognosis and treatment in the chronic stage has also begun to show real growth (15).

FUNCTIONAL LOCALIZATION

Functional localization of strokes and of the reduction of blood flow to the cerebral hemisphere depends on which of the major arteries are involved and on the laterality of the stroke and the reduced flow.

Anterior Cerebral Artery Infarction

Occlusion of the anterior cerebral artery **(ACA)** produces deficits related to destruction of the medial frontoparietal area and the corpus callosum. Infarction or ischemia of the paracentral lobule results in weakness and sensory loss in the contralateral leg. There may be forced grasping and groping of the contralateral hand. When the infarction extends to the upper convexity, there may be proximal arm weakness. When the proximal deep branches supplying the anterior limb and genu of the internal capsule are involved, weakness of the contralateral face and hand are present. Urinary incontinence—and, to a lesser extent, fecal incontinence—may be found with a unilateral or bilateral anterior cerebral artery stroke. Unilateral occlusion of the left **ACA** results in language disturbance in which there occurs marked reduction of spontaneous speech, sometimes to the point of muteness. Infarction of the corpus callosum may produce an interhemispheric disconnection syndrome with apraxia and agraphia of the left hand, with an inability to name objects palpated with the left hand without the aid of vision. With bilateral medial frontal lobe infarction, there occurs a state of akinetic mutism in which there is unresponsiveness to the environment in the absence of alterations of the sensorimotor mechanism or coma.

Left Middle Cerebral Artery Infarction

Total infarction in the territory of the left middle cerebral artery **(LMCA)** produces global aphasia with right hemiparesis and right hemisensory loss, often with right hemianopia and poor conjugate gaze to the right in the acute state. Involvement of the superior division of the **LMCA** produces a frontocentral parietal infarct with Broca's aphasia, hemiparesis, and apraxia of the unparalized left upper extremity. Broca's aphasia is characterized by relatively intact auditory comprehension, with severe reduction in the amount of grammatical complexity of speech. Involvement with the inferior division of the left middle cerebral artery produces temporal lobe infarction, with associated Wernicke's aphasia but without motor or sensory deficits. Right hemianopia—or more commonly, a superior quadrantanopia—is sometimes found. Wernicke's aphasia is characterized by poor auditory comprehension and copious fluent speech that contains little meaning. Focal involvement of the left parietal lobe produces agraphia, alexia, and aphasia in which the ability to name objects is the major deficit.

Right Middle Cerebral Artery

Occlusion of the right middle cerebral artery **(RMCA)**, in addition to producing left hemiparesis and hemisensory deficit, results in sensory neglect of the left visual space, difficulty in drawing and copying, left visual field deficit, and poor conjugate gaze to the right in the acute state. The area of the right hemisphere most apt to produce sensory neglect is the parietal lobe. Patients with severe sensory neglect may manifest anosognosia, a condition in which the patient denies the sensory motor deficit. Deep small lesions in the territory of the lenticulostriate arteries take the form of lacunar strokes that, because of the involvement of the internal capsule, produce varying degrees of hemiparesis of the contralateral side without major abnormalities of higher cortical function.

Posterior Cerebral Artery

Occlusion of the left posterior cerebral artery **(PCA)** results in infarction of the mesial occipital lobe and produces a right visual field defect, sometimes in association with alexia but without a concomitant writing disorder or aphasia. Involvement of the right **PCA** produces a left visual field defect sometimes accompanied by posopagnosia, the impaired ability to recognize familiar faces. Bilateral **PCA** lesions produce cortical blindness, often in association with severe memory disorder because of the involvement of inferior medial temporal lobe branches that supply the left and right hippocampi. When the penetrating branches of the PCA are involved, thalamic infarction may occur, with associated numbness or decreased sensibility of the opposite side of the body. Some patients with left thalamic strokes develop transient aphasia. Strokes may also involve the posterior fossa area including the cerebellar hemispheres.

EVALUATING CEREBRAL VASODILATORY RESERVE

The question of evaluating cerebrovascular reserve in patients with a history of TIAs who have negative CTs can be enhanced by the regional cerebral blood flow (rCBF)/ SPECT studies (16–19). This can be accomplished by studying vascular reactivity using the vasodilator acetazolamide. A carbonic anhydrase inhibitor, acetazolamide, acts to produce dilation of the cerebrovasculature indirectly by increasing carbon dioxide levels. In normal individuals there is typically a uniform rCBF increase associated with acetazolamide administration compared with a baseline (nonacetazolamide scan). This technique will therefore increase the contrast between regions of adequate vascular reserve and those in which there is inadequate reserve. Regions of poor vascular reserve will not demonstrate the expected increase in rCBF associated with acetazolamide administration. In fact, postacetazolamide SPECT studies may reveal defects of reserve not evident on baseline scans. In general, it is recommended that if this procedure is being considered the acetazolamide scan be performed first; if it is within the normal range, then a second baseline scan is not required. If an abnormality is found, then a second study should be performed to determine if there are abnormalities present during unenhanced flow states. In some instances it is possible to perform both studies in the same sitting. One such approach requires the availability of both HMPAO and IMP, plus an imaging system capable of evaluating the peaks of both isotopes simultaneously. An alternative approach employs a low and high dose of HMPAO.

INTERPRETING rCBF/SPECT IMAGES

Interpreting rCBF/SPECT images in CVD requires a firm understanding of three-dimensional anatomy of the brain and the pathophysiology of CVD. Tables 5.1 through 5.3, as well as Tables 6.1, 6.2, and 6.3 in Chapter 6 provide summaries of the major findings that are associated with rCBF/SPECT scans obtained on patients with CVD. They represent the most frequently seen characteristics. However, one should expect many variations in the patterns described in the tables.

TABLE 5.1. *Transient ischemic attacks (TIAs)*

CT findings often within normal limits
Focal or hemispheric reduction in tracer uptake
Abnormal findings in 20–30% of cases imaged when patient is asymptomatic
Abnormal findings in 70–80% of cases studied with Diamox
Reduced tracer uptake after acetazolamide, compared with baseline, indicates reduced to absent vascular reserve

TABLE 5.2. *Acute/subacute/chronic stroke*

CT findings often normal in acute phase
Focus of infarct appears as a wedge of absent tracer uptake corresponding to the appropriate vascular territory
Regions of reduced tracer uptake often surround the region of infarction
Very large lesions will often involve the basal ganglia
Crossed cerebellar diaschisis is present when motor cortex or motor pathways have been effected
Cortical diaschisis (reduced tracer uptake in the cerebral cortex) may accompany infarction or hemorrhage to subcortical structures

TABLE 5.3. *Crossed cerebellar diaschisis*

Reduced tracer uptake in the cerebellar hemisphere opposite the side of infarction
Not always present in cerebrovascular disease
Usually not clinically relevant
Represents deafferentation between cortical pathways and cerebellar hemisphere

REFERENCES

1. Hellman RS, Tikofsky RS. An overview of the contribution of regional cerebral blood flow studies in cerebrovascular disease: is there a role for single photon emission computed tomography? *Semin Nucl Med,* 1990;20:303–324.
2. Moretti J, Defer G, Cinotti L, et al. "Luxury perfusion" with ^{99m}Tc-HMPAO and ^{123}I-IMP SPECT imaging during the subacute phase of stroke. *Eur J Nucl Med.* 1990;16:17–22.
3. Bogousslavsky J, Delaloye-Bischof A, Regli F, Delaloye B. Prolonged hypoperfusion and early stroke after transient ischemic attack. *Stroke* 1990;21:40–46.
4. Smith FW, Donald RT, Morris AJ, et al. The study of regional cerebral blood flow in stroke patients using technetium 99m HMPAO. *Br J Radiol* 1988;61:358–361.
5. Holman BL, Hellman RS, Goldsmith SJ, et al. Biodistribution, dosimetry, and clinical evaluation of Tc-99m ethyl cysteinate dimer (ECD) in normal subjects and in patients with chronic cerebral infarction. *J Nucl Med* 1989;30:1018–1024.

6. Ell PJ, Hacknell JML, Jarrit PH, et al. A 99mTc radiotracer for the investigation of cerebral vascular disease. *Nucl Med Commun* 1985;6:431–437.
7. Yeh S, Lui RS, Hu HH, et al. Brain SPECT imaging with 99m Tc-hexamethylpropyleneamine oxime in the early detection of cerebral infarction: comparison with transmission computed tomography. *Nucl Med Commun* 1986;7:873–878.
8. Feldmann M, Voth E, Dressler D, et al. 99m-Tc-hexamethylpropylene amine oxime SPECT and x-ray CT in acute cerebral ischemia. *J Neurol* 1990;237:475–479.
9. Raynaud C, Rancurel G, Tzourio N, et al. SPECT analysis of recent cerebral infarction. *Stroke* 1989;20:192–204.
10. Davis S, Andrews J, Lichtenstein M, et al. A single-photon emission computed tomography study of hypoperfusion after subarachnoid hemorrhage. *Stroke* 1990;21:252–259.
11. Hino A, Mizukawa N, Tenjin H, et al. Postoperative hemodynamic and metabolic changes in patients with subarachnoid hemorrhage. *Stroke* 1989;20:1504–1510.
12. Defer G, Moretti J, Cesaro P, et al. Early and delayed SPECT using N-isopropyl p-iodoamphetamine iodine 123 in cerebral ischemia. A prognostic index for clinical recovery. *Arch Neurol* 1987;44: 715–718.
13. Hanson SK, Grotta JC, Rhoades HJ, et al. Value of single-photon emission computed tomography in acute stroke therapeutic trials. *Stroke* 1993;24:1322–1329.
14. Mountz JM, Modell JG, Foster NL, et al. Prognostication of recovery following stroke using the comparison of CT and technetium-99m HMPAO SPECT. *J Nucl Med* 1990;31:61–66.
15. Giubilei F, Lenzi GL, Di Piero V, et al. Predictive value of brain perfusion single-photon emission computed tomography in acute ischemic stroke. *Stroke* 1990;21:895–900.
16. Burt RW, Witt RM, Cikrit DF, Reddy RV. Carotid artery disease: evaluation with acetazolamide-enhanced 1Tc-99m HMPAO SPECT. *Radiology* 1992;182:461–466.
17. Burt RW, Witt RM, Cikrit DF, Carter J. Increased brain retention of Tc-99m HMPAO following acetazolamide administration. *Clin Nucl Med* 1991;16:568.
18. Chollet F, Celsis P, Clanet M, et al. SPECT study of cerebral blood flow reactivity after acetazolamide in patients with transient ischemic attacks. *Stroke* 1989;20:458–464.
19. Knop J, Thie A, Fuchs C, et al. Tc99m-HMPAO-SPECT with acetazolamide challenge to detect hemodynamic compromise in occlusive cerebrovascular disease. *Stroke* 1992;23:1733–1742.

SUGGESTED READINGS

Companioni JM, Lassen NA, Tfelt-Hansen P, Friberg L. Delayed reflow of an ischemic infarct after spontaneous thrombolysis studied by CBF tomography using SPECT and Tc-99m HMPA. *Am J Pysiol Imaging* 1991;6:167–171.

Hayashida K, Nishimura T, Imakita S, Uehara T. Filling out phenomenon with technetium-99m HMPAO brain SPECT at the site of mild cerebral ischemia. *J Nucl Med* 1989;30:591–598.

Hayman LA, Taber KH, Jhingran SG, et al. Cerebral infarction: diagnosis and assessment of prognosis by using ^{123}IMP-SPECT and CT. *AJNR* 1989;10:557–562.

Lewis DH, Eskridge JM, Newell DW, et al. Brain SPECT and the effect of cerebral angioplasty in delayed ischemia due to vasospasm. *J Nucl Med* 1992;32:1789–1796.

Limburg M, van Royen EA, Hijdra A, Verbeeten B Jr. rCBF-SPECT in brain infarction: when does it predict outcome? *J Nucl Med* 1991; 32:382–387.

Nakano S, Konoshita K, Jinnouchi S, et al. Comparative study of regional cerebral blood flow images by SPECT using xenon-133, iodine-123 IMP, and technetium-99m HMPAO. *J Nucl Med* 1989;30:157–164.

Perani D, Di Piero V, Lucignani G, et al. Remote effects of subcortical cerebrovascular lesions: a SPECT cerebral perfusion study. *J Cereb Blood Flow Metab* 1988;8:560–567.

Raynaud C, Rancurel G, Samson Y, et al. Pathophysiologic study of chronic infarcts with I-123 isopropyl iodo-amphetamine (IMP): the importance of periinfarct area. *Stroke* 1989;18:21–29.

Seiderer M, Krappel W, Moser E, et al. Detection and quantification of chronic cerebrovascular disease: comparison of MR imaging, SPECT, and CT. *Radiology* 1989;170:545–548.

Shinoda J, Kimura T, Funakoshi T, et al. Acetazolamide reactivity on cerebral blood flow in patients with subarachnoid hemorrhage. *Acta Neurochirurg* 1992;109:102–108.

Simonson TM, Ryals TJ, Yuh WT, et al. MR imaging and HMPAO scintigraphy in conjunction with balloon test occlusion: value in predicting sequelae after permanent carotid occlusion. *AJR* 1992;159: 1063–1068.

Tranquart F, Ades PE, Groussin P, et al. Postoperative assessment of cerebral blood flow in subarachnoid hemorrhage by means of 99mTc-HMPAO tomography. *Eur J Nucl Med* 1993;20:53–58.

CASE 5-1

Clinical Diagnosis:
Acute Left Middle Cerebral Artery Infarction

CONTRIBUTOR:	IMAGING DATA:	
Name: Ronald L. Van Heertum, M.D.	**Camera:** GE 400AC/T;STARII	**Collimator:** High resolution, parallel hole
Institution: St. Vincent's Hospital and Medical Center	**Isotope:** ^{123}I IMP	**Dose:** 3.0 mCi

This 76-year-old woman was referred for evaluation of an acute infarction of the left cerebral hemisphere. Her history was significant for an infarction of her right cerebral hemisphere a year earlier.

A CT scan (Fig. 5.1) showed a hypodensity in the right frontal and temporal lobes and basal ganglia, consistent with a previous infarction of the right middle cerebral artery. There was a loss of distinction between the gray and white matter in the left frontotemporal region; however, no definite abnormality was discerned.

The cerebral SPECT study (Fig. 5.2) in the transaxial **(A)** and coronal **(B)** planes revealed an absence of tracer uptake in a large area of the left frontal, temporal, and parietal lobes, a portion of the occipital lobe, and the left basal ganglia, and the thalamus.

Teaching Points:

1. The pattern of acute symptoms, the large, left-sided defect on the cerebral SPECT study (associated with the lack of a definitive abnormality of the left hemisphere on CT scan) is most consistent with an acute infarction of the left cerebral hemisphere.
2. A very large defect of the cerebral hemisphere is most likely the result of an occlusion of the internal carotid artery on the involved side.
3. A large defect in an acute stroke patient is, in general, indicative of a very poor short-term clinical outcome.

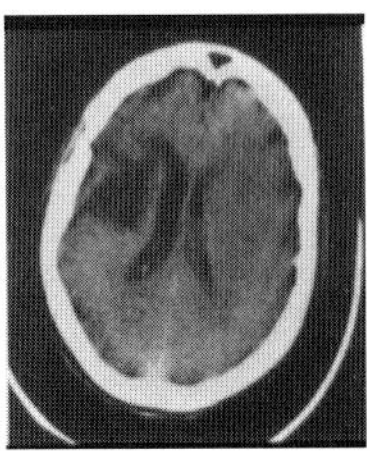

FIG. 5.1

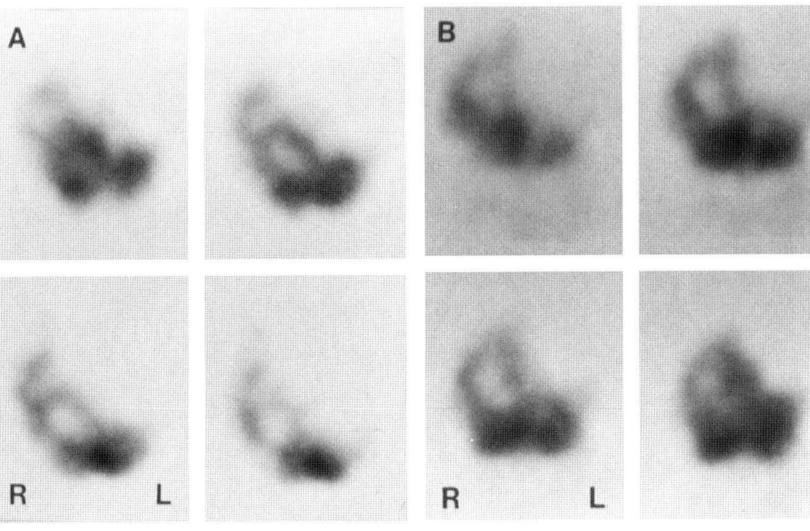

FIG. 5.2A **FIG. 5.2B**

CASE 5-2

Clinical Diagnosis: Acute Left Middle Cerebral Artery Infarction

CONTRIBUTOR:

Name: Anthony P. Yudd, PhD., M.D.
Institution: St. Vincent's Hospital and Medical Center

IMAGING DATA:

Camera: GE 3000 XCT
Isotope: ^{99m}Tc HMPAO

Collimator: Ultra-high resolution, parallel hole
Dose: 20.0 mCi

This 21-year-old woman was referred for evaluation after the acute onset of a combined receptive/expressive aphasia and a progressive right hemiparesis. The patient had no prior history of cerebrovascular disease and no associated risk factors.

An initial CT scan (Fig. 5.3) showed a focal area of increased density in the region of the horizontal segment of the left middle cerebral artery, raising the question of a hyperdense clot.

HMPAO SPECT in the transaxial plane (Fig. 5.4) revealed absent radiotracer uptake in the left frontotemporal region, corresponding to the anterior-superior distribution of the left middle cerebral artery.

A follow-up CT scan (Fig. 5.5) 7 days after the initial study demonstrated an evolving hypodensity in the left frontotemporal and ganglionic regions corresponding to the defect noted on the prior HMPAO SPECT study.

Published with permission: ***Appl Radiol*** **1993;22:35–44.**

Teaching Point:

In the first 24 hr following the onset of a stroke, cerebral SPECT, particularly when combined with CT, can be very helpful in detecting the presence of an infarction and also in defining the stroke subtype.

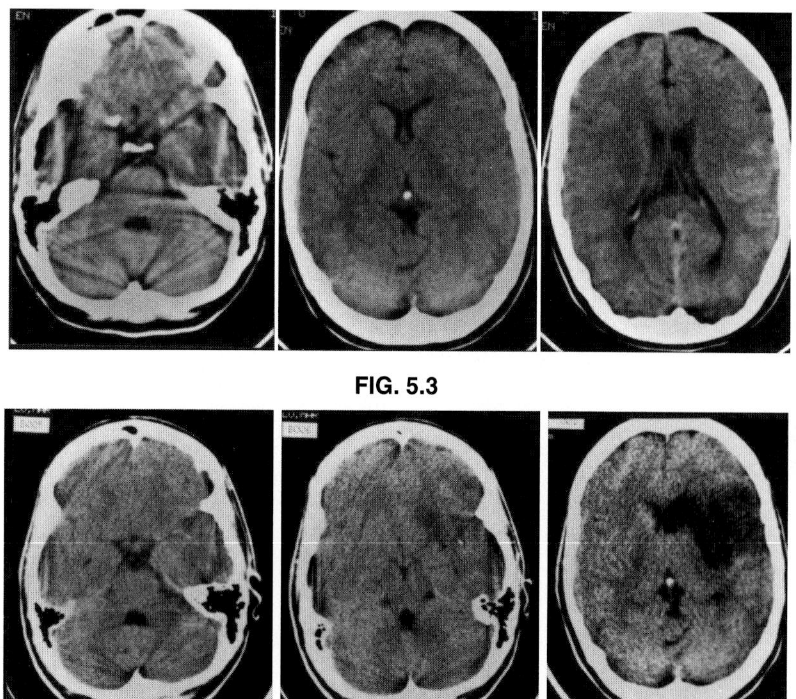

FIG. 5.3

FIG. 5.5

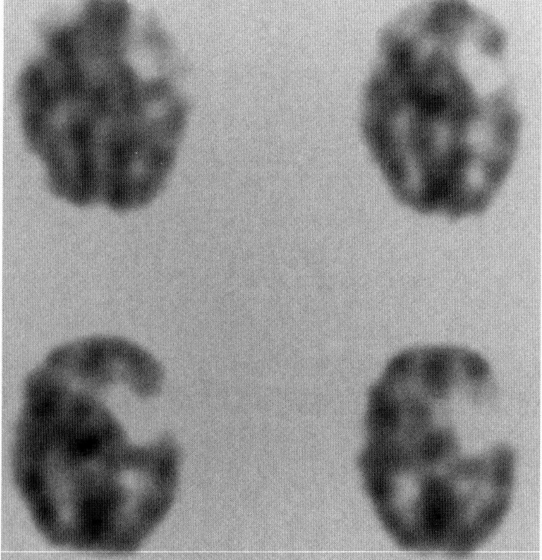

FIG. 5.4

CASE 5-3

Clinical Diagnosis:
Acute Right Middle Cerebral Artery Infarction

CONTRIBUTOR:

Name: Ronald L. Van Heertum, M.D.
Institution: St. Vincent's Hospital and Medical Center

IMAGING DATA:

Camera: GE 3000 XCT
Isotope: ^{99m}Tc ECD

Collimator: Ultra-high resolution, parallel hole
Dose: 21.8 mCi

This 38-year-old man with documented sickle cell trait presented with an acute progressive left-sided weakness and a severe headache in the right temporal area. A duplex Doppler study, performed 24 hr after initial clinical presentation, revealed a thrombus in the right middle cerebral artery with extension into the distal right internal carotid artery.

The initial CT scan, (Fig. 5.6), showed some loss of definition in the deep gray and white matter in the right posterior frontal and anterior temporal lobes and calcification of the horizontal portion of the right middle cerebral artery. No definite mass lesion was noted.

The ECD SPECT, transaxial plane (Fig. 5.7), revealed a large perfusion deficit in the right posterior frontal, anterior temporal, and basal ganglia regions.

A 10-day follow-up CT scan (Fig. 5.8) revealed a large well-defined (hypodensity) area of infarction corresponding in size and location to the cerebral SPECT study.

Teaching Point:

Cerebral SPECT is complementary to CT and duplex Doppler in the evaluation of acute cerebral infarction.

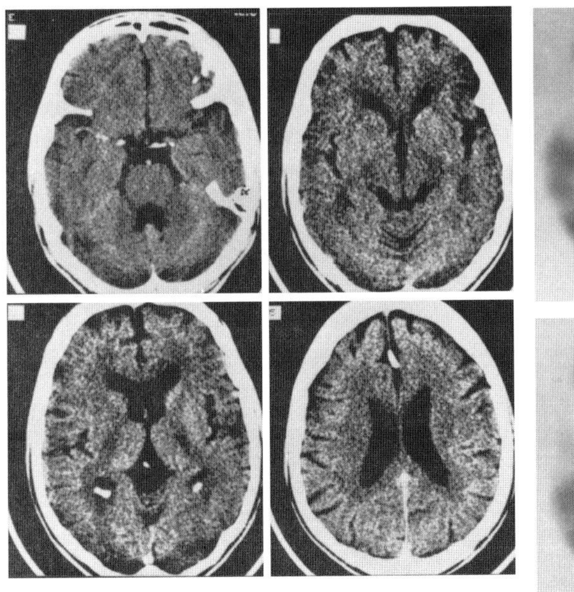

FIG. 5.6

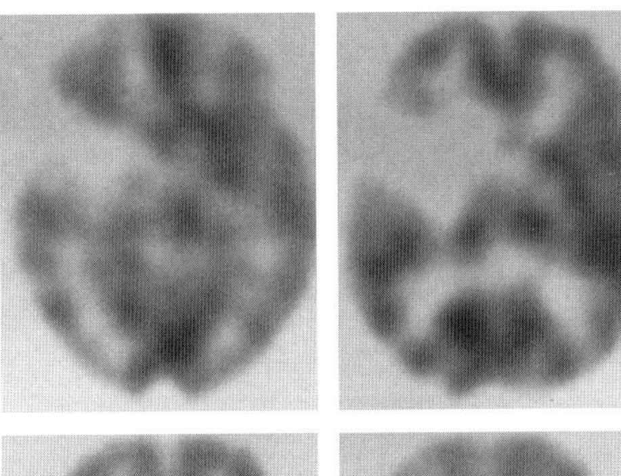

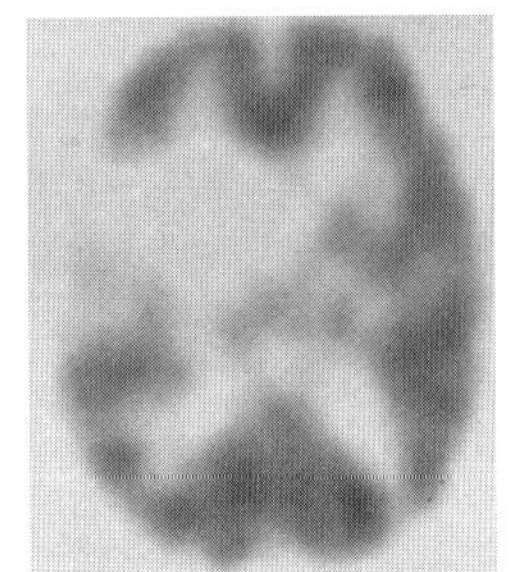

FIG. 5.7

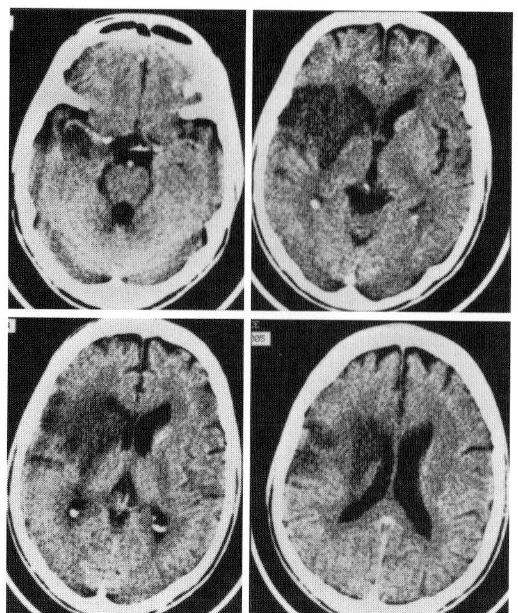

FIG. 5.8

CASE 5-4

Clinical Diagnosis: Acute Left Middle Cerebral Artery Infarction with Crossed Cerebellar Diaschisis

CONTRIBUTOR:	IMAGING DATA:	
Name: Ronald L. Van Heertum, M.D.	**Camera:** GE 3000 XCT	**Collimator:** Ultra-high resolution, parallel hole
Institution: St. Vincent's Hospital and Medical Center	**Isotope:** ^{99m}Tc ECD	**Dose:** 21.1 mCi

This 61-year-old man was referred for evaluation following the acute onset of an expressive aphasia and a progressive right hemiparesis. The patient had no prior history of stroke or significant risk factors.

An initial CT scan (Fig. 5.9) revealed effacement of the left sylvian fissure and some loss of anatomic detail in the region of the basal ganglia.

ECD SPECT in the transaxial plane (Fig. 5.10) revealed decreased radiotracer uptake in the right cerebellar hemisphere, consistent with crossed cerebellar diaschisis. In addition, the study demonstrated diffuse decreased radiotracer activity in the left basal ganglia and throughout the cerebral cortex corresponding to a left middle cerebral artery territory distribution.

A follow-up CT scan 7 days later (Fig. 5.11) revealed hypodensities compatible with evolving infarctions in the left middle cerebral artery territory.

Teaching Point:

Crossed cerebellar diaschisis, although not of great clinical significance, may be seen in patients with acute cortical and subcortical infarctions, particularly when the motor tracts are involved.

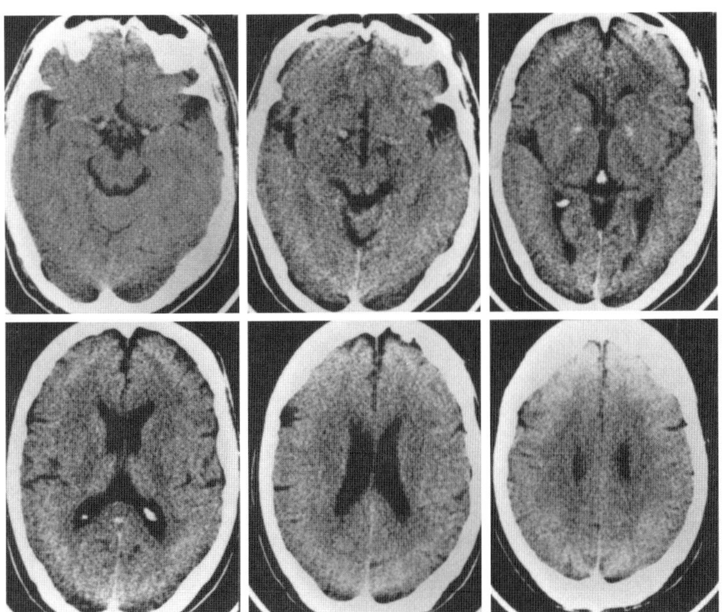

FIG. 5-9

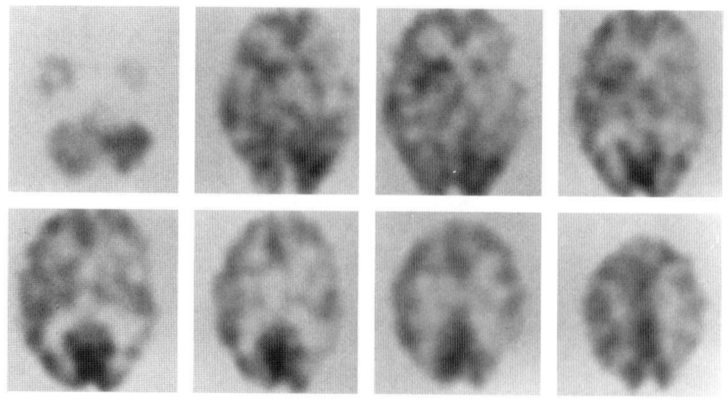

FIG. 5.10

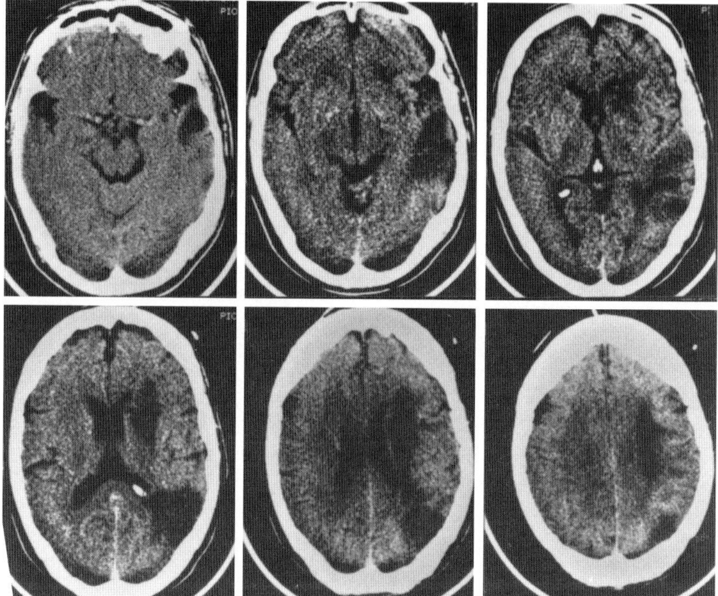

FIG. 5.11

CASE 5-5

Clinical Diagnosis:

Acute Infarction—Posterior Branch Left Middle Cerebral Artery

CONTRIBUTOR:	IMAGING DATA:	
Name: Ronald L. Van Heertum, M.D.	**Camera:** GE Neurocam	**Collimator:** Ultra-high resolution, parallel hole
Institution: Columbia-Presbyterian Medical Center	**Isotope:** ^{99m}Tc HMPAO	**Dose:** 21.7 mCi

This 73-year-old man was admitted to the hospital for evaluation and treatment of a major depressive episode (bipolar disorder). During his hospital stay, the patient was started on a course of electroconvulsive therapy (ECT) treatments. Soon after his 11th ECT treatment, the patient was observed to be confused and was thought to have a combined receptive and expressive aphasia and a right hemiparesis. Both the aphasia and hemiparesis were noted to be transient in nature.

An initial CT scan revealed mild diffuse atrophy and was otherwise unremarkable. An HMPAO SPECT study in the coronal (Fig. 5.12) and sagittal (Fig. 5.13) planes revealed a wedge-shaped area of absent radiotracer activity in the posterior-superior aspect of the left parietal lobe that was felt to be compatible with an infarction in this region.

A follow-up CT scan 4 days later revealed a hypodensity in the same region as the SPECT scan. The CT scan findings confirmed that the patient had sustained a left posterior branch occlusion most likely secondary to a thromboembolus, possibly secondary to an atherosclerotic plaque.

Teaching Point:

In some cases, post-ECT sequelae may be difficult to distinguish from an underlying evolving stroke or ischemia. Cerebral SPECT may be very helpful in such cases, particularly when the CT or MRI study is equivocal or negative.

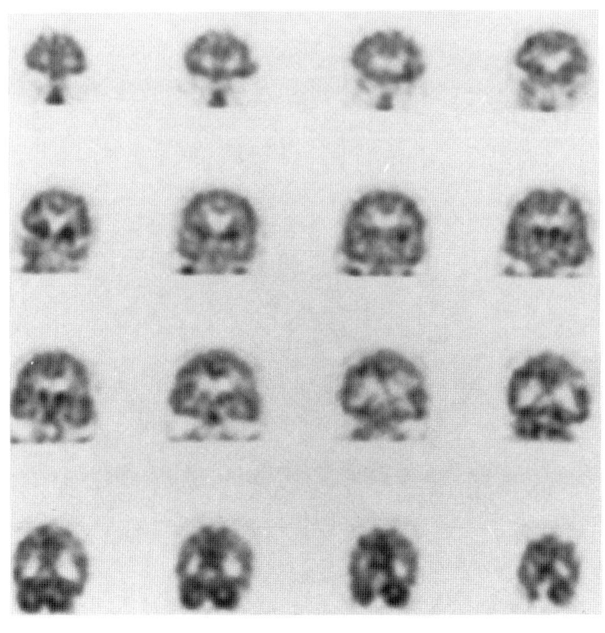

FIG. 5.12

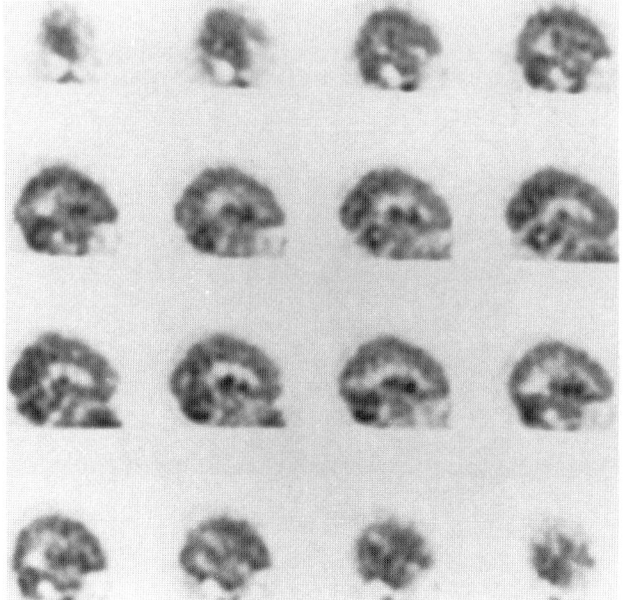

FIG. 5.13

CASE 5-6

Clinical Diagnosis: Progressive Right Hemisphere Stroke

CONTRIBUTOR:

Name: Ronald L. Van Heertum, M.D.
Institution: St. Vincent's Hospital and Medical Center

IMAGING DATA:

Camera: GE 3000 XCT
Isotope: ^{99m}Tc HMPAO
Collimator: Ultra-high resolution
Dose: 22.2 mCi

This 60-year-old woman, with a known history of chronic hypertension and diabetes, presented to the emergency room after having sustained a fall. Physical examination at that time revealed slurred speech, eyes deviated to the right, and a left hemiplegia.

An initial CT scan (Fig. 5.14) revealed hypodensities in the white matter in the right hemisphere consistent with changes related to a subcortical arteriosclerotic encephalopathy. In addition, an area of infarction in the right occipital lobe was observed.

An HMPAO SPECT study (Fig. 5.15) in the transaxial plane revealed focal absence of radiotracer activity in the right occipital lobe corresponding to the area of infarction noted on CT. Crossed cerebellar diaschisis with diminished radiotracer activity in the left cerebellar hemisphere was also noted. In addition, there was extensive decrease in radiotracer accumulation throughout the right cerebral hemisphere that was significantly greater than the area of abnormality noted on the CT scan. This latter finding was felt to be related to underlying carotid occlusive disease.

The patient's hospital course was relatively uneventful; however, at the time of discharge, the patient's left hemiplegia had not improved. Approximately 9 months after discharge from the hospital, the patient again presented to the emergency room. At that time, it was felt that the patient had sustained an extension of her prior stroke.

The CT scan (Fig. 5.16) performed at the time of her second hospital admission revealed an extensive infarction involving the right occipital, temporal, parietal, and frontal lobes.

The follow-up HMPAO SPECT study (Fig. 5.17) in the transaxial plane revealed an extensive area of absent radiotracer activity corresponding to the area of infarction noted on the CT scan.

Published with permission: ***Appl Radiol*** **1993;22:35–44.**

Teaching Point:

This case is an excellent example of the potential role for cerebral SPECT in the assessment of acute stroke. The initial SPECT study revealed hypoperfusion throughout the right cerebral hemisphere, suggesting the possibility of a low hemodynamic due to occlusion of the right internal carotid artery. In such a situation, the patient is at an increased risk of developing an extension of the area of infarction if left untreated.

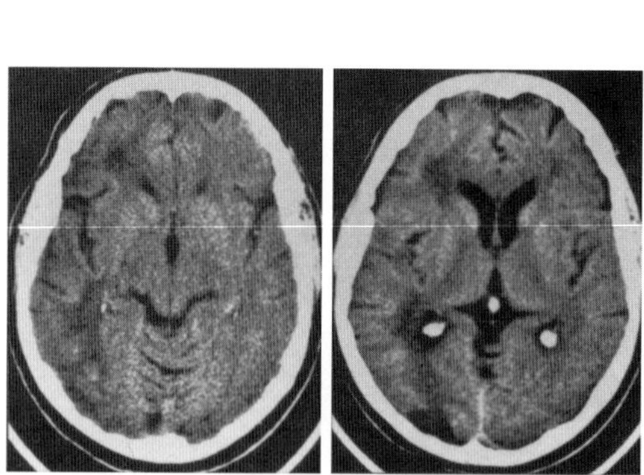

FIG. 5.14

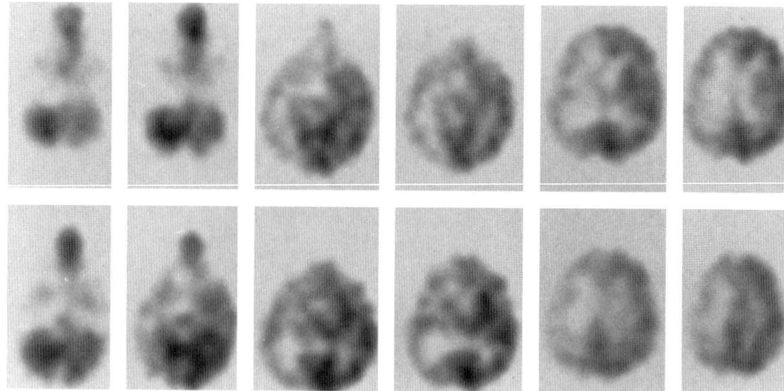

FIG. 5.15

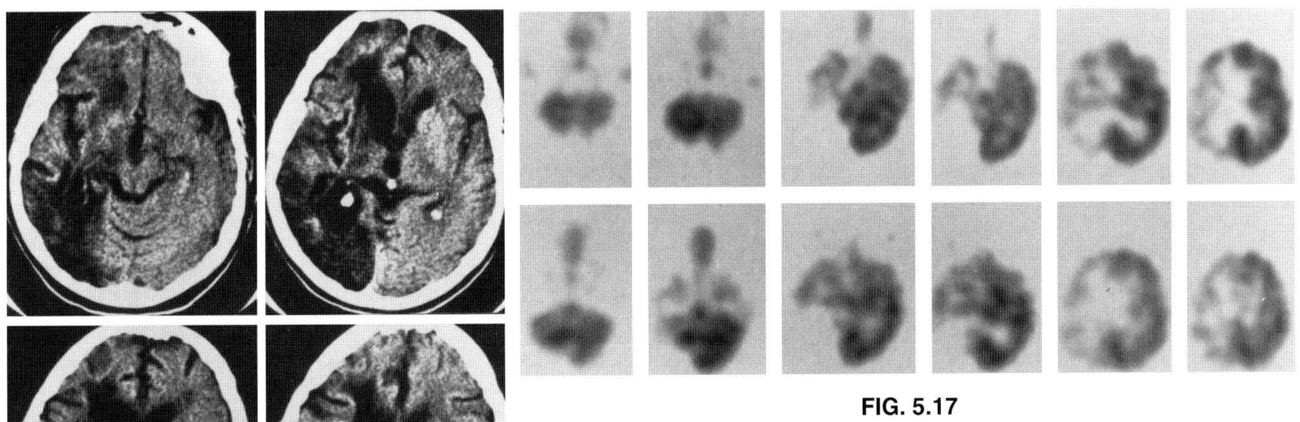

FIG. 5.16

FIG. 5.17

CASE 5-7

Clinical Diagnosis:
Progressive Stroke—Right Occipital Lobe

CONTRIBUTOR:

Name: Robert S. Hellman, M.D. and Ronald S. Tikofsky, Ph.D.
Institution: Medical College of Wisconsin

IMAGING DATA:

Camera: GE 400AC/T;STAR
Isotope: ^{123}I IMP
Collimator: High resolution
Dose: 5.0 mCi

This 29-year-old, right-handed woman was referred for evaluation of an episode of generalized weakness, slurring of speech, and blurring of vision associated with a migraine headache. Physical examination revealed a left visual field defect. Clinically, the patient was thought to have sustained an infarction of the right occipital lobe, possibly secondary to migrainous vasoconstriction.

An MRI study (Fig. 5.18) confirmed the diagnosis of a right occipital lobe infarction.

A cerebral SPECT study in the transaxial plane (Fig. 5.19), performed on the same day as the MRI examination, showed absent tracer deposition in the right occipital lobe *(arrow),* which represented a larger zone of abnormality than that seen on MRI.

A follow-up cerebral SPECT study (Fig. 5.20) performed 2 days later revealed a decrease in size of the abnormal area in the right occipital lobe *(arrow).* The overall findings were compatible with a combined pattern of infarction with a reversible ischemic zone surrounding the area of infarction.

Teaching Point:

Cerebral SPECT, in combination with MRI, may be useful in defining the penumbra surrounding an area of infarction. This type of observation can be made most reliably when precise image fusion (coregistration) of the MRI and SPECT studies can be performed.

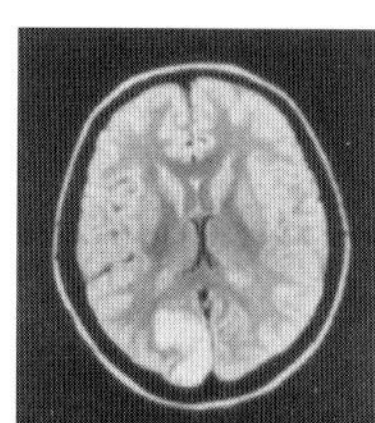

FIG. 5.18

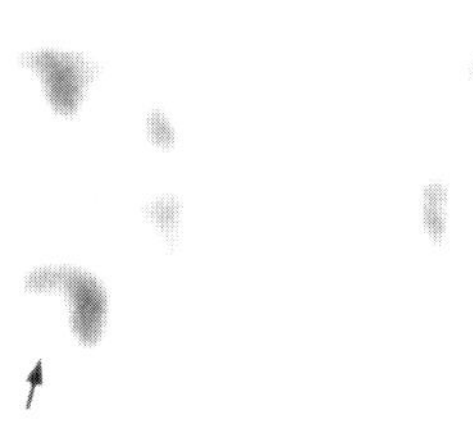

FIG. 5.19

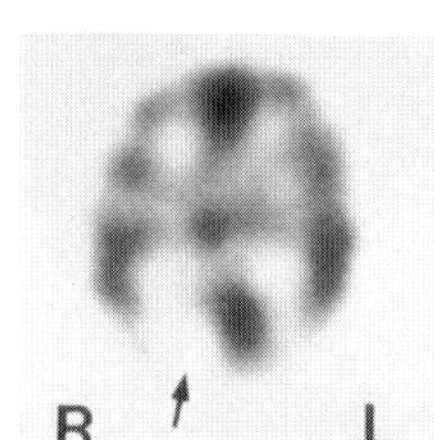

FIG. 5.20

CASE 5-8

Clinical Diagnosis: Acute Right Posterior Cerebral Artery Infarction

CONTRIBUTOR:	IMAGING DATA:	
Name: Ronald L. Van Heertum, M.D.	**Camera:** GE 400 AC/T;STAR II	**Collimator:** High resolution
Institution: Columbia-Presbyterian Medical Center	**Isotope:** ^{123}I IMP	**Dose:** 3.0 mCi

This 60-year-old woman was referred for evaluation of a single episode of occipital headache, loss of vision, and transient loss of consciousness.

The initial CT scan (Fig. 5.21) revealed an osteoma projecting from the inner table of the left parietal bone. The study was otherwise unremarkable.

The cerebral SPECT study (Fig. 5.22) in the transaxial **(A)**, coronal **(B)**, and sagittal **(C)** planes showed an area of absent tracer deposition in the right occipital lobe, with involvement of the visual cortex *(arrows.)* The adjacent posterior temporal lobe and posterior right thalamus were also involved.

A follow-up CT scan (Fig. 5.23) revealed an evolving infarction of the right occipital lobe, with involvement of the right temporal lobe and thalamus corresponding to the deficit seen on the cerebral SPECT study.

The overall findings are quite typical of an acute infarction in the right posterior cerebral artery territory.

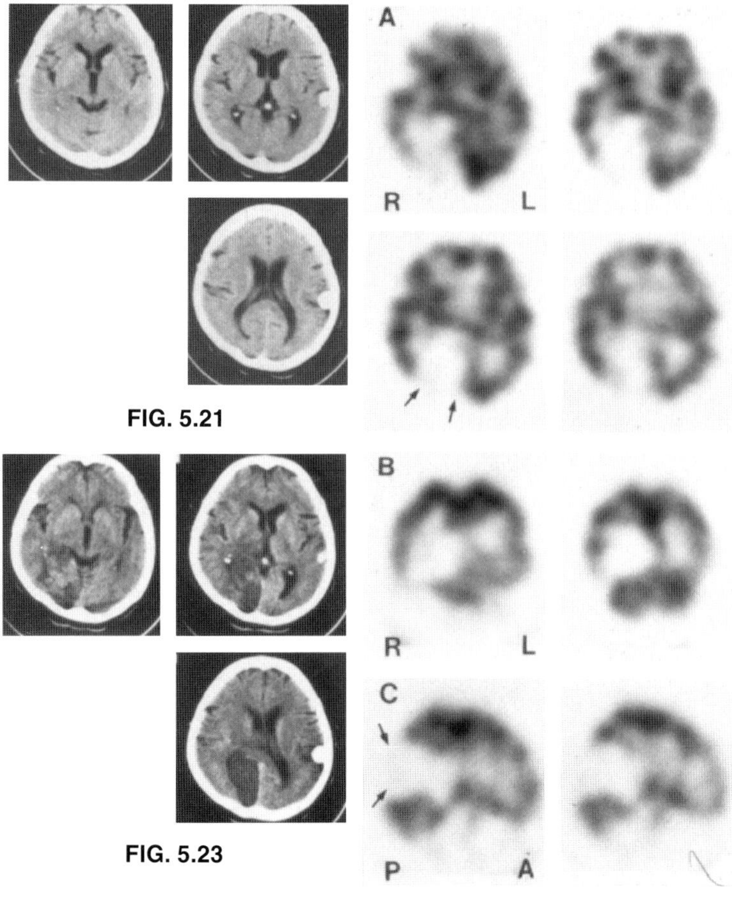

FIG. 5.21

FIG. 5.23

FIG. 5.22

CASE 5-9

Clinical Diagnosis: Acute Right Posterior Cerebral Artery Infarction

CONTRIBUTOR:

Name: Paul Hoffer, M.D. and David Moon, M.D.
Institution: Yale University School of Medicine

IMAGING DATA:

Camera: Picker PRISM 3000
Isotope: ^{99m}Tc HMPAO

Collimator: High resolution, fan beam
Dose: 20 mCi

This 69-year-old woman was referred for evaluation of the acute onset of a visual field deficit that developed immediately following a cerebral arteriogram.

An initial CT scan (Fig. 5.24) demonstrated an area of infarction in the right posterior occipital lobe with adjacent white matter changes felt to be secondary to ischemia.

The HMPAO SPECT study (Fig. 5.25) revealed absent radiotracer activity in the right occipital lobe corresponding to the combined area of infarction and ischemia noted on CT. Inaddition, diminished radiotracer activity was noted in the right anterior temporal lobe.

Teaching Point:

Highly valuable information can be obtained by comparing the size of the deficit on SPECT with CT. In this case the right occipital lobe deficit noted on the SPECT study corresponded to the combined areas of ischemia and infarction noted on CT. In addition, the SPECT study suggested that additional disease existed in the right middle cerebral artery territory distribution.

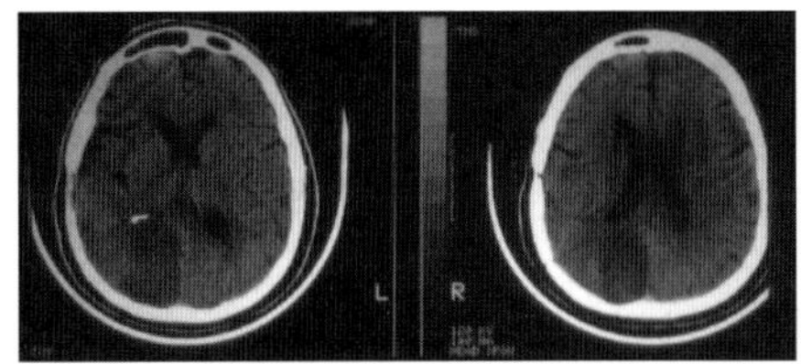

FIG. 5.24

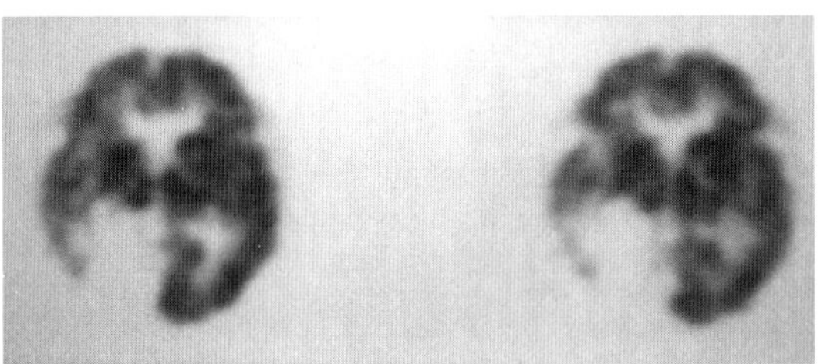

FIG. 5.25

CASE 5-10

Clinical Diagnosis: Acute Left Posterior Cerebral Infarction

CONTRIBUTOR:	**IMAGING DATA:**	
Name: Richard Rome, M.D.	**Camera:** Elscint Helix	**Collimator:** High resolution
Institution: Huguley Memorial Medical Center	**Isotope:** ^{123}I IMP	**Dose:** 2.6 mCi

The 59-year-old man with a long-standing history of labile hypertension presented for evaluation following a sudden loss of vision involving the nasal and temporal fields in his right eye. The visual fields in his left eye remained intact.

A CT scan at the time of presentation was negative.

An HMPAO SPECT study (Fig. 5.26) in the transaxial plane revealed markedly decreased radiotracer activity in the left occipital lobe.

Teaching Point:

Cerebral SPECT can be very useful differentiating acute infarction from other causes of acute presentation of visual field deficits. The SPECT study may be particularly helpful particularly when CT and MRI are negative or equivocal.

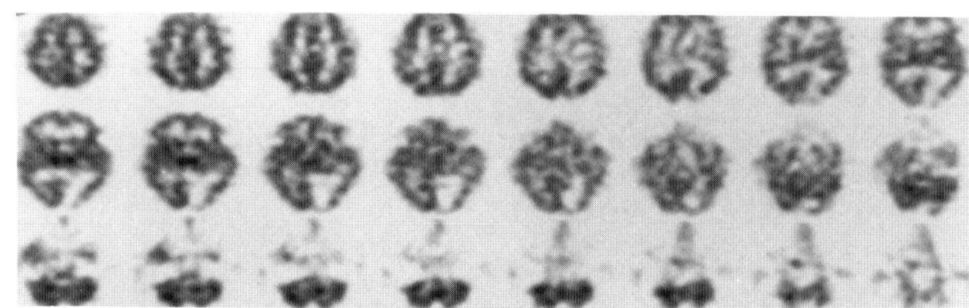

FIG. 5.26

CASE 5-11

Clinical Diagnosis: Balint Syndrome

CONTRIBUTOR:	IMAGING DATA:	
Name: Jean Luc Moretti, M.D.	**Camera:** GE 400AC	**Collimator:** LEAP
Institution: Hôpital Avicenne	**Isotope:** ^{123}I IMP	**Dose:** 10.0 mCi

This 77-year-old woman presented for evaluation of progressive symptoms of optic ataxia with altitudinal hemianopia and object agnosia. Physical examination revealed shrinking visual fields. The overall clinical findings were felt to be compatible with Balint syndrome secondary to a posterior stroke.

The HMPAO SPECT study (Fig. 5.27a) in the transaxial plane revealed bilateral decrease in radiotracer activity at 20 min post-IMP injection that remained unchanged on the follow-up SPECT study (Fig. 5.27b), at 200 min post-IMP injection. The findings were felt to be compatible with bilateral occipital lobe infarctions.

Teaching Point:

This case and the previous four cases demonstrate the spectrum of SPECT findings in patients presenting with acute visual field abnormalities due to underlying occipital lobe lesions of a cerebrovascular etiology.

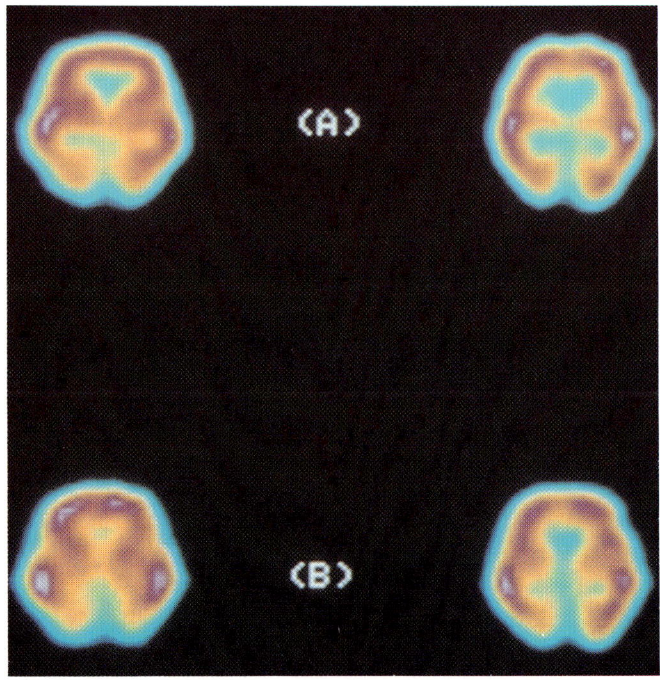

FIG. 5.27

CASE 5-12

Clinical Diagnosis:
Acute Left Hemisphere Stroke Before and After Tissue Plasminogen Activator

CONTRIBUTOR:

Name: Paul Hoffer, M.D. and David Moon, M.D.
Institution: Yale University of Medicine

IMAGING DATA:

Camera: Picker PRISM 3000
Isotope: ^{99m}Tc HMPAO

Collimator: High resolution, fan beam
Dose: 20 mCi

This 35-year-old man presented for evaluation immediately following the acute onset of right-sided weakness. An initial CT scan at the time of presentation was negative for acute hemorrhage or infarction.

The initial HMPAO SPECT study, performed on the same day as the CT scan (Fig. 5.28) in the transaxial plane, revealed a significant decrease in radiotracer activity throughout much of the left hemisphere, corresponding to the left middle cerebral artery territory. In addition, crossed cerebellar diaschisis, with diminished radiotracer activity in the right cerebellar hemisphere, was noted. Immediately following this study, tissue plasminogen activator was administered to the patient.

A follow-up HMPAO SPECT study performed 2 days later (Fig. 5.29) revealed an overall improvement in the radiotracer uptake throughout the left hemisphere. Focal increased activity, felt to be secondary to luxury perfusion, was observed in the left frontal temporal region. In addition, a focal deficit was observed in the left lenticular nucleus and adjacent left insular cortex corresponding to a residual area of infarction noted on a follow-up MRI exam.

Teaching Point:

This case illustrates the potential value of cerebral SPECT in the assessment of a variety of therapeutic interventions in patients with acute stroke.

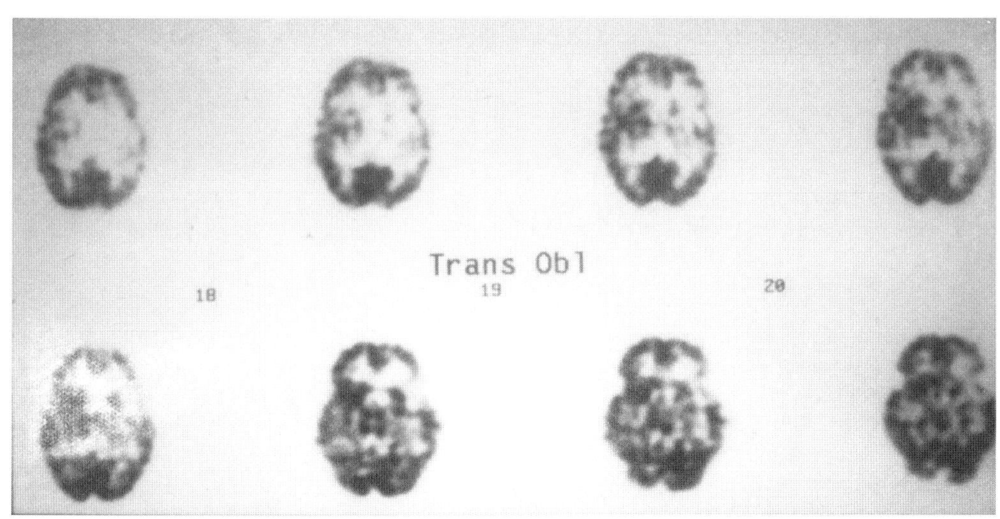

FIG. 5.28

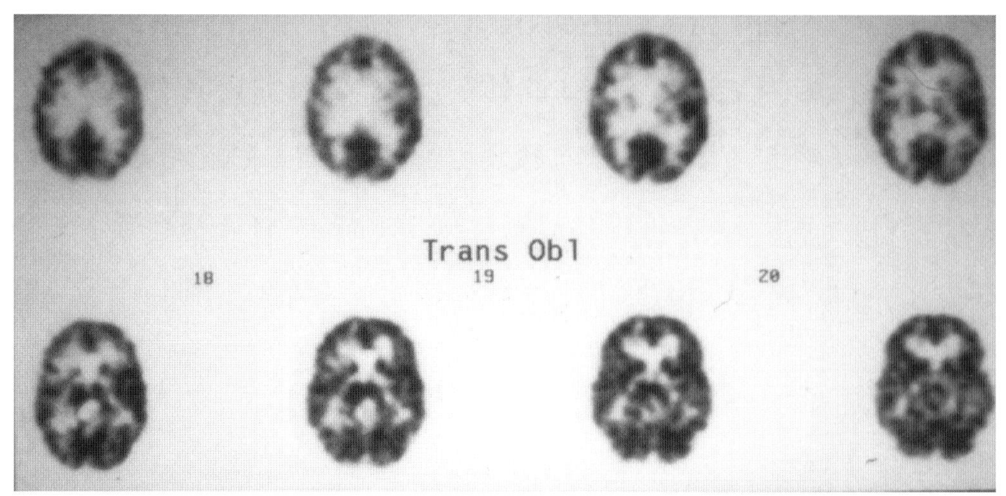

FIG. 5.29

CASE 5-13

Clinical Diagnosis:

Left Cerebellar Hemisphere Infarction

CONTRIBUTOR:	**IMAGING DATA:**	
Name: William L. Ashburn, M.D.	**Camera:** Elscint APEX 409AG-ECT; APEX 009 Precursor	**Collimator:** LEAP
Institution: UCSD Medical Center	**Isotope:** ^{123}I IMP	**Dose:** 3.0 mCi

This 57-year-old man was referred for evaluation of dizziness of 6 months' duration.

A CT scan was negative.

A cerebral SPECT study (Fig. 5.30) in the transaxial plane showed a marked decrease in tracer deposition in the left cerebellar hemisphere *(arrows)* that was compatible with ischemia or infarction in that region.

A follow-up cerebral arteriogram revealed absent flow to the left cerebellar hemisphere due to complete occlusion of the left vertebral artery and 60 percent stenosis of both internal carotid arteries.

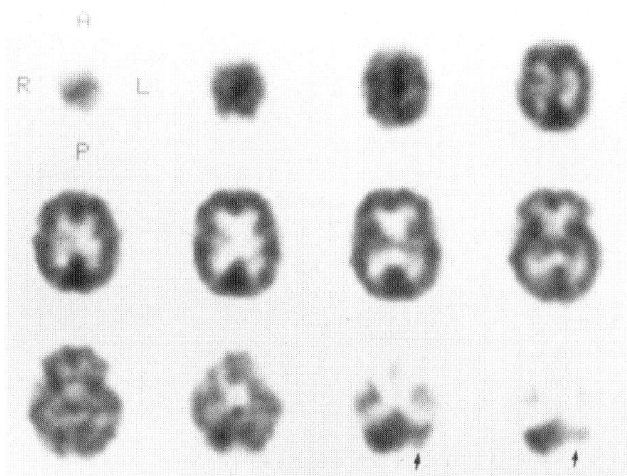

FIG. 5.30

CASE 5-14

Clinical Diagnosis:
Massive Left Cerebrovascular Accident Secondary to Cocaine Abuse

CONTRIBUTOR:

Name: Robert S. Hellman, M.D. and Ronald S. Tikofsky, Ph.D.
Institution: Medical College of Wisconsin

IMAGING DATA:

Camera: GE Neurocam
Isotope: ^{99m}Tc HMPAO

Collimator: High resolution, parallel hole
Dose: 30 mCi

This 32-year-old man presented for evaluation 1 day after having collapsed while walking. At that time, his family reported that the patient was confused and unable to communicate or move his right side. At the time of presentation to the emergency room, a urine screen for cocaine was positive. Other risk factors, in addition to cocaine abuse, included a long-term history of smoking.

The initial CT scan (Fig. 5.31) was unremarkable, with no evidence of mass effect, hemorrhage, or acute infarction.

The HMPAO SPECT study performed 1 day later (Fig. 5.32) in the transaxial plane showed a large area of absent radiotracer uptake in the left middle cerebral artery territory, consistent with an area of infarction. A second smaller area of absent radiotracer activity was also noted in the left posterior and superior parietal regions, suggesting an additional area of infarction. In addition, crossed cerebellar diaschisis with decreased radiotracer activity in the right cerebellar hemisphere was noted.

A follow-up HMPAO SPECT study 19 days later (Fig. 5.33) in the transaxial plane revealed a dramatic increase in radiotracer accumulation at the two sites of previously noted diminished uptake, which was felt to be secondary to luxury perfusion. In addition, crossed cerebellar diaschisis was no longer evident.

A third HMPAO SPECT study performed approximately 6 months following the initial presentation (Fig. 5.34) in the transaxial plane again revealed absent radiotracer activity in the left frontal, temporal, and parietal lobes along with crossed cerebellar diaschisis.

Teaching Points:

1. The HMPAO SPECT studies in this case illustrate one of the characteristic findings that may be seen in cocaine abuse, namely, cerebral infarction.
2. In addition, this case demonstrates the difficulties associated with luxury perfusion that may arise when initial studies are performed 3 to 5 days after ictus due to a loss of autoregulation. Similar patterns of increased radiotracer uptake may be seen with capillary hyperplasia (neovascularity) 14 to 21 days after ictus. When using ^{99m}Tc HMPAO, follow-up studies should be obtained at a time when luxury perfusion is not likely to be present, (i.e., 3 to 6 months after ictus).

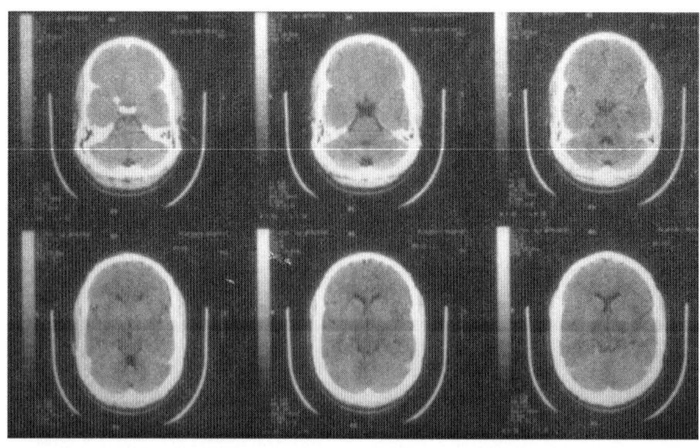

FIG. 5.31

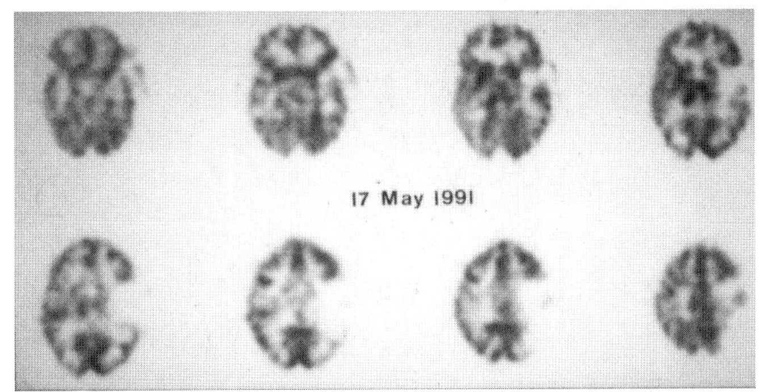

FIG. 5.32

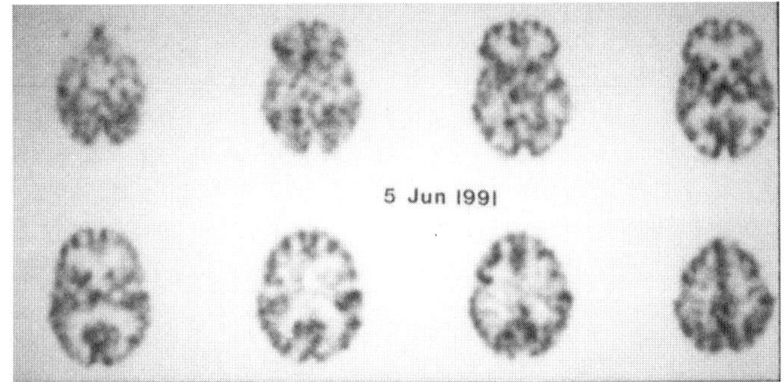

FIG. 5.33

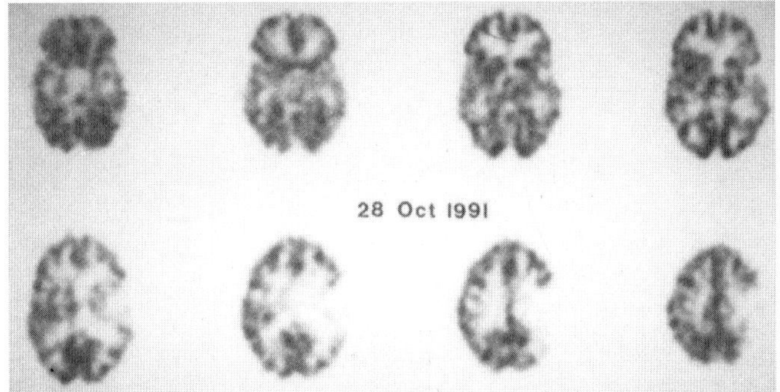

FIG. 5.34

CASE 5-15

Clinical Diagnosis:
Subacute Left Anterior Cerebral Infarction—Luxury Perfusion

CONTRIBUTOR:

Name: Ronald L. Van Heertum, M.D.
Institution: St. Vincent's Hospital and Medical Center

IMAGING DATA:

Camera: GE 300 XCT
Isotope: ^{99m}Tc HMPAO
Collimator: Ultra-high resolution, parallel hole
Dose: 20.8 mCi

This 78-year-old woman was referred for evaluation of a combined expressive/receptive aphasia and progressive right hemiparesis. The patient apparently first experienced symptoms five days prior to her presentation to the hospital.

A CT scan (Fig. 5.35) at the time the patient was evaluated in the hospital revealed a hypodensity in the left anterior cerebral artery territory consistent with a subacute infarction.

An HMPAO SPECT study (Fig. 5.36) in the transaxial plane revealed an increase in radiotracer activity, in the left anterior frontal region secondary to luxury perfusion.

Published with permission: ***Radiol Clin North Am* 1993;31:881–907.**

Teaching Point:

Cerebral SPECT studies may be difficult to interpret during the period when luxury perfusion is prominent. The difficulties with luxury perfusion are most problematic with ^{99m}Tc HMPAO and less of an issue with ^{123}I IMP or ^{99m}Tc ECD.

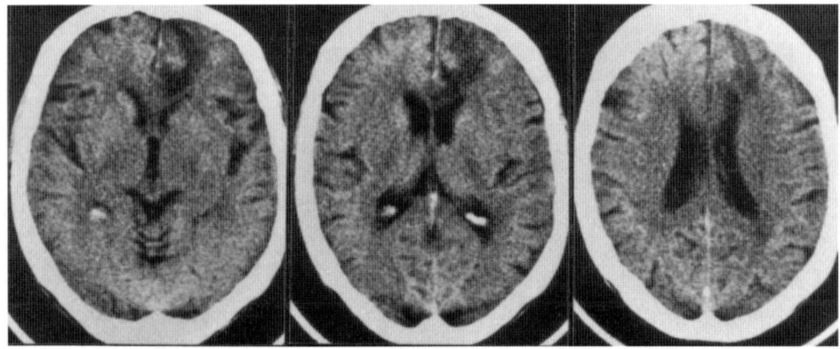

FIG. 5.35

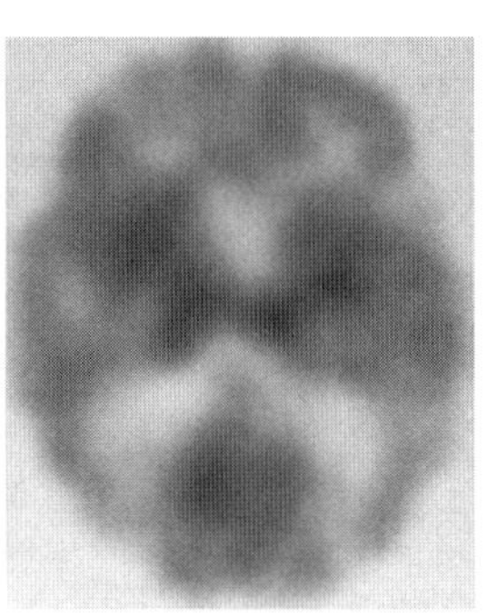
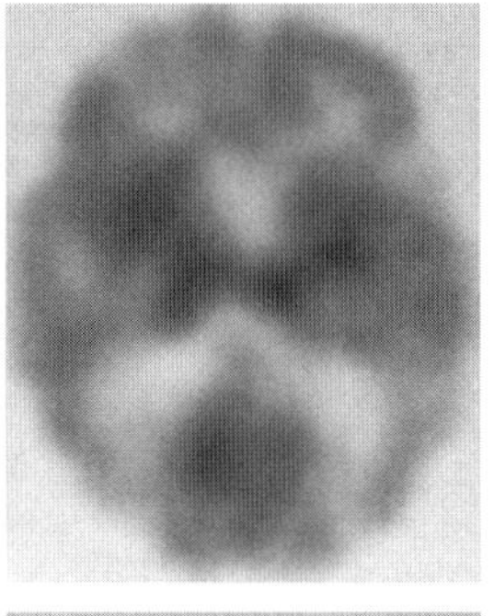
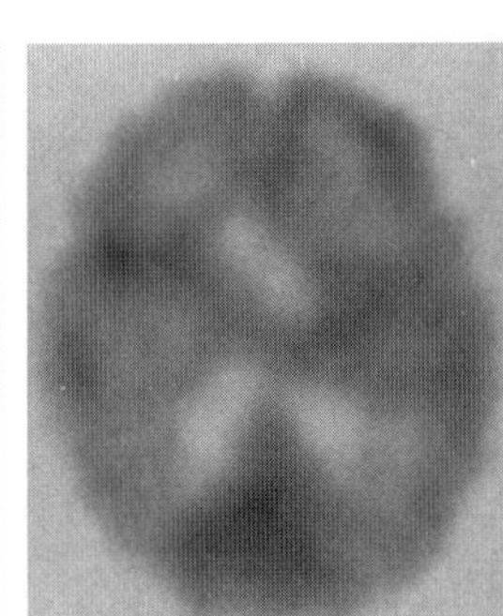
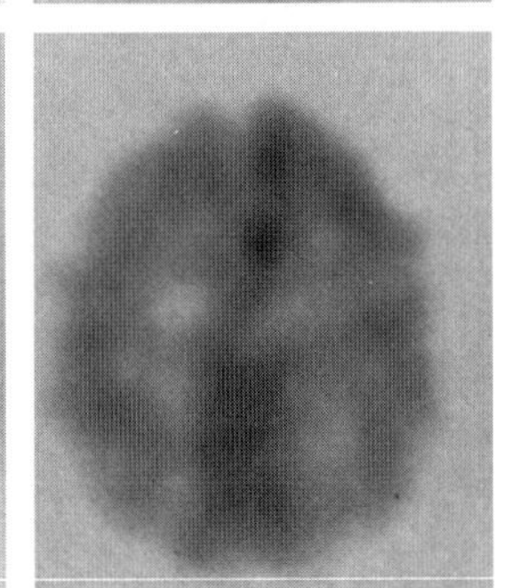

FIG. 5.36

CASE 5-16

Clinical Diagnosis:

Acute Right Anterior and Middle Cerebral Artery Infarction

CONTRIBUTOR:	**IMAGING DATA:**	
Name: Ronald L. Van Heertum, M.D.	**Camera:** GE 3000 XCT	**Collimator:** Ultra-high resolution, parallel hole
Institution: St. Vincent's Hospital and Medical Center	**Isotope:** ^{99m}Tc ECD	**Dose:** 20.2 mCi

This 82-year-old woman was admitted to the hospital for evaluation of a series of "falling down" episodes at home. Following admission to the hospital the patient developed a progressive left hemiplegia.

CT scan (Fig. 5.37) revealed hypodensities in the right frontal (parasagittal) lobe, right ganglionic region, and right frontal-temporal regions.

The ECD SPECT study (Fig. 5.38) performed several days after the CT scan, revealed markedly diminished radiotracer activity in the right frontal, temporal, and ganglionic regions corresponding in size to the area of infarction seen on the CT scan.

Teaching Point:

^{99m}Tc ECD may prove to be a useful radiopharmaceutical for evaluating stroke cases that are first studied more than 72 hr after ictus. Further case studies are needed to validate this observation.

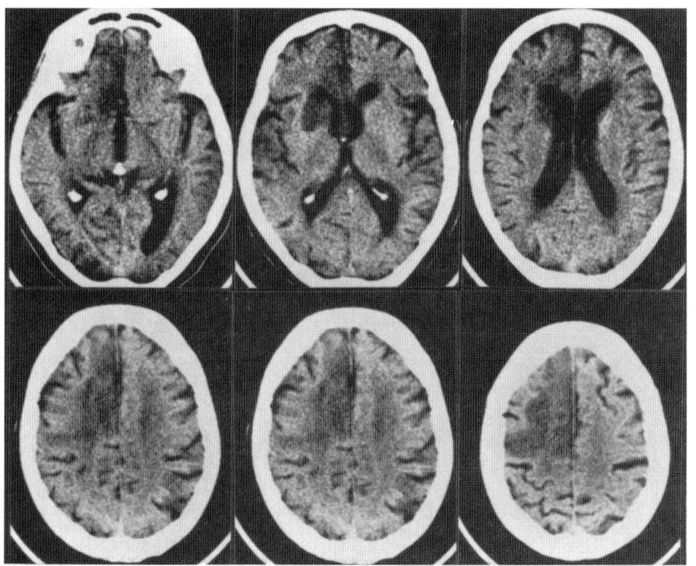

FIG. 5.37

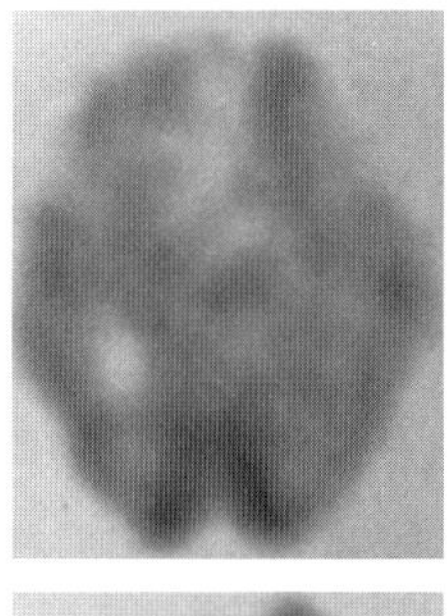
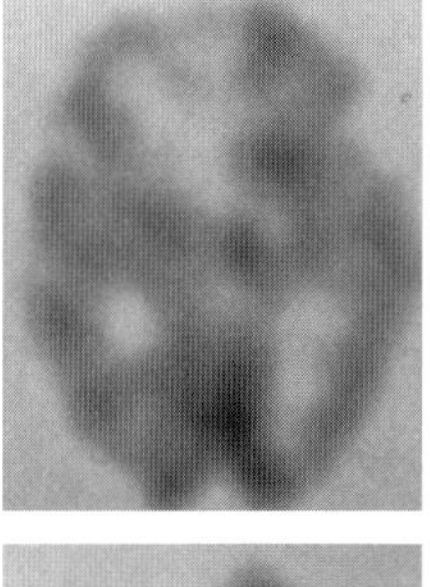
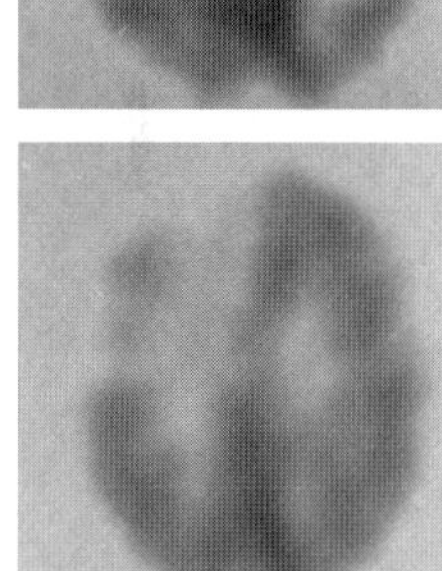
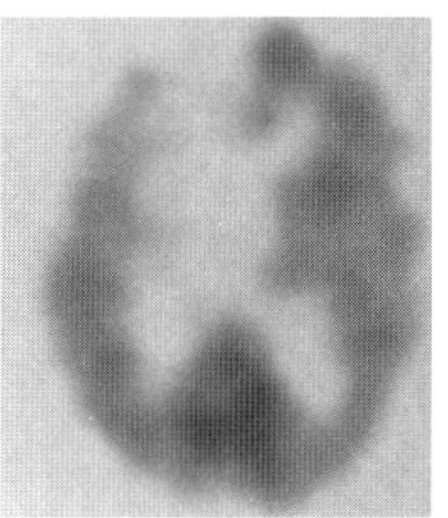
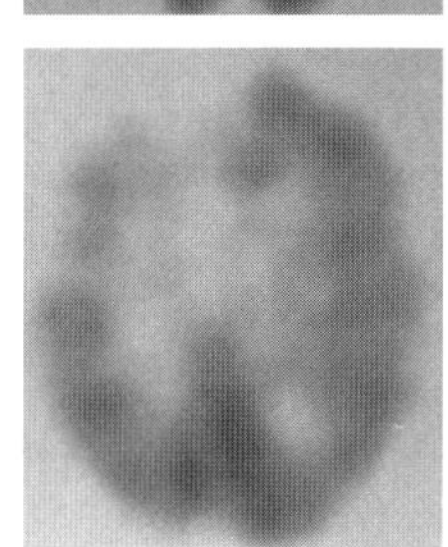

FIG. 5.38

CASE 5-17

Clinical Diagnosis:

Right Anterior Cerebral Artery Infarction

CONTRIBUTOR:	IMAGING DATA:	
Name: Robert S. Hellman, M.D. and Ronald S. Tikofsky, Ph.D.	**Camera:** GE 400AC/T;STAR	**Collimator:** High resolution
Institution: Medical College of Wisconsin	**Isotope:** ^{123}I IMP	**Dose:** 5.0 mCi

This 69-year-old man was referred for evaluation of progressive dementia, possibly of the Alzheimer's type.

A cerebral SPECT study (Fig. 5.39) in the transaxial **(A),** coronal **(B),** and sagittal **(C)** planes revealed decreased tracer uptake in the medial aspect of the right frontal lobe *(arrow).* This pattern is typical of an infarction of the anterior cerebral artery.

Teaching Point:

The pattern demonstrated in this case is quite different from the bilateral reduction of tracer uptake in the posterior temporal parietal lobe, which is typically associated with Alzheimer's disease. The pattern is much more compatible with infarction as a cause of the patient's dementia.

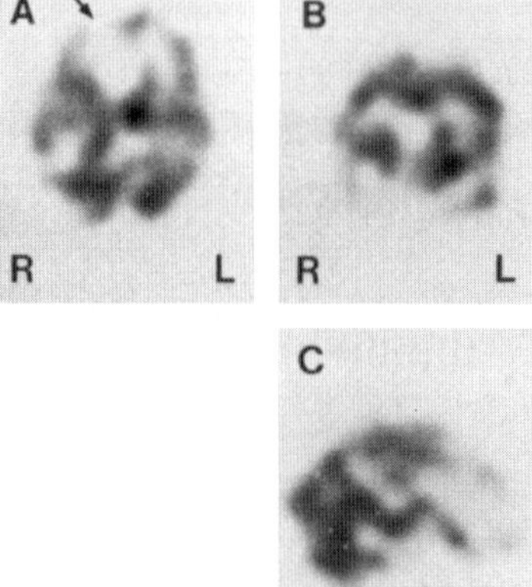

FIG. 5.39

CASE 5-18

Clinical Diagnosis: Remote Left Middle Cerebral Artery Infarction

CONTRIBUTOR:	IMAGING DATA:	
Name: Robert S. Hellman, M.D. and Ronald S. Tikofsky, Ph.D.	**Camera:** GE 400AC/T;STAR	**Collimator:** High resolution
Institution: Medical College of Wisconsin	**Isotope:** ^{123}I IMP	**Dose:** 5.0 mCi

Approximately 2 years after sustaining a left cerebrovascular accident, this 30-year-old, right-handed man was referred for evaluation. At the time of referral, the patient had a right hemiparesis, expressive aphasia, lingual dyspraxia, and a right homonymous hemianopsia.

A CT scan (Fig. 5.40) showed a large infarction of the left frontal, temporal, and anterior parietal lobes.

A cerebral SPECT study (Fig. 5.41) in the transaxial **(A),** coronal **(B),** and sagittal **(C)** planes demonstrated absent tracer deposition in the region of the left middle cerebral artery. The extent of the abnormality appears greater on the SPECT study than on the CT.

Teaching Point:

When CT or MRI examinations do not explain the cause of the neurologic deficit in stroke patients, a cerebral SPECT study is an additional useful, noninvasive approach.

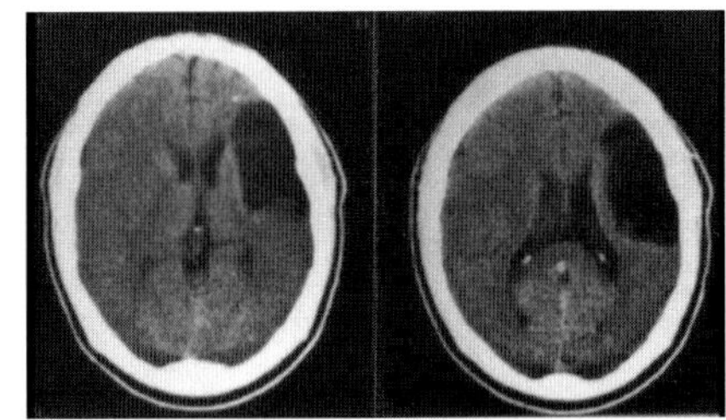

FIG. 5.40

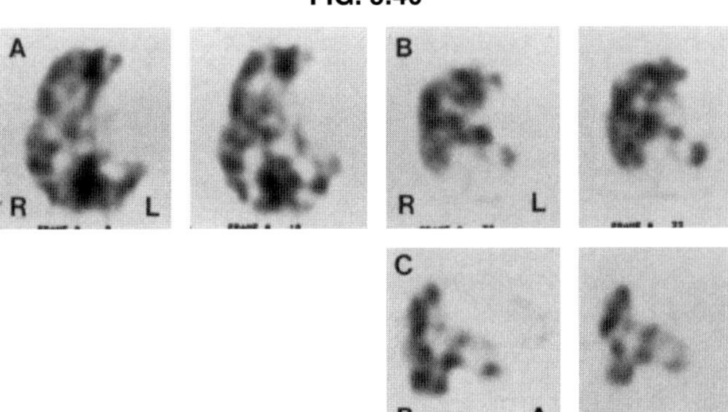

FIG. 5.41

CASE 5-19

Clinical Diagnosis:
Left Basal Ganglia Infarction

CONTRIBUTOR:

Name: Thomas C. Hill, M.D.
Institution: New England Deaconess Hospital

IMAGING DATA:

Camera: Strichman SME-810
Isotope: ^{123}I IMP
Collimator: High resolution
Dose: 3.0 mCi

This patient was referred for evaluation of an acute left cerebrovascular accident.

A CT scan (Fig. 5.42), performed without intravenous contrast, showed an oval low-density area involving the left basal ganglia and internal capsule.

A cerebral SPECT study (Fig. 5.43) in the transaxial plane showed that tracer deposition was absent in the left caudate nucleus *(arrow)*. In addition, there was a slight decrease of tracer activity in the adjacent cortical gray matter *(arrowhead)*. The overall findings were consistent with a left lacunar infarction, and a concomitant decrease in the adjacent cerebral cortex felt to be secondary to cortical diaschisis.

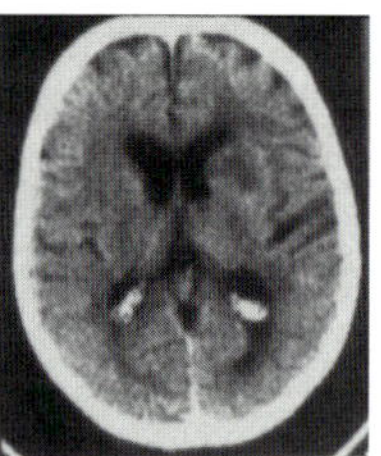

FIG. 5.42

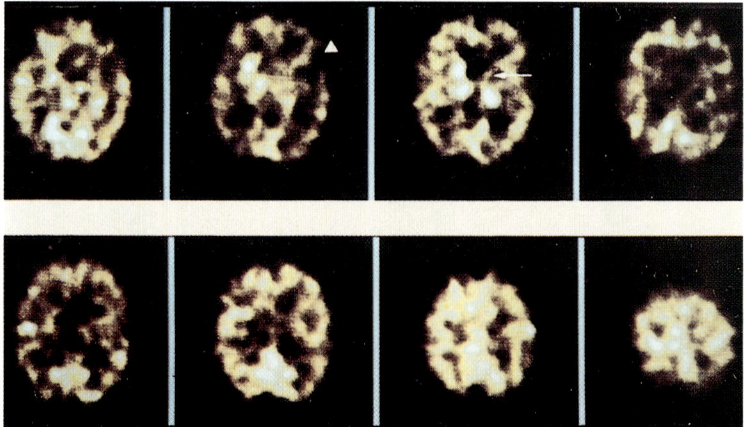

FIG. 5.43

CASE 5-20

Clinical Diagnosis: Acute Left Caudate Nucleus Infarction

CONTRIBUTOR:	**IMAGING DATA:**	
Name: Ronald L. Van Heertum, M.D.	**Camera:** GE 400AC/T;STAR II	**Collimator:** High resolution
Institution: St. Vincent's Hospital and Medical Center	**Isotope:** ^{123}I IMP	**Dose:** 3.0 mCi

This 62-year-old man was referred for evaluation of an acute onset of right-sided weakness, paresthesia, slurred speech, and decreased sensation on the right side of his face.

The CT scan (Fig. 5.44) showed a hypodensity in the region of the left caudate nucleus.

A cerebral SPECT study (Fig. 5.45) in the transaxial plane revealed decreased tracer deposition in the left caudate nucleus *(arrow)*. The combined findings are consistent with an acute left lacunar infarction.

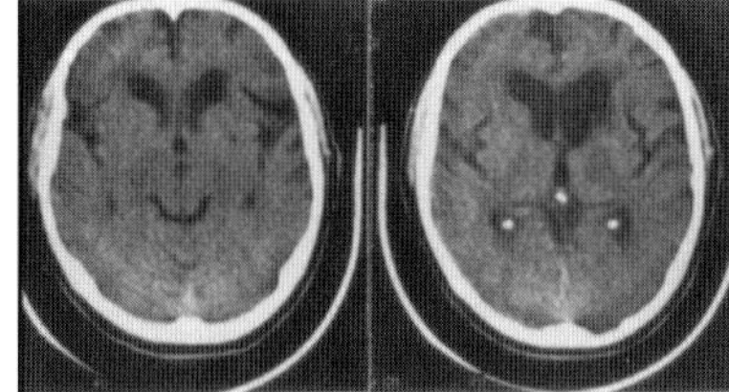

FIG. 5.44

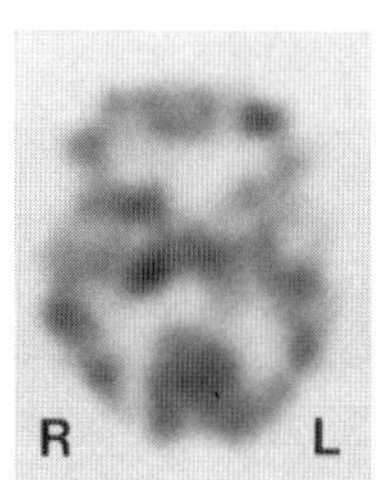

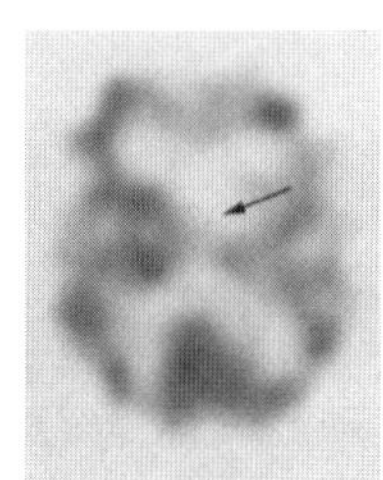

FIG. 5.45

CASE 5-21

Clinical Diagnosis: Left Thalamic Intracerebral Hemorrhage

CONTRIBUTOR:

Name: Robert S. Hellman, M.D. and Ronald S. Tikofsky, Ph.D.
Institution: Medical College of Wisconsin

IMAGING DATA:

Camera: GE 400AC/T;STAR
Isotope: ^{123}I IMP
Collimator: High resolution
Dose: 5.0 mCi

This 45-year-old, right-handed woman had sustained a cerebrovascular accident of the left hemisphere 2 months before the cerebral SPECT study. At the time of the SPECT examination, she had a mild expressive/receptive aphasia and a moderate right hemiparesis in which the effect on the upper extremity was greater than that on the lower.

A CT scan (Fig. 5.46) revealed a large hemorrhage involving the lateral aspect of the left thalamus and adjacent subcortical structures.

The cerebral SPECT study (Fig. 5.47) in the transaxial plane demonstrated an absence of tracer uptake at the site of the hemorrhage *(arrow).* In addition, a larger zone of decreased tracer deposition, involving most of the left cerebral hemisphere *(arrowheads),* was observed. This findings was felt to be compatible with a larger area of associated ischemia.

Teaching Point:

This case is a good example of the complementary role of cerebral SPECT, when used in conjunction with CT and MRI, in the assessment of subcortical cerebrovascular disease.

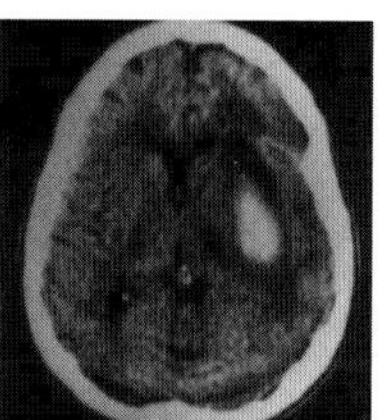

FIG. 5.46

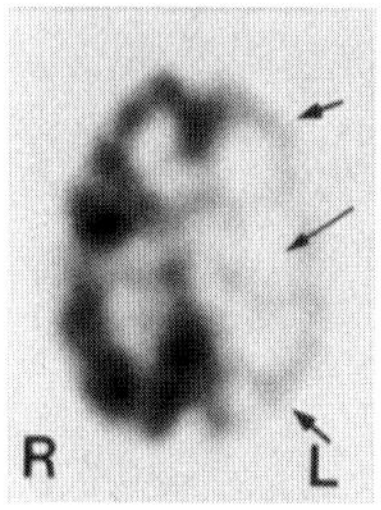

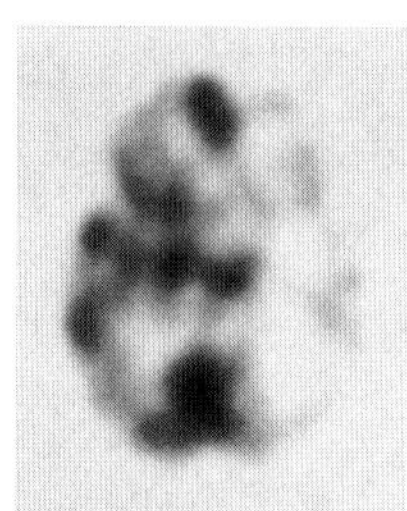
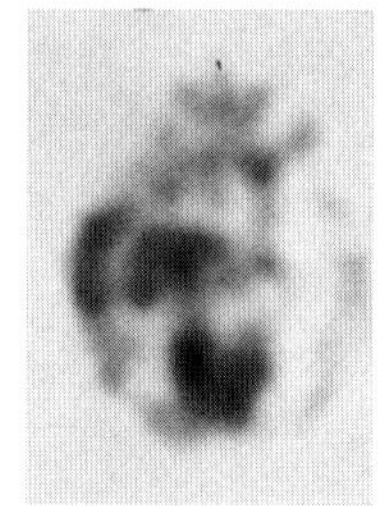

FIG. 5.47

CASE 5-22 Clinical Diagnosis: Left Thalamic Intracerebral Hemorrhage

CONTRIBUTOR:	IMAGING DATA:	
Name: Matthew Bloom, M.D.	**Camera:** Picker Prism 3000	**Collimator:** Ultra-high resolution, fan beam
Institution: Columbia-Presbyterian Medical Center	**Isotope:** ^{99m}Tc HMPAO	**Dose:** 21.5 mCi

This 72-year-old woman, with a history of long-standing hypertension, was referred for evaluation of the acute onset of dysarthria. At the time of presentation, the patient was extremely agitated, and a progressive weakness in her right upper extremity was noted.

The initial CT scan (Fig. 5.48) revealed an intracerebral hemorrhage involving the left thalamus.

The HMPAO SPECT (Fig. 5.49) in the transaxial plane demonstrated a deficit corresponding to the site of the left thalamic hemorrhage. In addition, decreased radiotracer activity was noted in the region of the left anterior temporal and posterior frontal lobes.

Published with permission: *Appl Radiol* 1993;22:35–44.

Teaching Point:

Subcortical hemorrhage or infarctions may produce changes that can be observed on SPECT scans in cortical radiotracer uptake (cortical diaschisis); such changes help to explain the patient's clinical symptoms of impaired cortical function. The finding of cortical diaschisis is particularly significant when the CT and MRI scans are equivocal or negative.

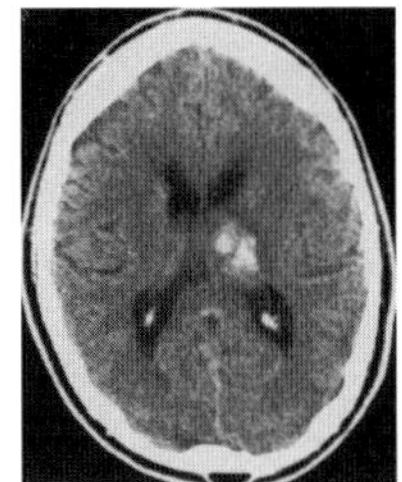

FIG. 5.48

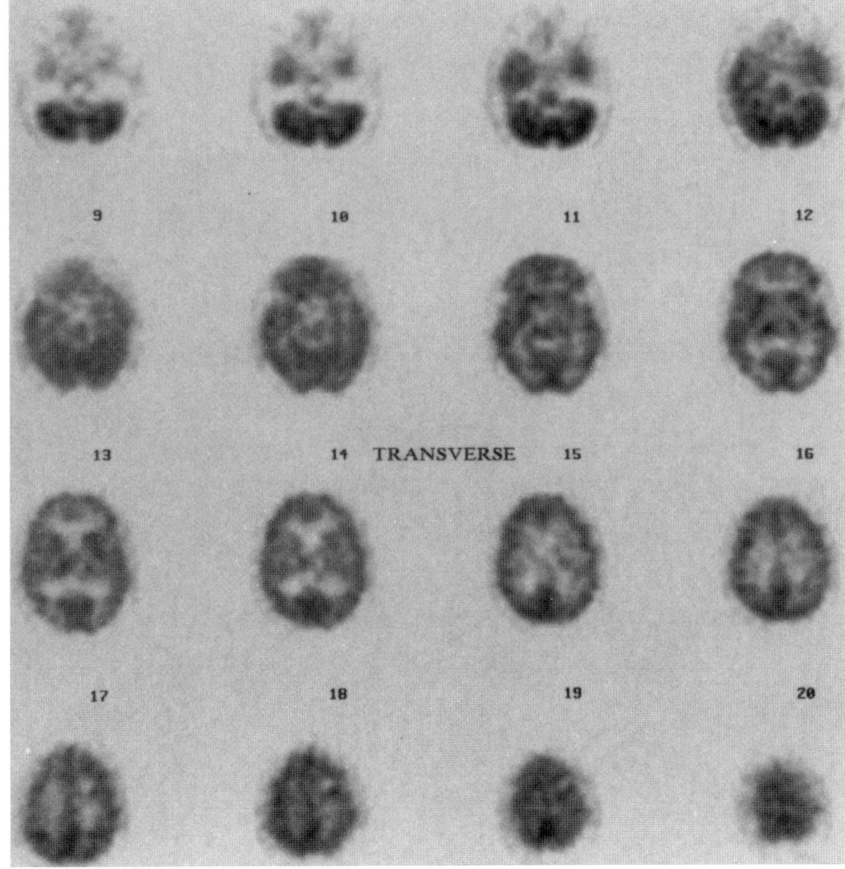

FIG. 5.49

CASE 5-23

Clinical Diagnosis:

Hypertensive Intracerebral Hemorrhage

CONTRIBUTOR:	IMAGING DATA:	
Name: Robert S. Hellman, M.D. and Ronald S. Tikofsky, Ph.D.	**Camera:** GE Neurocam	**Collimator:** High resolution, parallel hole
Institution: Medical College of Wisconsin	**Isotope:** ^{99m} Tc HMPAO	**Dose:** 30 mCi

On the morning of admission, this 66-year-old woman, with a 30-year history of hypertension, began to experience a severe headache along with a transient syncopal episode. At the time of presentation to the hospital, the patient was noted to have a rapidly progressive left hemiparesis.

The initial CT scan (Fig. 5.50) revealed a large right-sided intracerebral hematoma with extension into the right basal ganglia and associated midline shift to the left.

The HMPAO SPECT study (Fig. 5.51) in the transaxial plane showed a large deficit involving the right posterior frontal, temporal, and parietal lobes. The SPECT deficit was noted to be significantly larger than the area of hemorrhage noted on CT. In addition, decrease in left frontal radiotracer activity was noted.

A 2 month follow-up CT scan (Fig. 5.52) revealed a hypodensity involving the deep right parietal and basal ganglia regions consistent with the residual of an evolving intracerebral bleed. In addition, a left basal ganglia hypodensity, secondary to a prior infarction, was also noted.

Teaching Point:

SPECT deficits associated with intracerebral hemorrhages may be significantly larger than the area of hemorrhage noted on CT scan. The larger deficit on SPECT is due to a penumbra zone surrounding the area of hemorrhage. This penumbra zone may be due to edema, selective neuronal loss, ischemia, or diaschisis.

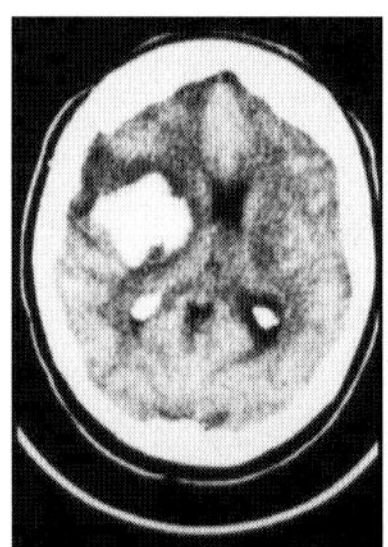

FIG. 5.50

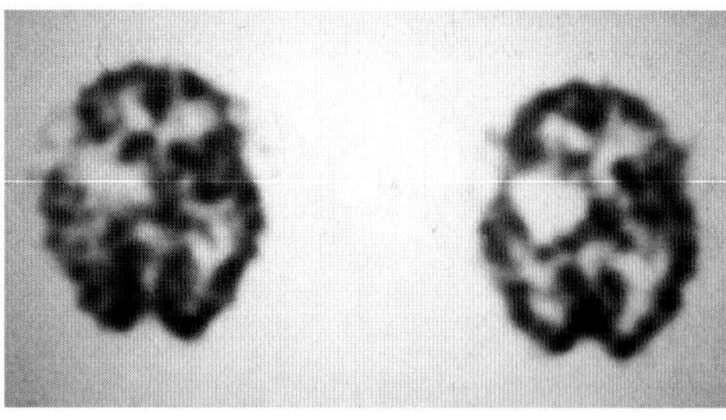

FIG. 5.51

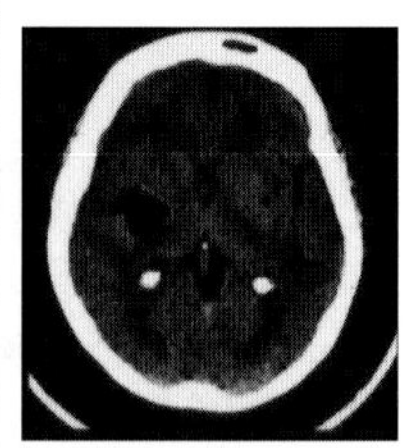

FIG. 5.52

CASE 5-24

Clinical Diagnosis:

Intracerebral Hemorrhage—Left Occipital Lobe

CONTRIBUTOR:	IMAGING DATA:	
Name: Kazufumi Kimura, M.D.	**Camera:** SPECT 2000H-40 (Hitachi)	**Collimator:** High resolution
Institution: Osaka University Medical School	**Isotope:** ^{123}I IMP	**Dose:** 3.0 mCi

This patient was referred for evaluation of a known intracerebral hemorrhage in the left occipital lobe.

The immediate cerebral SPECT study (Fig. 5.53) in the transaxial and sagittal planes showed absent tracer deposition in the left occipital lobe *(arrows)*.

The delayed study (Fig. 5.54) revealed a smaller area of absent tracer deposition of tracer *(arrowhead)*, suggesting the presence of a zone of ischemia surrounding the area of infarction.

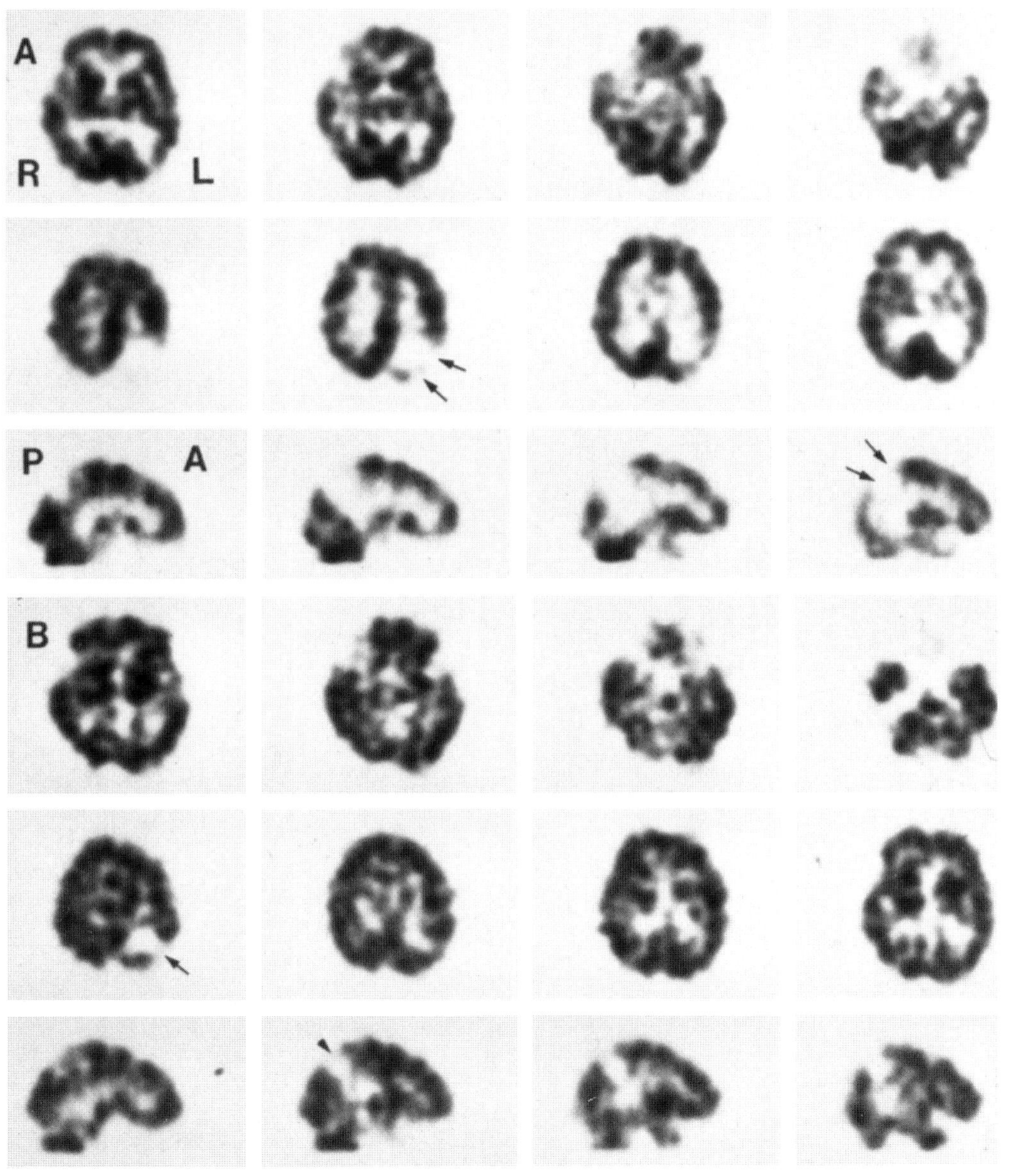

FIG. 5.53 (top) and **FIG. 5.54** (bottom)

CASE 5-25

Clinical Diagnosis: Vasospasm after Clipping of a Left Posterior Communicating Artery Aneurysm

CONTRIBUTOR:	IMAGING DATA:	
Name: David H. Lewis, M.D.	**Camera:** GE 400 AT	**Collimator:** LEAP
Institution: Harborview Medical Center	**Isotope:** ^{99m}Tc HMPAO	**Dose:** 30.0 mCi

This 46-year-old woman became progressively more lethargic 4 days following the surgical clipping of a left posterior communicating artery aneurysm. A CT scan at that time revealed residual subarachnoid hemorrhage.

On the day of the first SPECT study, the patient was observed to be severely obtunded. The initial HMPAO SPECT study (Fig. 5.55) revealed a diffuse decrease in radiotracer activity that was more marked on the left.

A transcranial Doppler (TCD) study revealed marked decrease in the velocity of flow bilaterally consistent with severe vasospasm in both the internal carotid and middle cerebral arteries bilaterally.

A bilateral cerebral arteriogram (Fig. 5.56A) confirmed the presence of severe vasospasm involving multiple segments in the right and left internal carotid *(arrows)* and middle cerebral arteries *(arrows)*. Repeat bilateral cerebral arteriograms (Fig. 5.56B), following balloon angioplasty revealed significant decrease in the degree of vasospasm.

Following the balloon angioplasty, the patient's clinical status rapidly improved. At the time of the follow-up SPECT study, she was alert and without evidence of focal neurologic deficits.

The follow-up HMPAO SPECT (Fig. 5.57) study revealed markedly improved radiotracer uptake bilaterally.

Published with permission: ***J Nucl Med*** **1992;33:1789–1796.**

Teaching Point:

Cerebral SPECT imaging can be extremely useful in the pre- and postoperative evaluation of subarachnoid hemorrhage. In particular, SPECT is complementary to TCD in the noninvasive assessment of patients with vasospasm.

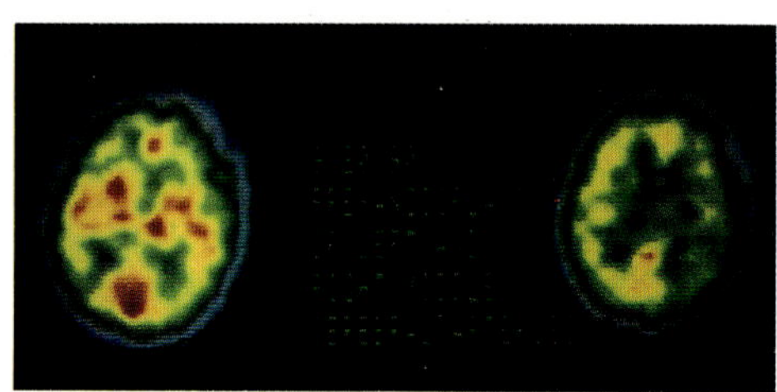

FIG. 5.55

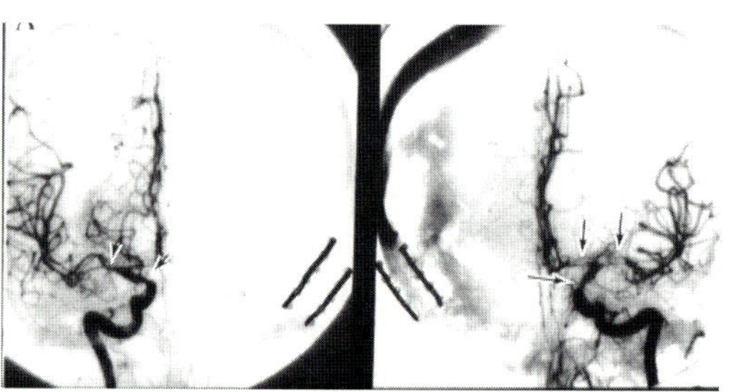

FIG. 5.56A

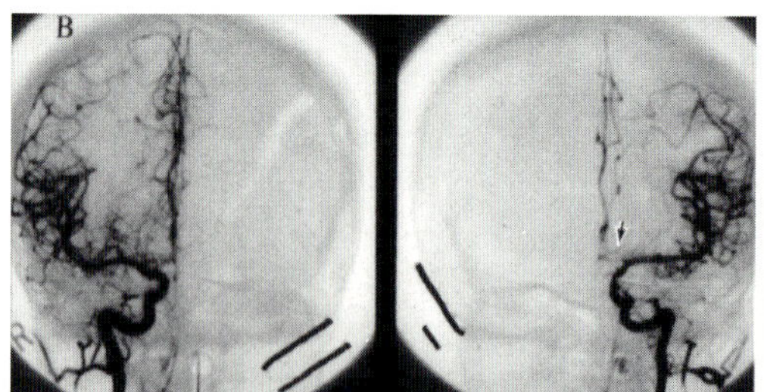

FIG. 5.56B

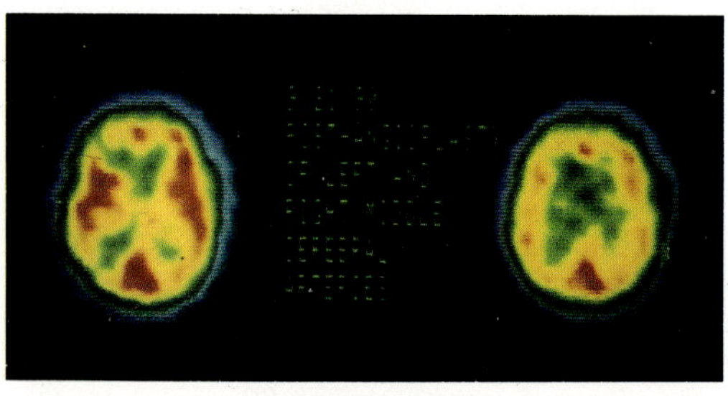

FIG. 5.57

CASE 5-26

Clinical Diagnosis:
Subarachnoid Hemorrhage

CONTRIBUTOR:	IMAGING DATA:	
Name: Robert S. Hellman, M.D. and Ronald S. Tikofsky, Ph.D.	**Camera:** GE 400AC/T;STAR	**Collimator:** High resolution
Institution: Medical College of Wisconsin	**Isotope:** ^{123}I IMP	**Dose:** 5.0 mCi

This 38-year-old, right-handed woman was admitted for continued management of a subarachnoid hemorrhage secondary to a basilar tip aneurysm. During the course of her hospitalization, she had intermittent elevations of blood pressure, with peak systolic blood pressure >200 mm and diastolic blood pressure of 80 to 110 mm Hg. The patient remained neurologically intact until the fourth day after admission. At that time, she was first observed to be confused and later to develop a marked aphasia and right hemiparesis.

A CT scan (Fig. 5.58) on the sixth day after admission showed the residual of a subarachnoid hemorrhage, mild ventricular dilation, and a basilar tip aneurysm *(arrow).*

The initial cerebral SPECT study (Fig. 5.59) in the transaxial plane was done on the same day as the initial CT scan. This study showed decreased tracer deposition in the left posterior parietal-occipital region and in the left posterior temporal lobe *(arrowheads),* suggesting either infarction or severe ischemia.

A follow-up CT scan (Fig. 5.60) on the tenth day after admission revealed a large, posterior parietal-occipital infarction of the left hemisphere and persistent, mild ventricular dilation.

A second cerebral SPECT study, with both immediate (Fig. 5.61A) and delayed (Fig. 5.61B) phases, was performed 4 days later. This study showed a "fixed" region (in the left posterior parietal occipital area) of decreased tracer deposition that was compatible with infarction *(arrowheads).* In addition, decreased tracer deposition was noted throughout the remainder of the left hemisphere, with improved tracer deposition on the delayed images *(arrows).* This latter finding was felt to be compatible with extensive ischemia.

Teaching Points:

Cerebral SPECT studies are often useful in the follow-up of patients with subarachnoid hemorrhage, as the studies supply information that is complimentary to CT scans.

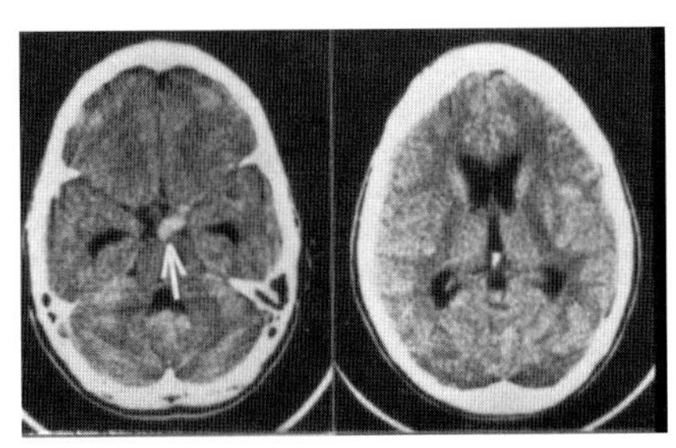

FIG. 5.58

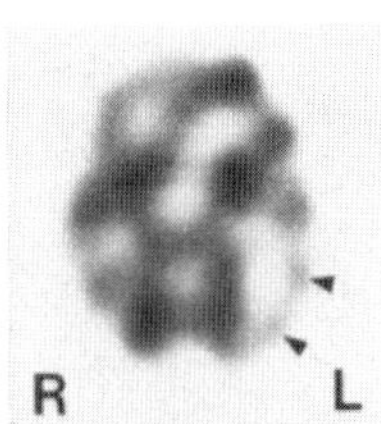

FIG. 5.59

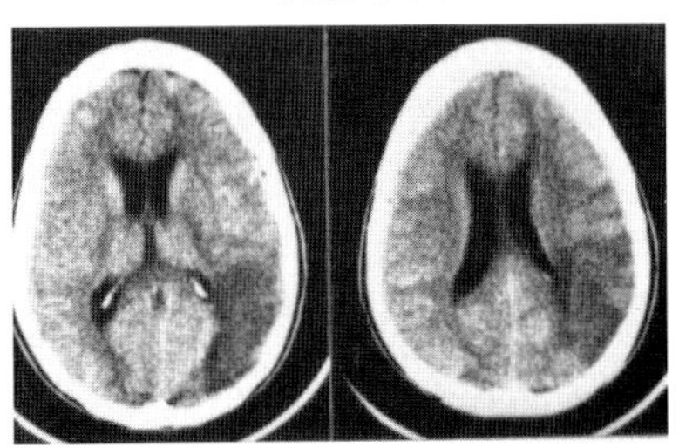

FIG. 5.60

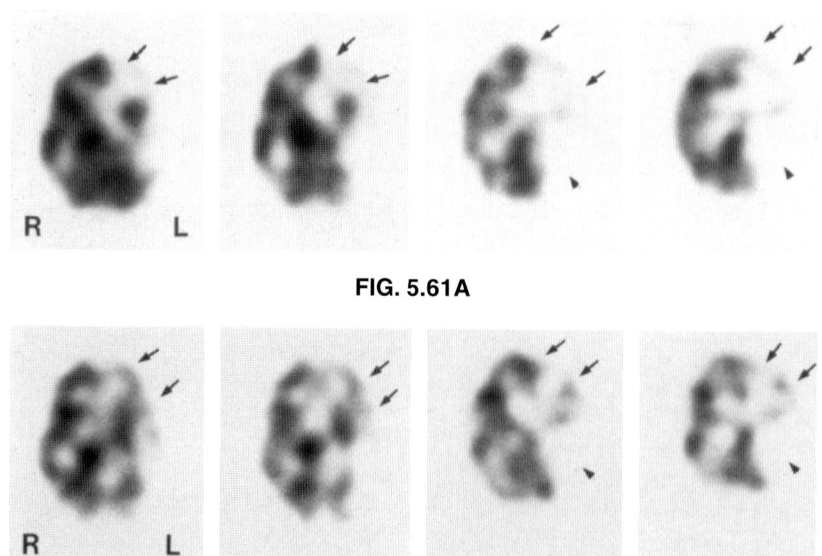

FIG. 5.61A

FIG. 5.61B

CASE 5-27

Clinical Diagnosis:

Combined Ischemia (Vasospasm) and Infarction after Surgical Clipping of an Aneurysm

CONTRIBUTOR:	IMAGING DATA:	
Name: Joji Nagawara, M.D.	**Camera:** Shimadzu Headtome Set-031	**Collimator:** High resolution
Institution: Nakamura Memorial Hospital	**Isotope:** ^{123}I IMP	**Dose:** 3.0 mCi

This 44-year-old man presented with complaints of headaches, vomiting, and feeling faint. Physical examination revealed a left upper extremity paresis, and subsequent workup disclosed a ruptured aneurysm arising from the right middle cerebral artery. Following surgical clipping of the aneurysm, the patient's left-sided paresis increased in severity.

Serial cerebral SPECT studies in the transaxial plane (Fig. 5.62) revealed a progressive decrease in the size of a defect in the right middle cerebral artery territory *(arrowheads)*. A residual pattern defect persisted at 90 days.

The overall pattern was compatible with combined ischemia (vasospasm) and infarction.

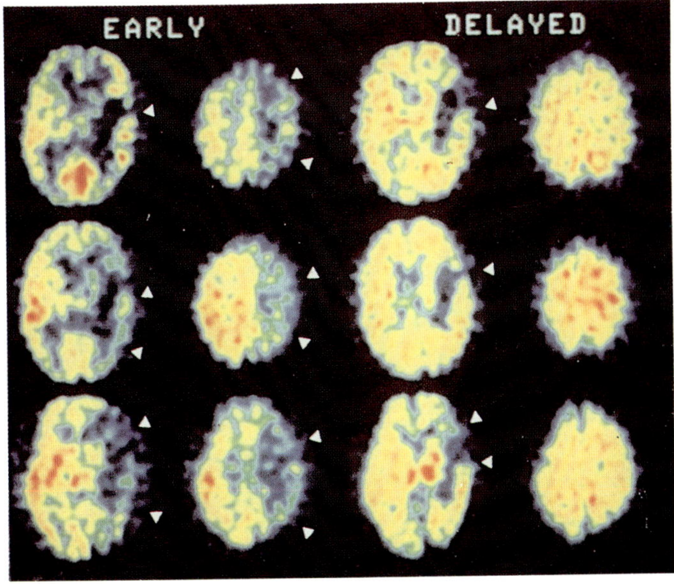

FIG. 5.62

CASE 5-28

Clinical Diagnosis:
Occlusion of the Left Internal Carotid Artery

CONTRIBUTOR:	IMAGING DATA:	
Name: Kazufumi Kimura, M.D.	**Camera:** SPECT 2000 H-40	**Collimator:** High resolution
Institution: Osaka University Medical School	**Isotope:** ^{123}I IMP	**Dose:** 3.0 mCi

This patient had a known occlusion of the left internal carotid artery, with an infarction in the distribution of the left middle cerebral artery.

The cerebral SPECT study (Fig. 5.63) in the transaxial plane indicated an absence of tracer uptake throughout most of the left cerebral hemisphere. This tracer distribution pattern was consistent with an internal carotid artery occlusion.

Teaching Point:

A pattern of absence radiotracer activity throughout a hemisphere is generally indicative of internal carotid occlusive disease, as demonstrated in this case.

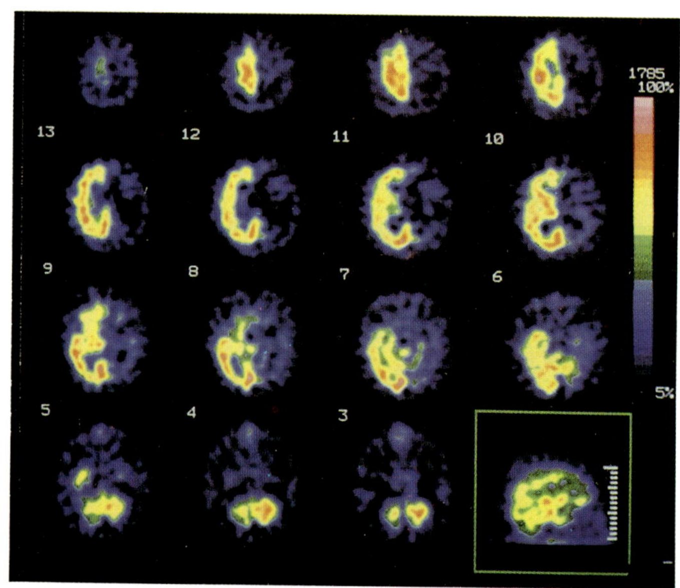

FIG. 5.63

CASE 5-29

Clinical Diagnosis:

Hemodynamic Insufficiency Secondary to Nifedipine Therapy

CONTRIBUTOR:	**IMAGING DATA:**	
Name: Jean Luc Moretti, M.D.	**Camera:** GE 400AC	**Collimator:** LEAP
Institution: Hôpital Avicenne	**Isotope:** ^{99m}Tc HMPAO	**Dose:** 20.0 mCi

This 77-year-old man with known arterial hypertension and gait disturbance was referred for evaluation of progressive cognitive impairment, dysarthria, and worsening of his gait disturbance. The patient's symptoms had commenced approximately 4 months previously, soon after he had been started on nifedipine.

An HMPAO SPECT study, (Fig. 5.64a), in the transaxial plane revealed a diffuse decrease in radiotracer activity in the frontal lobes as well as throughout the entire left hemisphere.

Following the SPECT study, the nifedipine treatment was stopped. Soon after discontinuing nifedipine, the patient began to show dramatic clinical improvement in his gait and reversal of his cognitive disturbances.

A follow-up HMPAO SPECT study (Fig. 5.64B) in the transaxial plane revealed improved radiotracer activity in the frontal lobes. Some decrease is still seen in the left hemisphere, presumably due to underlying atherosclerotic disease.

Teaching Point:

Antihypertensive therapy may, on occasion, give rise to clinically significant cerebral hemodynamic insufficiency, particularly in cases with underlying clinically significant atheromatous vessels. In such cases, brain SPECT may be useful for identifying regional or more generalized changes in cerebral perfusion.

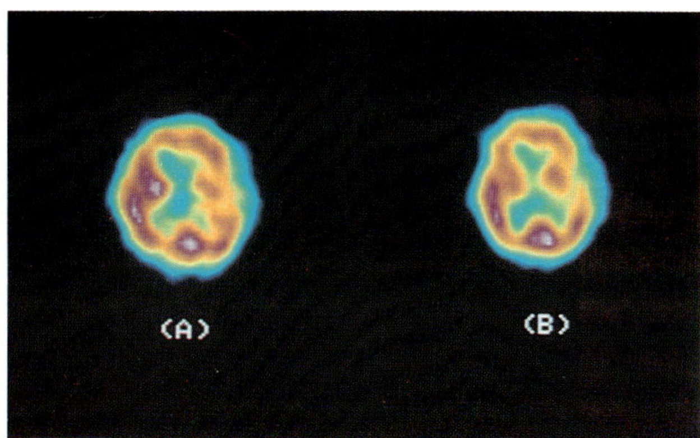

FIG. 5.64

CASE 5-30

Clinical Diagnosis: Transient Ischemic Attack

CONTRIBUTOR:	IMAGING DATA:	
Name: Allan H. Maurer, M.D.	**Camera:** GE STARCAM	**Collimator:** LEAP
Institution: Temple University School of Medicine	**Isotope:** ^{123}I IMP	**Dose:** 3.0 mCi

This 64-year-old man presented following an episode of left upper extremity weakness and an occasional episode of blurred vision.

A CT scan (Fig. 5.65) revealed an old lacunar infarction in the region of the right external capsule.

An aortic arch arteriogram (Fig. 5.66) revealed a 50 percent stenosis, with an irregular and probably ulcerated plaque of the right common carotid artery *(large arrow)* and shallow, irregular plaques involving the right innominate *(small arrow)* and left subclavian arteries.

IMP SPECT images (Fig. 5.67, *upper row*) in the transaxial plane, in the immediate phase *(upper row),* demonstrated decreased radiotracer activity in the right posterior parietal occipital region *(doubled arrows)* that filled in *(arrow)* on the 4-hr delay SPECT images (Fig. 5.67, *lower row*) in the transaxial plane.

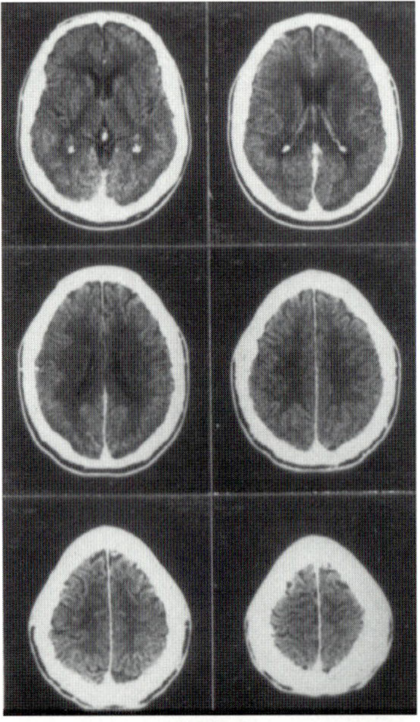

FIG. 5.65

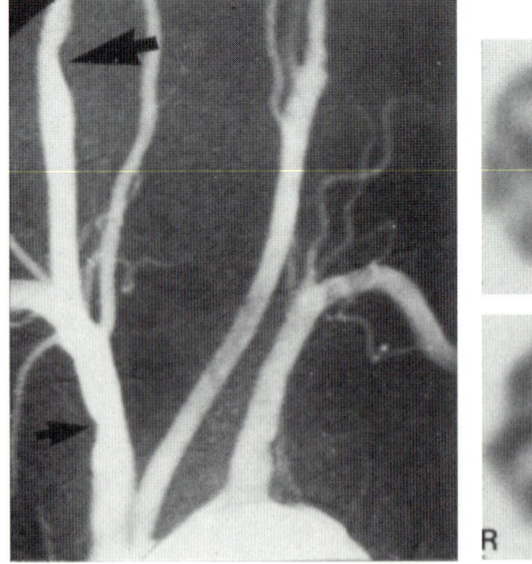

FIG. 5.66

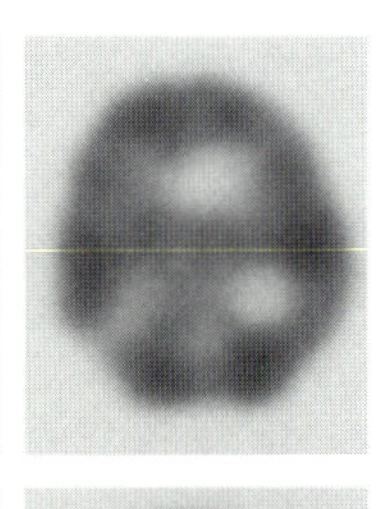

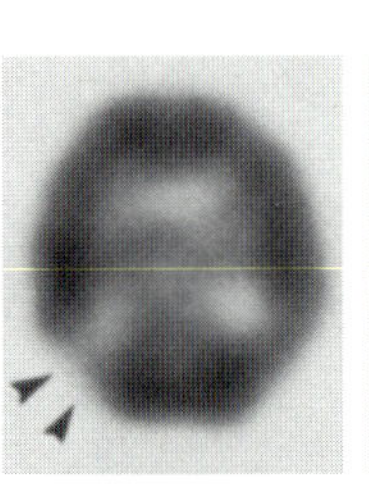

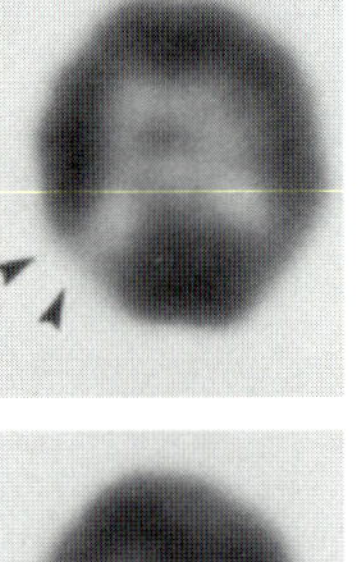

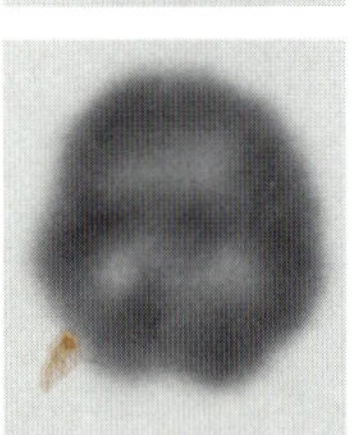

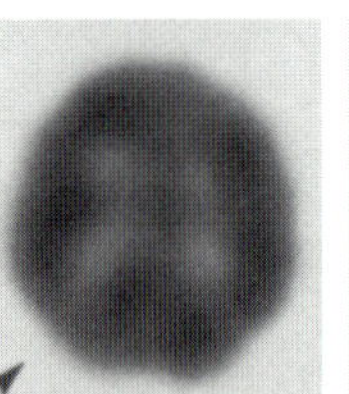

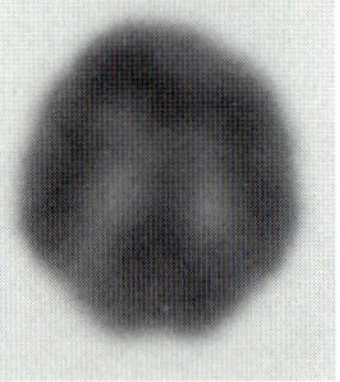

FIG. 5.67

CASE 5-31

Clinical Diagnosis: Left Internal Carotid Artery Stenosis

CONTRIBUTOR:	**IMAGING DATA:**	
Name: Alice Scheff, M.D.	**Camera:** GE ACT	**Collimator:** LEAP
Institution: Albert Einstein Medical Center	**Isotope:** ^{123}I IMP	**Dose:** 3.0 mCi

This 70-year-old woman was referred for evaluation of amaurosis fugax and a bruit in the left carotid artery.

A CT scan was reported to be negative.

An early phase IMP SPECT study (Fig. 5.68) in the transaxial plane revealed a large deficit in the distribution of the left internal carotid territory. Follow-up 3-hr delay SPECT images (Fig. 5.69) in the transaxial plane revealed filling in of most of the left-sided defect consistent with an area of ischemia.

Teaching Point:

Cerebral SPECT imaging with IMP has the potential for identifying areas of ischemia. Further large-scale studies are needed to verify the utility of this phenomenon.

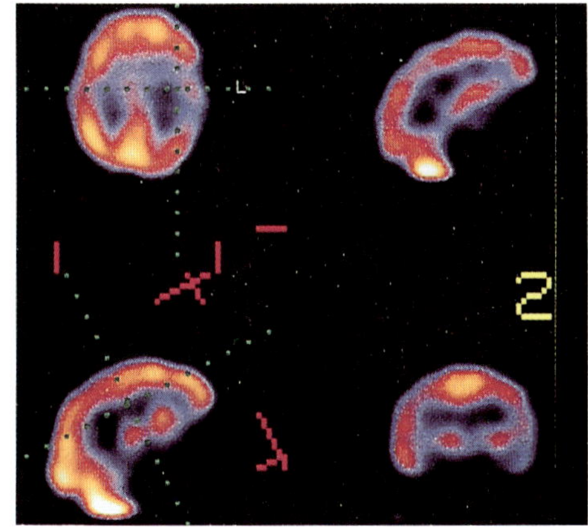

FIG. 5.68

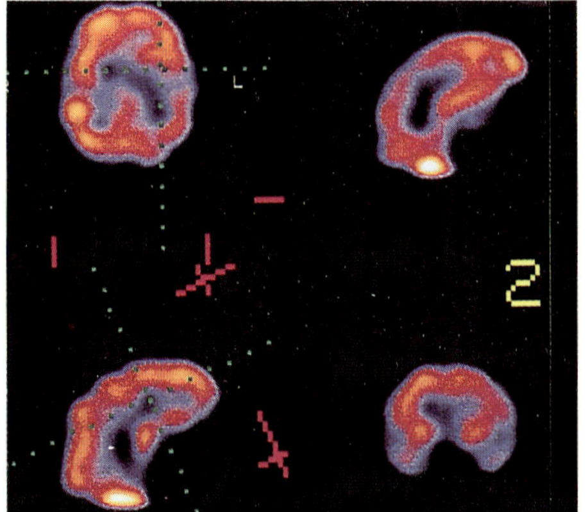

FIG. 5.69

CASE 5–32

Clinical Diagnosis:
Recurrent Transient Ischemic Attacks

CONTRIBUTOR:

Name: Robert S. Hellman, M.D. and Ronald S. Tikofsky, Ph.D.
Institution: Medical College of Wisconsin

IMAGING DATA:

Camera: GE Neurocam
Isotope: ^{99m}Tc HMPAO
Collimator: High resolution
Dose: 30.4 mCi

This 80-year-old woman was referred for evaluation of recurrent episodes of suspected transient ischemia manifested as vertigo attacks. At the time of referral, she had experienced a well-defined TIA while undergoing a cerebral arteriogram. During the episode, she developed a right hemiplegia and aphasia and became progressively more unresponsive. Her symptoms lasted for approximately 5 min, after which she slowly returned to her baseline neurological status.

An MRA study revealed an aneurysm of the right internal carotid artery near the origin of the posterior communicating artery measuring approximately 12 mm in diameter. A cerebral arteriogram confirmed the presence of an aneurysm of the right internal carotid artery with evidence of plaque involving the origin of the right internal carotid artery. No hemodynamically significant lesion was seen on the left side; however, the study was abbreviated due to the patient developing symptoms of a TIA.

An HMPAO SPECT study (Fig. 5.70) in the transaxial plane, which was performed soon after her TIA in the angiography suite, showed decreased radiotracer activity in the left temporal and posterior parietal lobes. In addition, an adjacent area of increased radiotracer activity was seen in the left anterior temporal lobe extending superior and posterior into the parietal lobe.

At 24 hr, a follow-up HMPAO SPECT study (Fig. 5.71) in the transaxial plane revealed an overall improvement in radiotracer activity in the left temporal and posterior parietal lobes that correlated with the patient's improved neurologic status. A small deficit persisted in the left posterior temporal lobe.

Teaching Point:

Cerebral SPECT imaging is a highly sensitive technique for documenting regional perfusion abnormalities in patients experiencing a TIA. Perfusion deficits seen on SPECT scan will generally resolve within 24 to 48 hr following the TIA. Patients with persistent defects at 72 hr after TIA appear to be at greater risk for developing a progressive stroke and therefore should be evaluated for potential surgery on a more emergency basis.

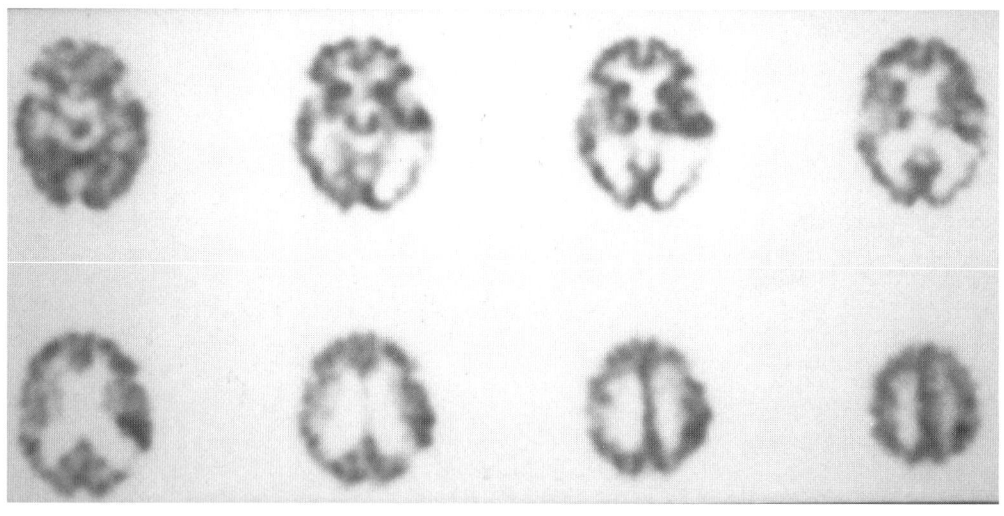

FIG. 5.70

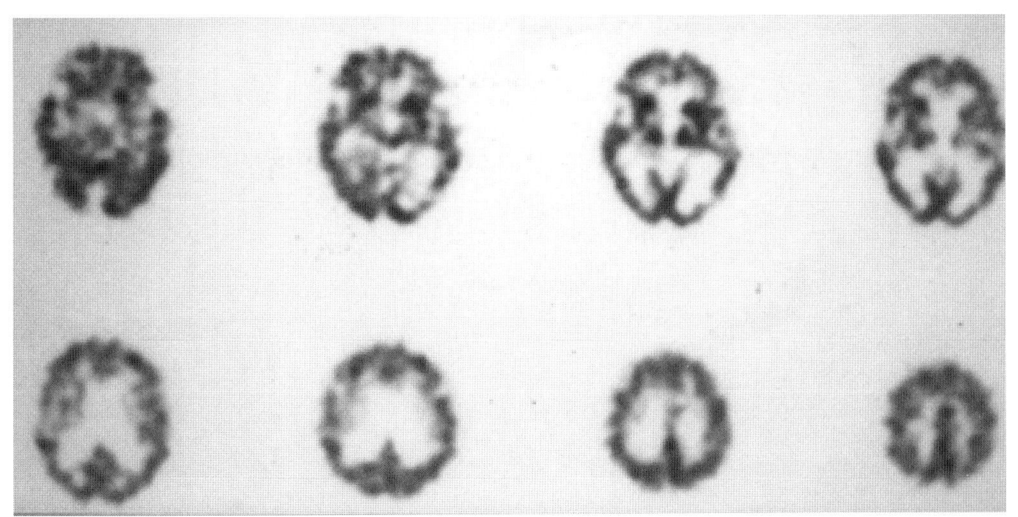

FIG. 5.71

CASE 5-33

Clinical Diagnosis: Left Internal Carotid Artery Stenosis

CONTRIBUTOR:	IMAGING DATA:	
Name: Paul Katz, M.D. and Janet Lan, M.D.	**Camera:** Trionix-Triad	**Collimator:** Ultra-high resolution
Institution: Montefiore Medical Center	**Isotope:** ^{99m}Tc HMPAO	**Dose:** 20 mCi

This 70-year-old man was referred for further evaluation of monocular blindness (OS) secondary to an occlusion of the central retinal artery. The neurologic examination was otherwise within normal limits. There was no prior history of neurologic disease or symptoms; however, the patient did have a long-standing history of hypertension.

A CT scan (Fig. 5.72A and B) was normal. A cerebral arteriogram revealed a high-grade stenosis of the left internal carotid artery (Fig. 5.73A and B) with collateral flow from the right side via the anterior communicating artery.

An HMPAO SPECT (Fig. 5.74) in the transaxial, sagittal, and coronal planes, was performed to assess the hemodynamic significance of the stenosis. The SPECT study revealed a normal symmetrical pattern of radiotracer uptake indicative of an intact and adequate collateral circulation at rest.

Teaching Point:

Cerebral SPECT imaging can be a useful predictor of a competent intracranial collateral circulation pathway.

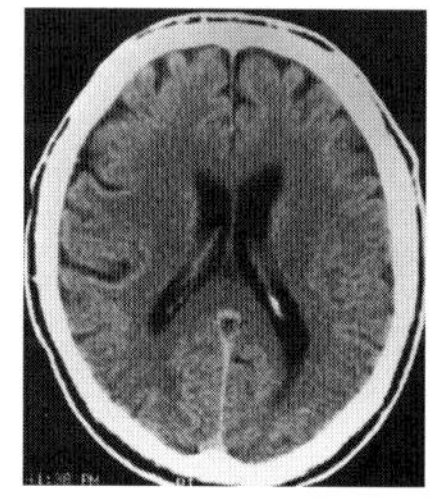

FIG. 5.72A

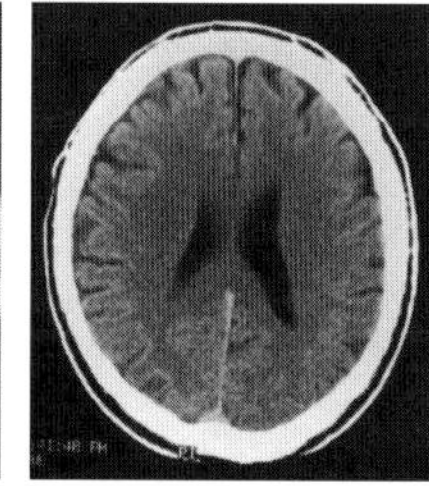

FIG. 5.72B

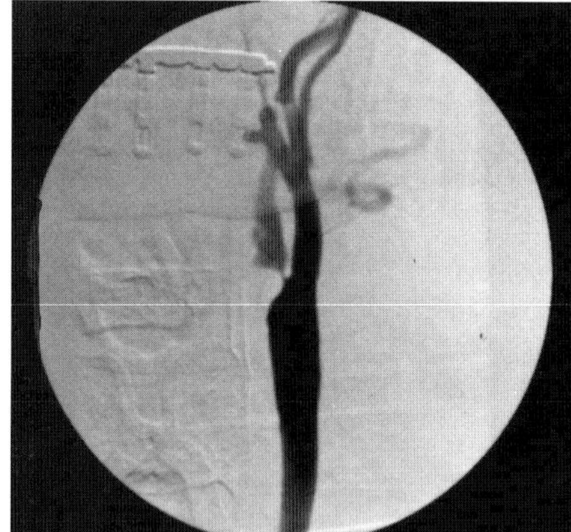

FIG. 5.73A

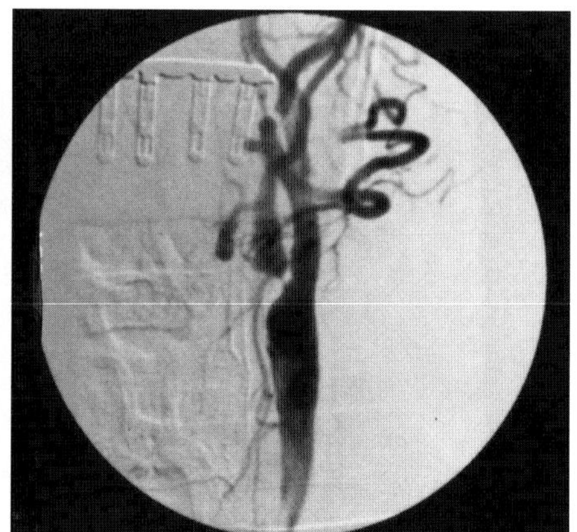

FIG. 5.73B

9 10 11 12 13 14 15
17 18 19 20 21 22 23
28 29 30 31 32 33 34
36 37 38 39 40 41 42
25 26 27 28 29 30 31
35 36 37 38 39

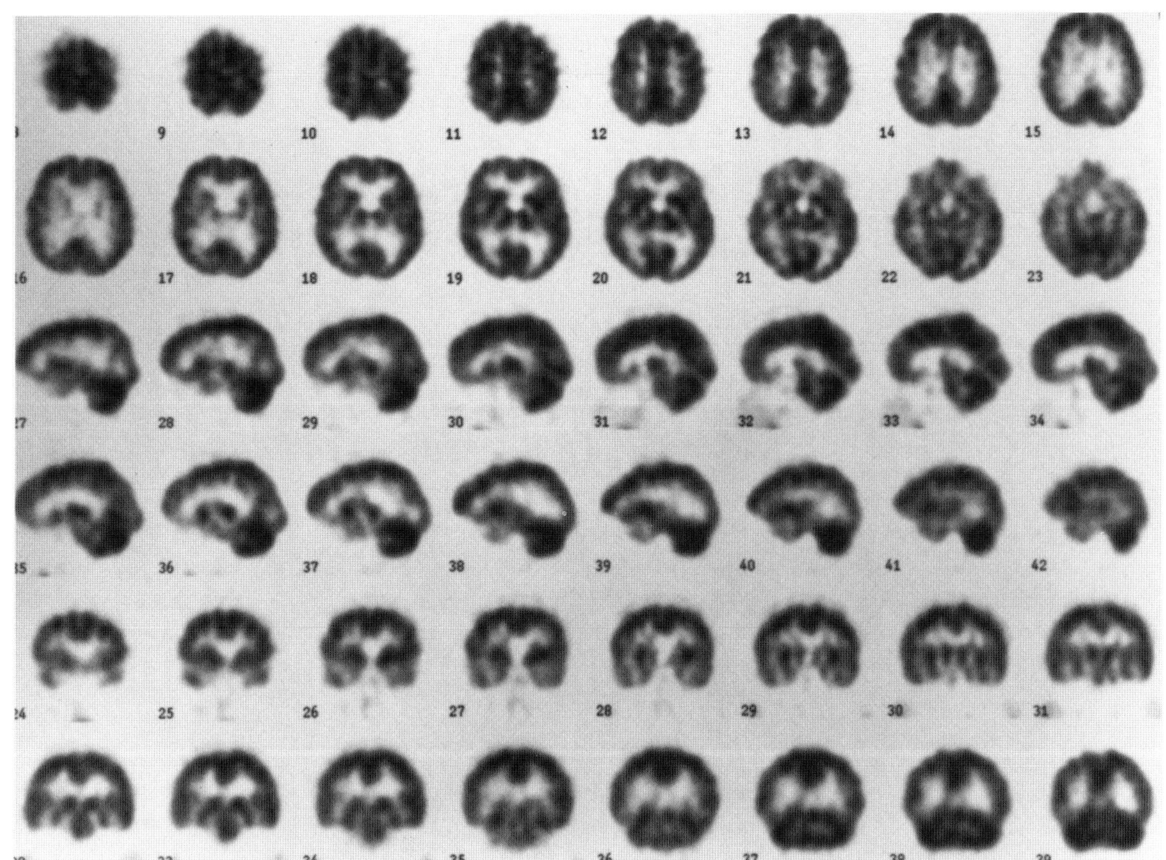

FIG. 5.74

CASE 5-34 Clinical Diagnosis: Bilateral Carotid Artery Stenoses

CONTRIBUTOR:

Name: Paul Katz, M.D. and Janet Lan, M.D.
Institution: Montefiore Medical Center

IMAGING DATA:

Camera: Trionix-Triad
Isotope: ^{99m}Tc HMPAO
Collimator: Ultra-high resolution
Dose: 20 mCi

This 58-year-old woman with known atherosclerotic aortoiliac disease was referred for evaluation of suspected bilateral carotid artery stenoses.

A CT scan (Fig. 5.75A–C) revealed hypodensities in the cortex of the left frontal lobe and the white matter of the left parietal lobe. Carotid arteriography confirmed the presence of complete occlusion of the left internal carotid artery and a moderate (70 to 80 percent) stenosis of the right internal carotid artery. In addition, there was collateral flow from the anterior communicating artery (Fig. 5.76), with incomplete filling of the distal left anterior and middle cerebral artery territories.

HMPAO SPECT (Fig. 5.77) showed diffuse decrease radiotracer activity throughout the left hemisphere, most marked in the high parietal region, corresponding to the angiographic finding of decreased distal perfusion.

Teaching Point:

Cerebral SPECT imaging, as shown in this case, can be very useful in assessing distal hemodynamic (watershed territory) hypoperfusion.

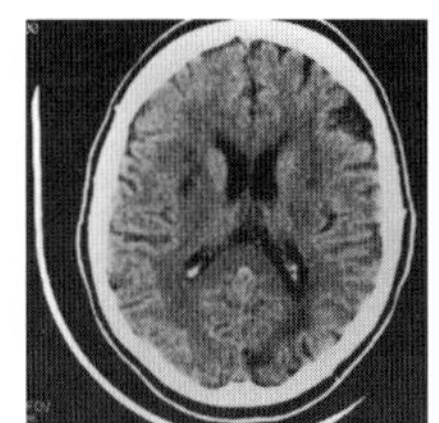

FIG. 5.75A

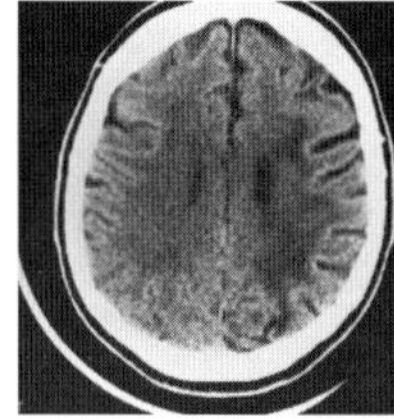

FIG. 5.75B

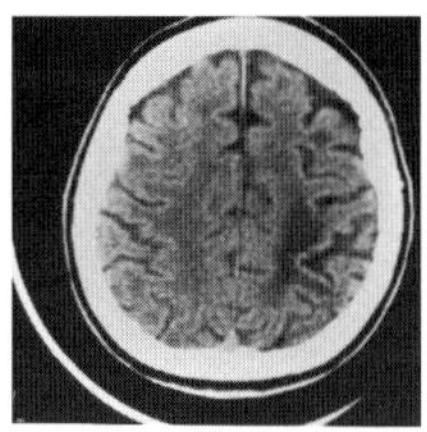

FIG. 5.75C

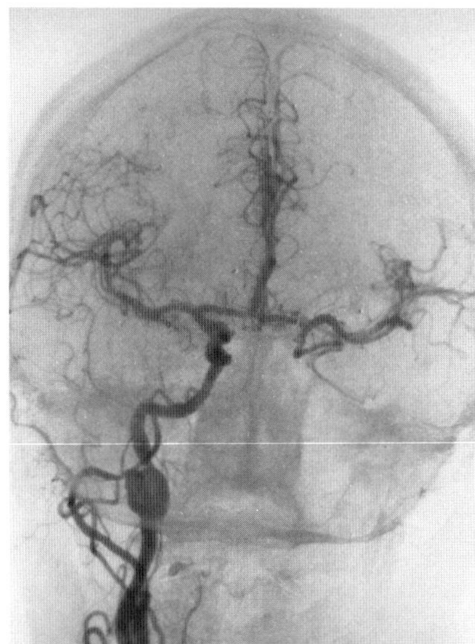

FIG. 5.76

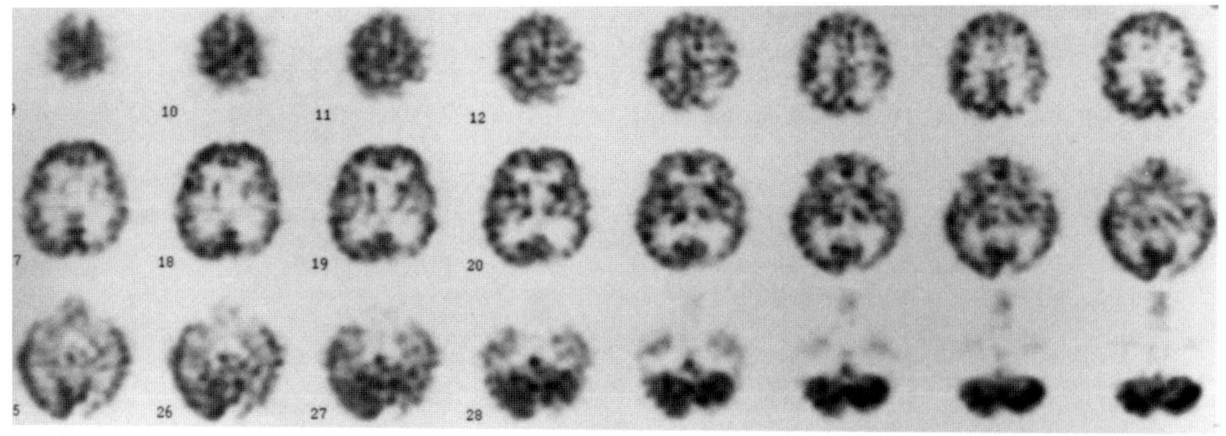

FIG. 5.77

CASE 5-35 Clinical Diagnosis: Transient Ischemic Attack

CONTRIBUTOR:	IMAGING DATA:	
Name: Paul F. Hoffer, M.D. and David Moon, M.D.	**Camera:** Picker Prism 3000	**Collimator:** High resolution
Institution: Yale University School of Medicine	**Isotope:** ^{99m}Tc HMPAO	**Dose:** 20.0 mCi

This 85-year-old man was referred for evaluation of a suspected TIA.

A CT scan (Fig. 5.78) demonstrated a hypodensity in the left posterior frontal and anterior temporal lobes compatible with an evolving infarction. In addition, mild diffuse cortical atrophy was evident.

An HMPAO SPECT study in the transaxial plane (Fig. 5.79) and coronal plane (Fig. 5.80) revealed decreased radiotracer activity in the left posterior frontal lobe and the left temporal lobe, representing a larger area than the area of abnormality noted on the CT scan.

Teaching Point:

Not all clinically manifest TIAs are in reality solely due to reversible ischemia. As shown in this patient, some cases may actually represent combined ischemia and infarction.

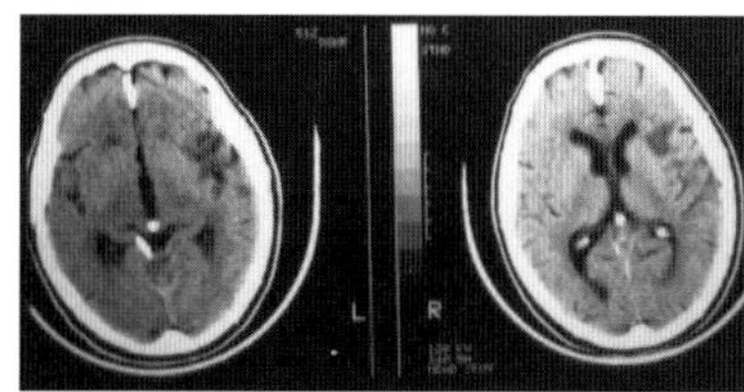

FIG. 5.78

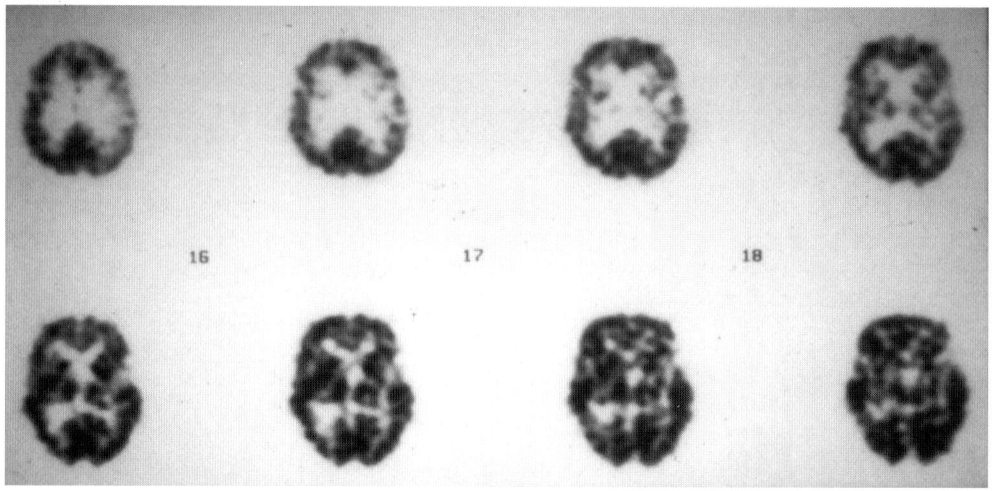

FIG. 5.79

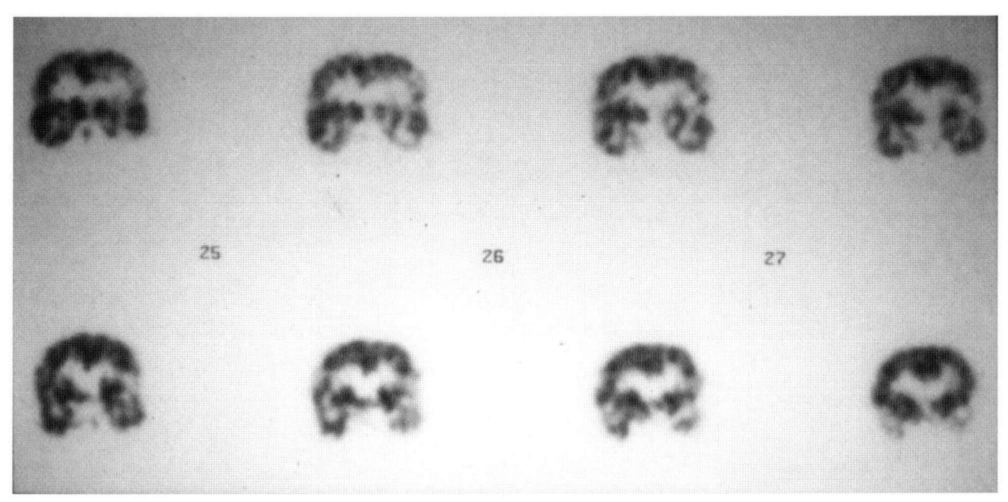

FIG. 5.80

CASE 5-36

Clinical Diagnosis:
Transient Ischemic Attack

CONTRIBUTOR:	IMAGING DATA:	
Name: Ronald L. Van Heertum, M.D.	**Camera:** Picker Prism 3000	**Collimator:** Ultra-high resolution, fan beam
Institution: Columbia-Presbyterian Medical Center	**Isotope:** ^{99m}Tc HMPAO	**Dose:** 18.0 mCi

This 73-year-old man, with known long-standing insulin-dependent diabetes mellitus, was referred for evaluation of suspected TIAs. Specifically, the patient complained of three separate episodes of transient dizzy spells lasting approximately 30 to 40 min.

Duplex doppler and MRI studies revealed bilateral severe (85%) stenoses of the internal carotid arteries.

An HMPAO SPECT study in the transaxial plane (Fig. 5.81) and coronal plane (Fig. 5.82) after intravenous acetazolamide administration revealed diminished radiotracer activity throughout the right cerebral hemisphere consistent with a loss of cerebrovascular reserve in the region of the right internal carotid artery territory.

Teaching Point:

In cases with bilateral carotid stenoses, cerebral SPECT can be very useful for identifying which lesion is of greatest hemodynamic significance.

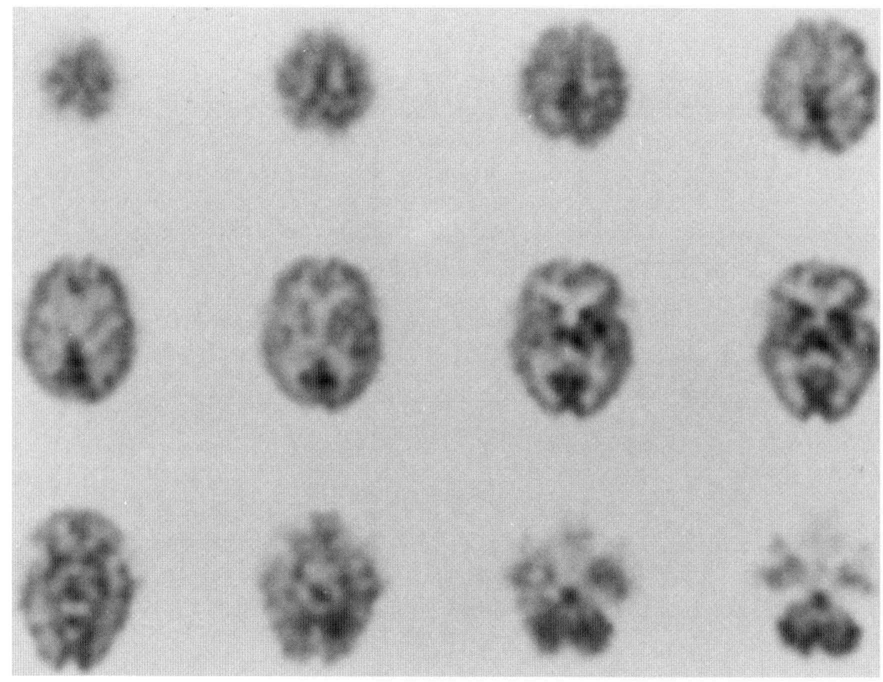

FIG. 5.81

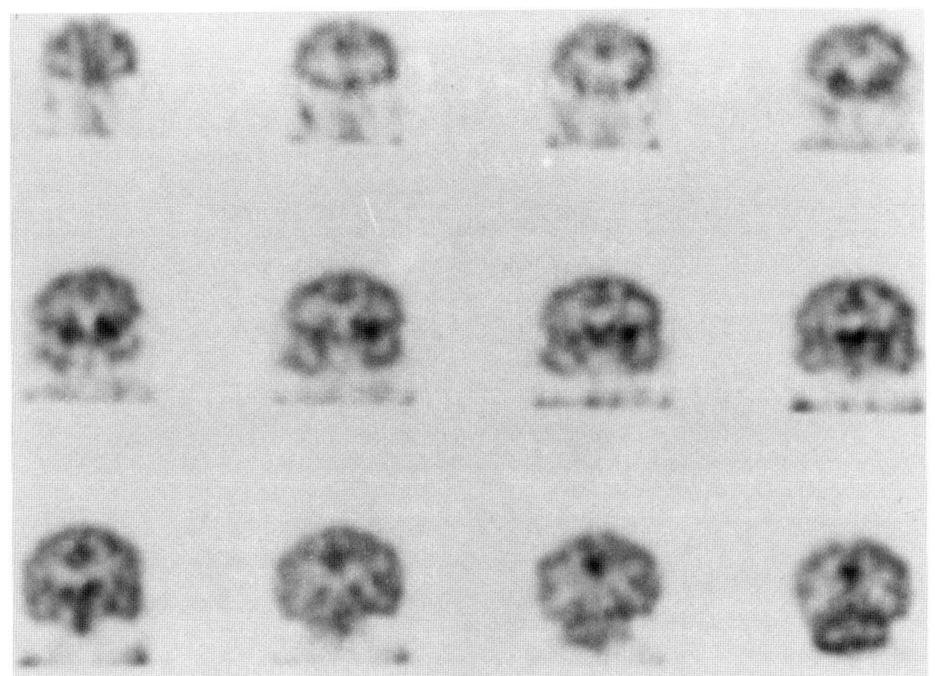

FIG. 5.82

CASE 5-37

Clinical Diagnosis: Moyamoya Disease

CONTRIBUTOR:	IMAGING DATA:	
Name: Matthew Bloom, M.D.	**Camera:** Picker Prism 3000	**Collimator:** Ultra-high resolution
Institution: Columbia-Presbyterian Medical Center	**Isotope:** ^{99m}Tc HMPAO	**Dose:** 20.5 mCi

This 34-year-old woman presented for evaluation following the acute onset of a progressive left hemiplegia and dysarthria. The patient had experienced similar symptoms approximately 3 years prior to her current presentation. At that time, her symptoms were transient and felt to be related to a TIA.

A CT scan (Fig. 5.83A and B) revealed a large area of infarction in the right basal ganglia and sulcal effacement in the right frontal-temporal region.

A subsequent MRI scan confirmed the right basal ganglia infarction along with smaller areas of infarction in the right frontal-parietal region. An MRA study (Fig. 5.84) and a cerebral arteriogram revealed bilateral occlusions of the internal carotid arteries in a pattern compatible with moyamoya disease.

An HMPAO SPECT study (Fig. 5.85) in the transaxial plane revealed a diffuse decrease in radiotracer activity throughout the right cerebral hemisphere.

A follow-up HMPAO study after intravenous acetazolamide (Fig. 5.86) in the transaxial plane revealed a more marked decrease in radiotracer activity in the right cerebral hemisphere as well as significant decrease in radiotracer uptake in the left hemisphere. The overall findings are consistent with a significant bilateral loss of cerebrovascular reserve.

Teaching Point:

Acetazolamide-enhanced cerebral SPECT imaging is very useful for identifying which areas of the brain are most hemodynamically impaired, as demonstrated in this case with bilateral carotid occlusive disease.

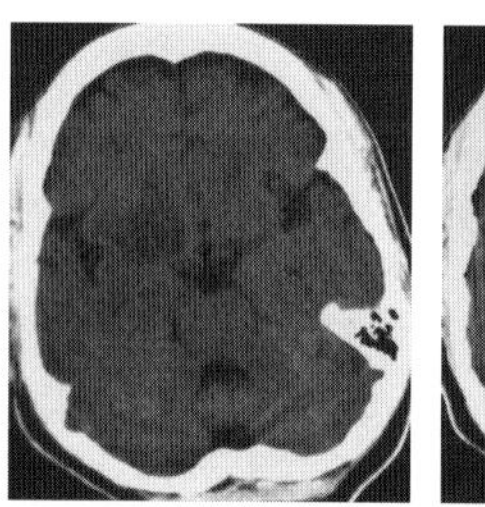

FIG. 5.83A

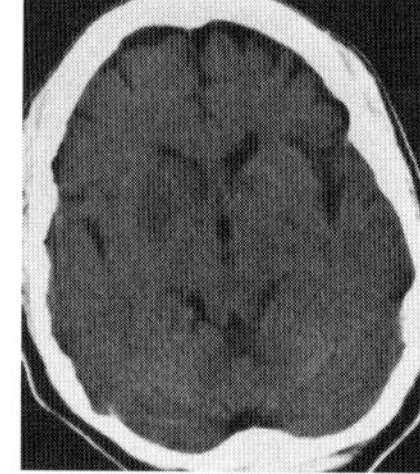

FIG. 5.83B

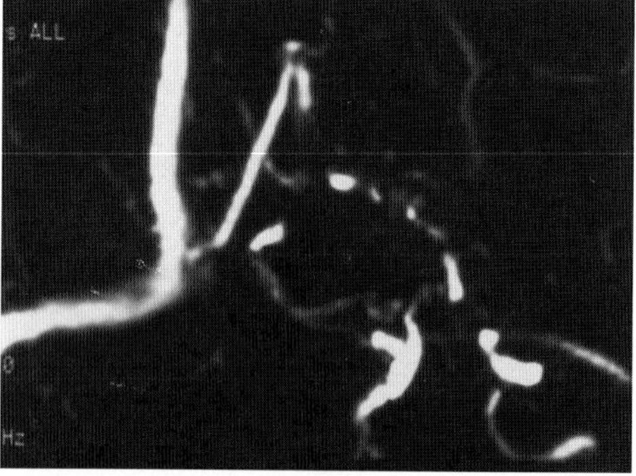

FIG. 5.84

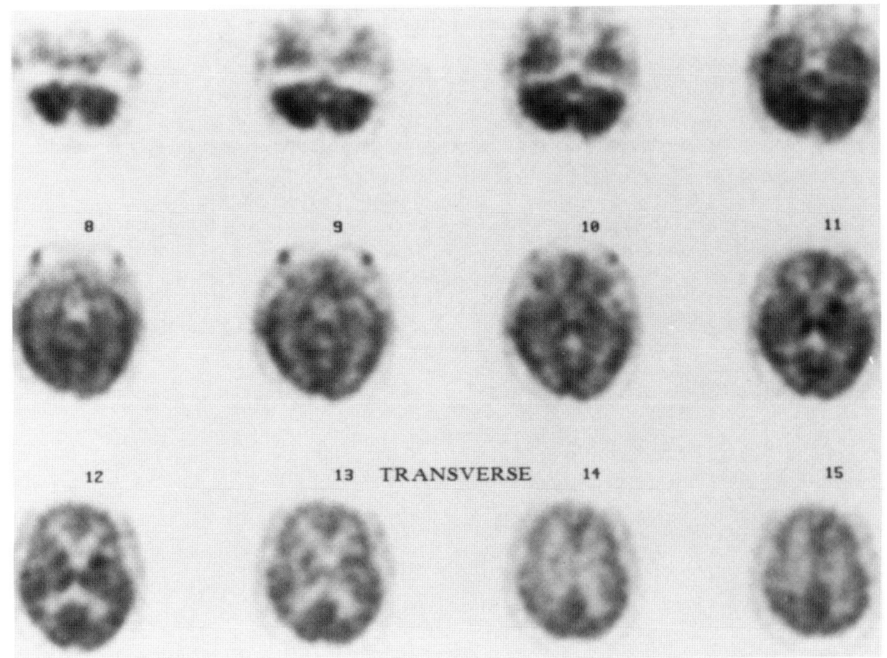

FIG. 5.85

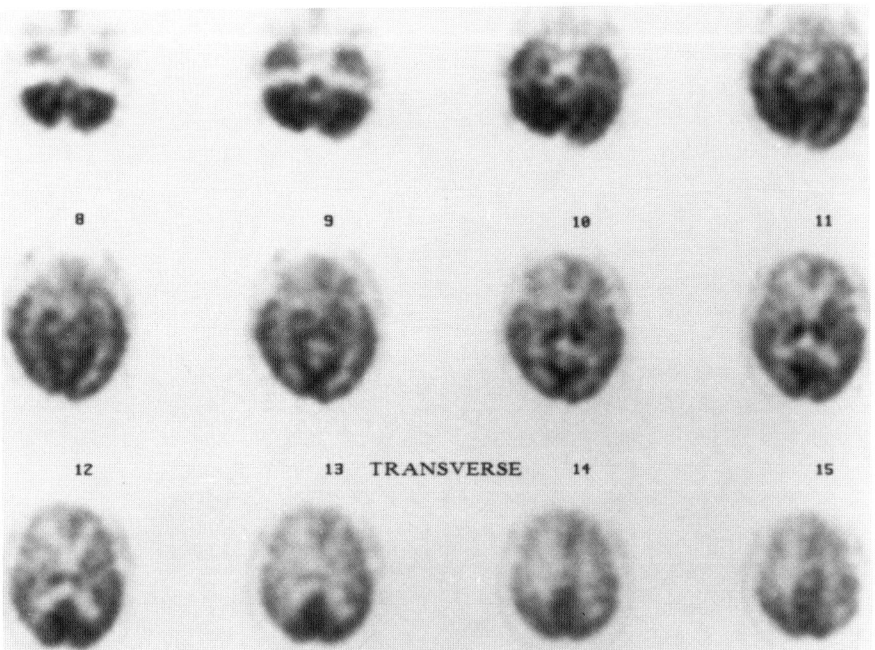

FIG. 5.86

CASE 5-38

Clinical Diagnosis:

Left (Petrosal Cavernous) Carotid Artery Aneurysm

CONTRIBUTOR:	**IMAGING DATA:**	
Name: Ronald L. Van Heertum, M.D.	**Camera:** GE Neurocam	**Collimator:** Ultra-high resolution
Institution: Columbia-Presbyterian Medical Center	**Isotope:** ^{99m}Tc HMPAO	**Dose:** 21.0 mCi

This 31-year-old female school teacher was referred for further evaluation of a left internal carotid (cavernous) artery aneurysm. The patient had previously sustained left facial bone fracture in a motor vehicle accident several years prior to her current presentation.

An MRA study revealed a left internal carotid (cavernous) artery aneurysm.

The patient was injected with ^{99m}Tc HMPAO at the time of a temporary balloon occlusion of the left internal carotid artery. The HMPAO SPECT study (Fig. 5.87) in the transaxial plane revealed an overall decrease in radiotracer uptake in the left cerebral hemisphere. In addition, a focal area of decreased radiotracer activity was noted in the right frontal cortex.

Teaching Point:

Performing cerebral SPECT at the time of temporary balloon occlusion of the internal carotid artery can be useful for determining whether patients will be able to tolerate permanent carotid artery occlusion. In this particular case, the study demonstrated decreased radiotracer activity in the left cerebral hemisphere after balloon occlusion, indicative of an inadequate collateral circulation supply from the right side. As a result, a decision was made to change the clinical management from carotid occlusion to obliteration of the aneurysm with GDC coils. This decision was based on the SPECT results coupled with the observation of a very small ophthalmic collateral on a subsequent cerebral arteriogram.

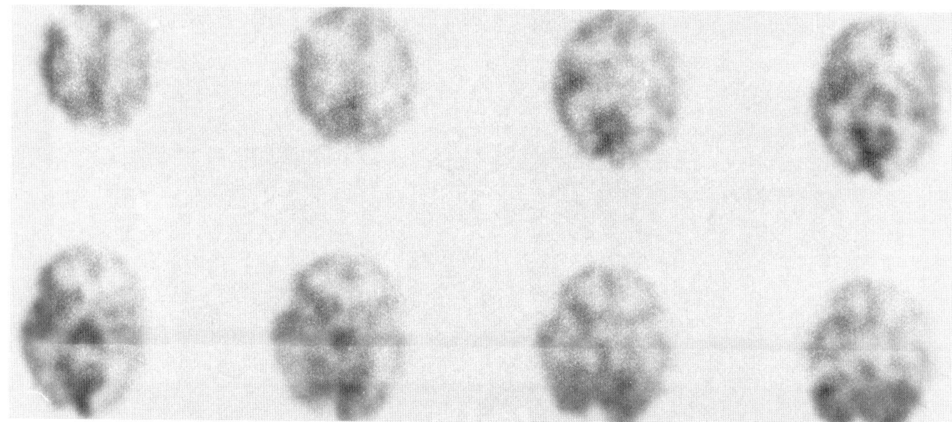

FIG. 5.87

CASE 5-39

Clinical Diagnosis: Right Cavernous Carotid Artery Aneurysm

CONTRIBUTOR:	IMAGING DATA:	
Name: Frederick J. Bonte, M.D.	**Camera:** Toshiba GCA 9300	**Collimator:** High resolution, fan beam
Institution: University of Texas-Southwestern Medical Center	**Isotope:** ^{99m}Tc HMPAO	**Dose:** 21.0 mCi

This 59-year-old woman was referred for evaluation of double vision associated with right third and fourth nerve palsies.

CT and MRI were both reported to be negative. However, a cerebral arteriogram showed a small aneurysm of the right cavernous carotid artery. After angiography, the patient was observed to be lethargic, aphasic, and hemiparetic on the right side but recovered uneventfully.

An HMPAO SPECT study (Fig. 5.88A, *upper row*) revealed slight reduction of radiotracer uptake in the distribution of the right internal carotid artery.

A follow-up HMPAO SPECT study (Fig. 5.88B, *lower row*) performed at the time of a test balloon occlusion of the right internal carotid revealed a marked decrease in radiotracer activity throughout the right internal carotid artery territory with concomitant decrease in radiotracer activity in the left cerebellar hemisphere consistent with crossed cerebellar diaschisis, which was thought to have occurred immediately following the cessation of input from the corticopontine cerebellar tracts.

At the time of the test balloon occlusion, the patient lost consciousness for approximately 15 sec while the balloon was inflated.

Published with permission: *AJNR* 1992;13:55–57.

Teaching Points:

1. Crossed cerebellar diaschisis can be observed immediately following the loss of an afferent stimulus (deafferentation).
2. Cerebral SPECT in conjunction with temporary balloon occlusion of the carotid artery is a very useful technique for accurately assessing the integrity of the collateral cerebral circulation.

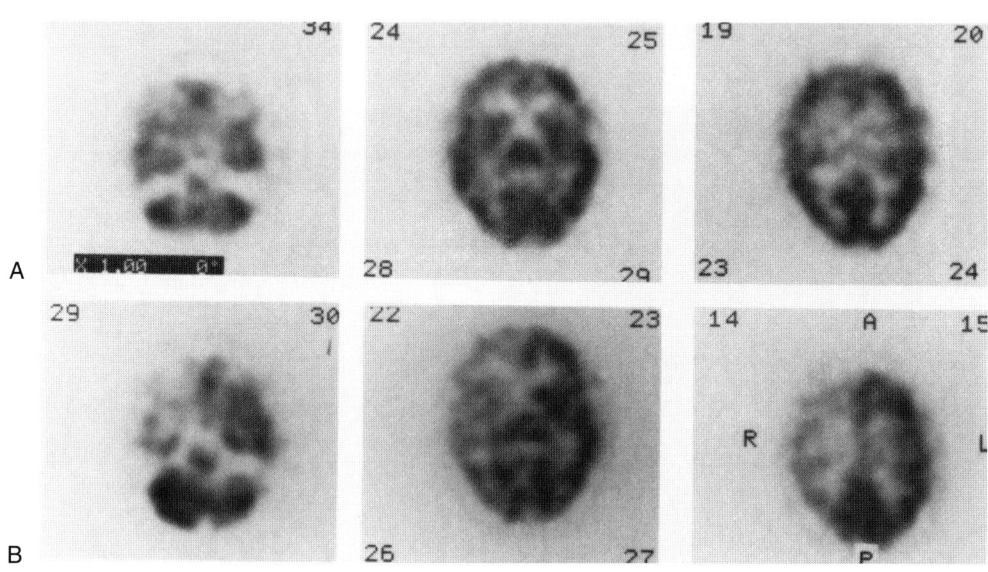

FIG. 5.88

CASE 5-40

Clinical Diagnosis: Right Cavernous Carotid Artery Aneurysm

CONTRIBUTOR:	IMAGING DATA:	
Name: Andrew Taylor, M.D.	**Camera:** Toshiba GCA 9300	**Collimator:** High resolution, fan beam
Institution: Emory University School of Medicine	**Isotope:** ^{99m}Tc HMPAO	**Dose:** 21.0 mCi

This 39-year-old man was referred for evaluation of headaches and diplopia.

A right common carotid arteriogram (Fig. 5.89) revealed a large cavernous carotid artery aneurysm. A left common arteriogram (Fig. 5.90) at the time of a test balloon occlusion of the right carotid revealed adequate filling of the right hemisphere via collateral flow from the left side. Neurologic examination at the time of balloon occlusion was normal.

An HMPAO SPECT study (Fig. 5.91) in the transaxial plane, which had been injected at the time of temporary balloon occlusion of the right carotid, revealed diffuse decrease radiotracer activity in the right internal carotid territory distribution.

A follow-up HMPAO SPECT study (Fig. 5.92) in the transaxial plane revealed a normalization of the radiotracer uptake bilaterally.

The patient went on to have a temporary vascular clipping of the right internal carotid artery during surgery to clip the cavernous carotid aneurysm. At that time, electroencephalographic monitoring showed ipsilateral ischemic changes that resolved after the carotid clips were removed.

Published with permission: ***AJNR*** **1991;12:1035–1041 (Case 2).**

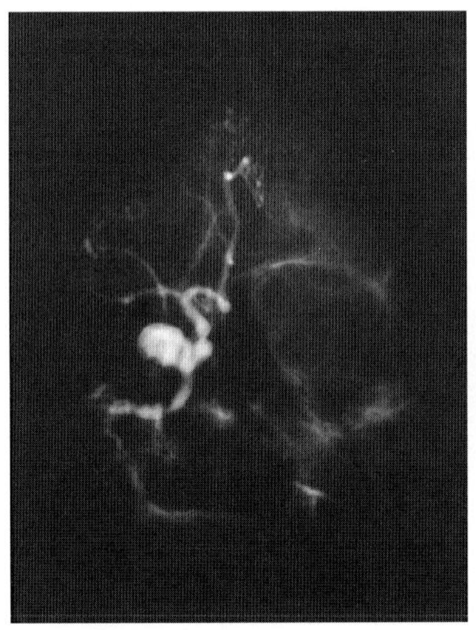

FIG. 5.89

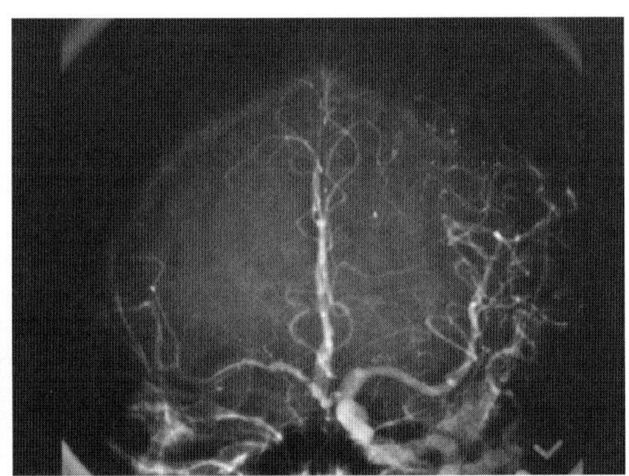

FIG. 5.90

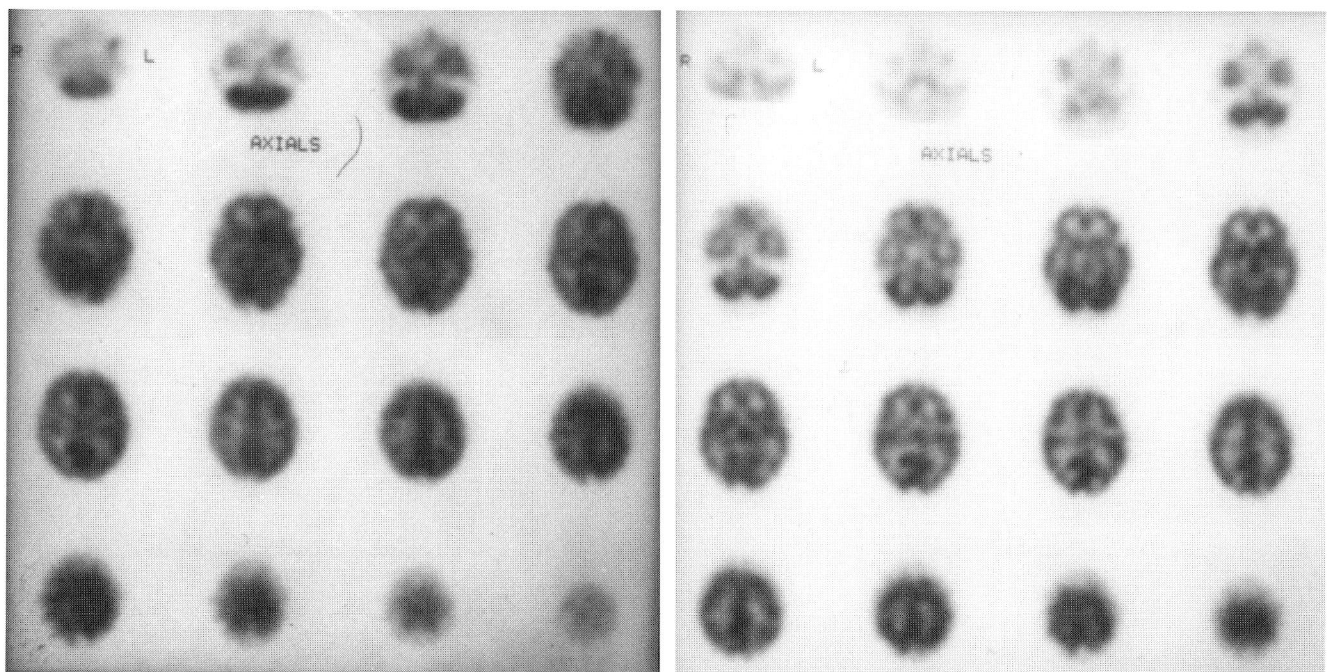

FIG. 5.91

FIG. 5.92

CASE 5-41

Clinical Diagnosis:

Luxury Perfusion Following a Migraine Attack

CONTRIBUTOR:

Name: Jacques Dacourt, M.D., Ph.D. and Ismael Mena, M.D.
Institution: University of Nice (France) and Harbor-UCLA Medical Center

IMAGING DATA:

Camera: GE 400T
Isotope: ^{99m}Tc HMPAO
Collimator: LEAP
Dose: 20.0 mCi

This 24-year-old woman was referred for evaluation of a migraine headache with an associated left hemiplegia. At the time of evaluation, the patient's migraine headache had resolved, but the patient remained hemiplegic.

MRI examination (Fig. 5.93, *right*), was normal.

An HMPAO SPECT study (Fig. 5.93, *left*) revealed an intense increase in radiotracer uptake throughout the right hemisphere, which was most marked in the frontal lobe. Overall the SPECT pattern was felt to be most compatible with luxury perfusion following a migraine crisis.

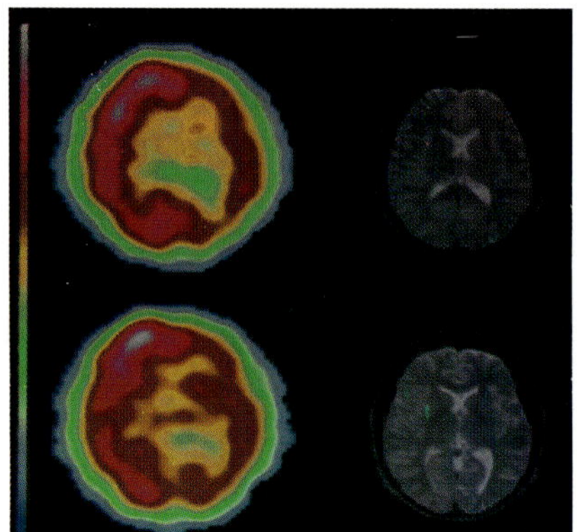

FIG. 5.93

Cerebral SPECT Imaging, Second Edition,
edited by R.L. Van Heertum and R.S. Tikofsky.
Raven Press, Ltd., New York © 1995.

CHAPTER 6

Dementia

Alan B. Rubens and Ronald S. Tikofsky

There has been a rapid increase in the utility of SPECT scanning in the diagnosis and understanding of dementia and its underlying, disordered brain function (1). Positron emission tomography (PET) imaging has demonstrated characteristic alterations in cerebral perfusion and metabolism in Alzheimer's disease, but its expense and lack of availability prevent it from being used routinely.

SPECT imaging is widely available and demonstrates the same patterns of perfusion and metabolic alteration as those seen with PET imaging (2,3). SPECT distinguishes Alzheimer's disease from other types of dementia, such as multi-infarct dementia, hydrocephalus, progressive supranuclear palsy, and various frontal lobe dementias (4–9). It also helps differentiate Alzheimer's disease from the cognitive impairments associated with depression.

The pattern of abnormality seen in regional cerebral blood flow (rCBF)/SPECT images generally associated with the presence of dementia is that of reduced tracer uptake. However, in certain types of dementia, i.e., multi-infarct dementia, regions of absent tracer uptake are observed. Unless there is a prior history of seizures, it is extremely rare to find increased tracer uptake. The distribution of decreased uptake provides information relative to the severity of disease and most prevalent type of cognitive impairment seen on clinical and neuropsychological examination (10–14). In almost all cases, except for Huntington's disease, dementia associated with Parkinson's disease, and human immunodeficiency virus (HIV) dementia, the basal ganglia, thalamus, sensorimotor cortex, occipital cortex, and cerebellum will show normal perfusion.

Tables 6.1 through 6.6 describe the rCBF/SPECT findings most often observed in the various forms of dementia. It should be noted that there are wide variations in the patterns. These variations are related to the patient's presenting status.

The typical finding in Alzheimer's disease is bilateral parietotemporal hypoperfusion and hypometabolism, with sparing of the sensorimotor and occipital regions. Frontal lobe hypoperfusion and hypometabolism are also found in more advanced cases. In a smaller proportion of patients, the SPECT abnormalities are primarily unilateral, and they frequently correspond to the signs of unilateral function disturbances that are found on neuropsychological tests.

The second most common type of dementia is multi-infarct or vascular dementia. This dementia is characterized by a random, multifocal distribution of infarcts and abnormalities associated with specific vascular territories. It may also be characterized by unilateral hemispheric reductions of tracer uptake.

Other types of dementia include the pseudodementia of depression; normal pressure hydrocephalus (NHP); Huntington's disease; alcohol or other substance abuse; frontal lobe disease (such as Pick's); and, more recently, acquired immunodeficiency syndrome (AIDS)-related dementia. SPECT imaging is helpful in the differentiation of the pathophysiologic patterns seen in the various forms of dementia. It is also useful in establishing physiological subgroups that correlate with the different clinical presentations seen in patients with Alzheimer's and other diseases.

The resolving power and radiopharmaceuticals of PET imaging are superior, but the availability, relative simplicity, and affordability of SPECT make it a valuable technique in the assessment of patients with dementia. It will play a significant role in the early diagnosis and longitudinal study of such patients.

At present the majority of reports in the literature indicate that rCBF/SPECT is a reliable tool for differentiating persons with moderate-to-severe dementia from normals (15). In addition, the scans reflect the type and severity of the cognitive deterioration associated with the dementing

A. B. Rubens: Department of Neurology, University of Arizona College of Medicine, Tucson, Arizona 85721.

R. S. Tikofsky: Department of Radiology, Section of Nuclear Medicine, Medical College of Wisconsin, Milwaukee, Wisconsin 53226.

disease process. Even with the newer SPECT instruments, it is still unclear as to whether the minimal changes in rCBF that may be associated with early onset of dementing disease can be detected. The development of new methods for assessing radioreceptor uptake, cognitive activation, and quantitative SPECT should help in this differentiation. Thus rCBF/SPECT is a valuable diagnostic tool for the assessment of persons with suspected dementia. At present, it also appears that quantitative rCBF/ SPECT has the potential to assess the effects of pharmacological treatments on dementia patients.

TABLE 6.1. *Alzheimer's disease*

Bilaterally reduced tracer uptake in the temporoparietal regions in moderate-to-severe disease
Very early or minimally impaired patients may have normal rCBF/SPECT scans
In the early stages of AD the reduced uptake may have a unilateral appearance
Frontal lobes show reduced tracer uptake as the disease progresses
Motor/sensory cortex, basal ganglia, thalamus, occipital lobes, and cerebellum typically show normal tracer uptake for age

TABLE 6.2. *Multi-infarct dementia*

Focal regions of absent and/or reduced tracer uptake that occur in typical vascular distribution
Regions of abnormality may be unilateral or bilateral
New lesions appear as the disease progresses, but the progression is stepwise as opposed to the continuous progression of Alzheimer's disease
MRI is the most appropriate diagnostic imaging procedure

TABLE 6.3. *Vascular dementia*

Unilateral reduced tracer uptake often following the distribution of the middle cerebral artery
Impairment of intellectual and cognitive functions correlate with regions showing reduced tracer uptake
CT/MRI may be normal for age

TABLE 6.4. *HIV-related dementia*

Global reduction in tracer uptake
Patchy (heterogenous) appearance in the cortical gray matter with superimposed (random) focal deficits
Decreased tracer uptake in white matter disproportionate to ventricular size
Focal decreases in basal ganglia and/or thalami

TABLE 6.5. *Pick's disease*

Significant reduction of tracer uptake bilaterally in the anterior frontal and inferior temporal lobes
Motor/sensory cortex and regions posterior to the motor/sensory cortex are within normal range
Rapid progression of decreased but not absent tracer uptake to the frontal lobes but not including motor/sensory cortex and to the remainder of the anterior and inferior temporal lobes bilaterally

TABLE 6.6. *Pseudodementia (depression in the elderly)*

Often initially diagnosed clinically as Alzheimer's disease
May appear near normal rCBF/SPECT scan for age
Decreased tracer activity in the frontal lobes may be seen

REFERENCES

1. Tikofsky RS, Hellman RS, Parks RW. Single photon emission computed tomography and applications to dementia. In: Parks RW, Zec RF, Wilson RS, eds. *Neuropsychology of Alzheimer's disease and other dementias.* New York: Oxford University Press; 1993:489–510.
2. Johnson KA, Holman BL, Rosen J, et al. Iofetamine I-123 single photon emission computed tomography is accurate in the diagnosis of Alzheimer's disease. *Arch Intern Med* 1990;150:752–756.
3. Holman BL, Johnson KA, Gerada B, et al. The scintigraphic appearance of Alzheimer's disease: a prospective study using technetium-99m-HMPAO SPECT. *J Nucl Med* 1992;33:181–185.
4. Neary D, Snowden JS, Shields RA, et al. Single photon emission tomography using ^{99m}Tc-HMPAO in the investigation of dementia. *J Neurol Neurosurg Psychiatry* 1987;50:1101–1109.
5. Jagust WJ, Budinger TF, Reed BR. The diagnosis of dementia with single photon emission computed tomography. *Arch Neurol* 1987;44: 258–262.
6. Antuono PG, Tikofsky RS, Hellman RS, Bexena VK. Single photon emission computed tomography (SPECT) in the evaluation of the dementias. *Mind* 1990;4:6–8.
7. Bartolini A, Gasparetto B, Loeb C. Assessment of SPECT features in the differential diagnosis between degenerative and multi-infarct dementia. In: Battistin L, Gerstenbrand F, eds. *Aging and dementia: new trends in diagnosis and therapy.* New York: Wiley-Liss; 1990: 441–438.
8. Cohen MB, Graham LS, Lake R, et al. Diagnosis of Alzheimer's disease and multiple infarct dementia by tomographic imaging of iodine-123 IMP. *J Nucl Med,* 1986;27:769–774.
9. Masdeu JC, Yudd A, Van Heertum RL, et al. Single-photon emission computed tomography in human immunodeficiency virus encephalopathy: a preliminary report. *J Nucl Med* 1991;32:1471–1475.
10. Goldenberg G, Podreka I, Suess E, Deecke L. The cerebral localization of neuropsychological impairment in Alzheimer's disease: a SPECT study. *J Neurol* 1989;236:131–138.
11. Hellman RS, Antuono PG, Tikofsky RS, et al. Correlation between regional reductions in cerebral blood flow (SPECT/IMP) and neuropsychological test scores in dementia patients. *J Nucl Med* 1990; 31:731(abst).
12. Johnson KA, Mueller ST, Walshe TM, et al. Single photon emission computed tomography in Alzheimer's disease: abnormal iofetamine I-123 uptake reflects dementia severity. *Arch Neurol* 1988;45: 392–396.

13. Montaldi D, Brooks DN, McColl JH, et al. Measurements of regional cerebral blood flow and cognitive performance in Alzheimer's disease. *J Neurol Neurosurg Psychiatry* 1990;53:33–38.
14. Tikofsky RS, Hellman RS, Antuono PA, et al. Boston naming test (ENT) enhanced quantitative SPECT HMPAO in Alzheimer's disease. *Radiology* 1991;181P:174(abst).
15. Hellman RS, Tikofsky RS, Van Heertum RL, et al. A multi-institutional study of inter-observer agreement in the evaluation of dementia with rCBF/SPECT technetium-^{99m} exametazime (HMPAO) *J. Eur Nucl Med* 1994; 21:306–313.

SUGGESTED READINGS

Devan MJ, Gupta S. Toward a definite diagnosis of Alzheimer's disease. *Compr Psychiatry* 1992;33:282–290.

Eberling JL, Reed BR, Baker MG, Jagust WJ. Cognitive correlation of regional cerebral blood flow in Alzheimer's disease. *Arch Neurol* 1993; 50:761–766.

Holman BL, Nagel JS, Johnson KA, Hill TC. Imaging dementia with SPECT. *Ann NY Acad Sci* 1991;629:165–174.

Launes J, Sulkava R, Erkinjuntti T, et al. 99Tcm-HMPAO SPECT in suspected dementia. *Nucl Med Commun* 1991;12:757–765.

Ohnishi T, Hoshi H, Nagamachi S, et al. Regional cerebral blood flow study with 123-IMP in patients with dementia. *Am J Neurorad,* 1991; 12:513–520.

Pearlson GD, Harris GJ, Powers RE, et al. Quantitative changes in medial temporal volume, regional cerebral blood flow, and cognition in Alzheimer's disease. *Arch Gen Psychiatry* 1992;49:402–408.

Rosci MA, Figorini F, Bernabei A, et al. Methods for detecting early signs of AIDS dementia complex in asymptomatic HIV-1-infected subjects. *AIDS* 1992;6:1309–1316.

Tranquart F, Ades PE, Groussin P, et al. Postoperative assessment of cerebral blood flow in subarachnoid hemorrhage by means of 99mTc-HMPAO tomography. *Eur J Nucl Med* 1993;20:53–58.

Tozzi V, Narciso P, Galgani S, et al. Effects of zidovudine in 30 patients with mild to end-stage AIDS dementia complex. *AIDS* 1993;7: 683–692.

Wyper D, Teasdale E, Patterson J, et al. Abnormalities in rCBF and computed tomography in patients with Alzheimer's disease and in controls. *Br J Radiol* 1993;66:23–27.

CASE 6-1 Clinical Diagnosis: Alzheimer's Disease

CONTRIBUTOR:	**IMAGING DATA:**	
Name: Ronald L. Van Heertum, M.D.	**Camera:** GE 400 AC/T;Star II	**Collimator:** High resolution
Institution: St. Vincent's Hospital and Medical Center	**Isotope:** ^{123}IMP	**Dose:** 3.0 mCi

This 58-year-old woman presented with a 2-year history of progressive deterioration of cognitive function.

A computed tomography (CT) scan (Fig. 6.1) showed a moderate degree of diffuse cortical atrophy.

The cerebral SPECT study (Fig. 6.2), in the transaxial **(A),** coronal **(B),** and sagittal **(C)** planes, revealed bilateral decreased tracer deposition in the posterior parietal, temporal, and occipital lobes, and in the anterior frontal lobes. There was relatively normal deposition in the subcortical areas, the motor strip cortex, and the cerebellum. These findings are typical of the pattern seen with dementia of the Alzheimer's type.

Published with permission: ***J Neuropsychiatry Clin Neurosci*** **1989;1:145–153, American Psychiatric Press.**

Teaching Point:

The pattern of bilateral posterior parietal-occipital temporal radiotracer reduction, particularly when associated with relative sparing of the sensory-motor cortex, subcortical (basal ganglia and thalamus) structures, and cerebellum is highly characteristic of Alzheimer's disease.

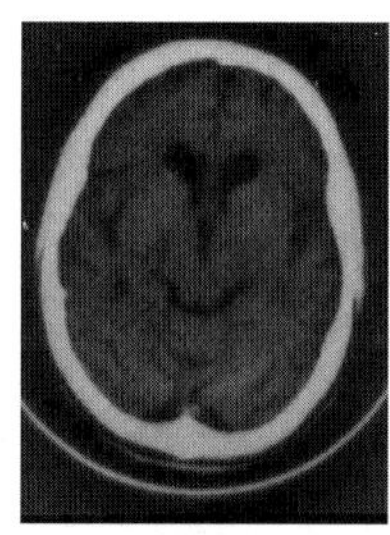

FIG. 6.1

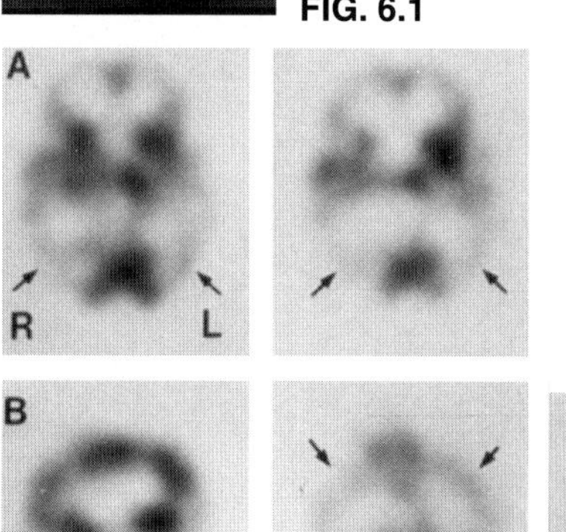

FIG. 6.2

CASE 6-2

Clinical Diagnosis: Senile Dementia of the Alzheimer's Type

CONTRIBUTOR:

Name: Ronald L. Van Heertum, M.D.
Institution: St. Vincent's Hospital and Medical Center

IMAGING DATA:

Camera: GE 400 AC/T;Star II
Isotope: ^{123}IMP
Collimator: High resolution
Dose: 3.0 mCi

This 78-year-old man was referred for evaluation of a progressive dementia of 6 years' duration.

The CT scan (Fig. 6.3) revealed diffuse cortical atrophy.

The cerebral SPECT study (Fig. 6.4), in the transaxial **(A),** coronal **(B),** and sagittal **(C)** planes, revealed reduced tracer deposition throughout the cerebral cortex, with a relatively normal pattern in the cerebellum and subcortical regions. The decrease in cortical activity of the tracer was most pronounced in the posterior parietal-occipital areas *(arrows),* with relative sparing of the motor strip area. This pattern is most consistent with senile dementia of the Alzheimer's type.

Published with permission: Volume 8: ***Directions in psychiatry.*** **Hatherleigh; New York: 1989:1–8.**

Teaching Point:

The decreased tracer deposition in such areas as the posterior parietal region may be asymmetric, as demonstrated in this case. The areas of greatest deficit typically correlate with the dominant area of cognitive dysfunction manifest on clinical neuropsychological testing.

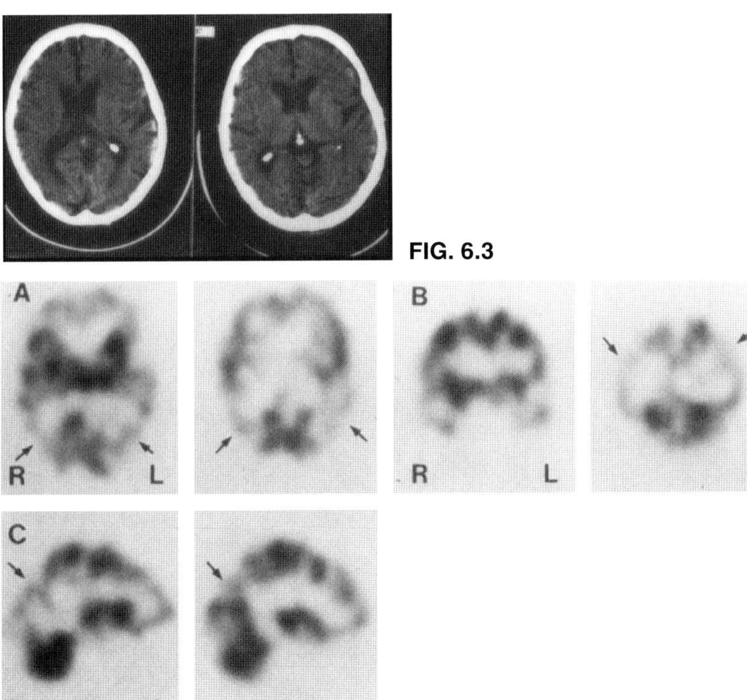

FIG. 6.3

FIG. 6.4

CASE 6-3 Clinical Diagnosis: Dementia, Possible Alzheimer's Disease

CONTRIBUTOR:

Name: Robert S. Hellman, M.D. and Ronald S. Tikofsky, M.D.
Institution: Medical College of Wisconsin

IMAGING DATA:

Camera: GE Neuro CAM
Isotope: ^{99m}Tc HMPAO
Collimator: High resolution
Dose: 30.0 mCi

This 79-year-old woman was referred by the Memory Disorders Clinic for evaluation of signs and symptoms of dementia. At the time of evaluation, her Mini-Mental Status Examination score was 17/30. The patient's symptoms, which had started 2 years previously, began with mood changes and hallucinations, inability to handle finances, and the progressive inability to operate her TV remote control.

No CT or magnetic resonance imaging (MRI) studies had been performed

A hexamethylpropyleneamine-okime (HMPAO) SPECT study (Fig. 6.5), in the transaxial **(A),** coronal **(B),** and sagittal **(C)** planes, revealed decreased radiotracer in the right frontal, temporal parietal, and left posterior parietal regions. These findings are consistent with Alzheimer's disease.

Teaching Point:

HMPAO SPECT can be useful in the evaluation of suspected Alzheimer's disease. The pattern of reduced radiotracer uptake is similar to ^{123}I IMP SPECT and F-18 fluorodeoxyglucose PET studies.

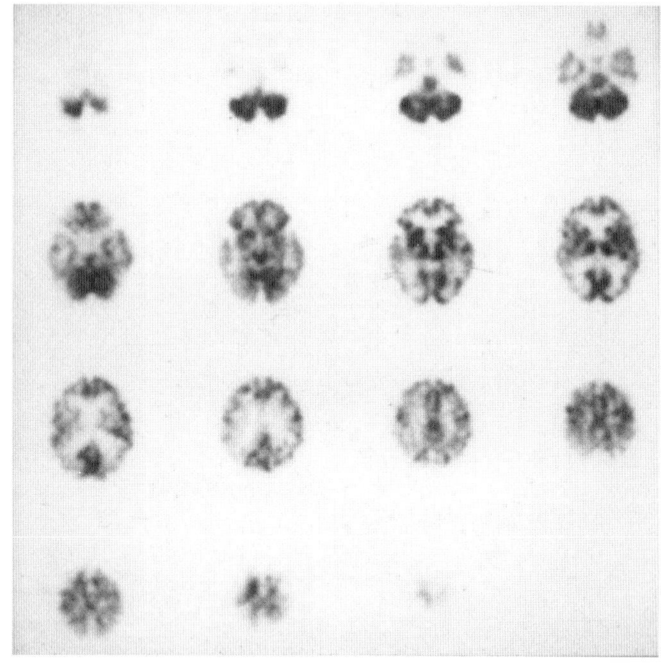

FIG. 6.5A

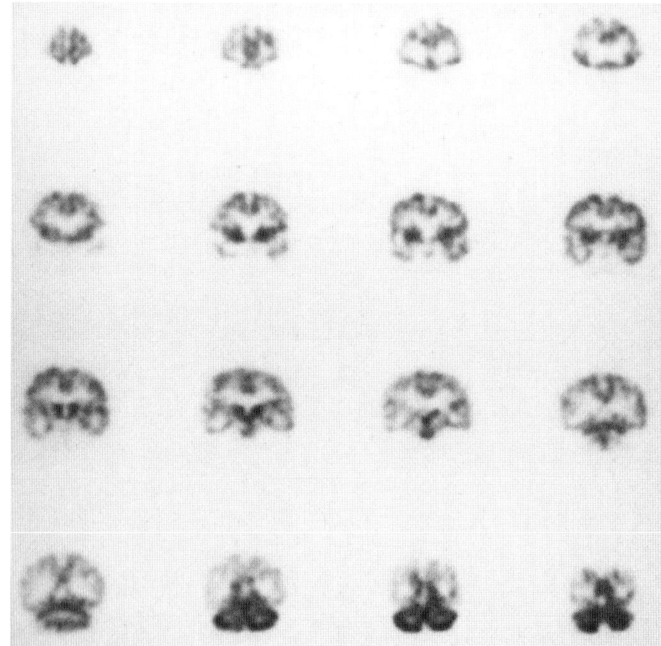

FIG. 6.5B

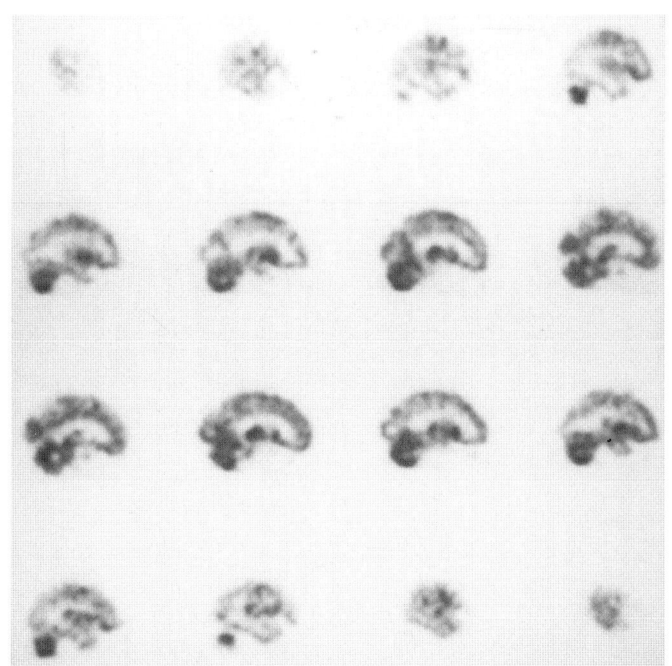

FIG. 6.5C

CASE 6-4

Clinical Diagnosis: Dementia, Probable Alzheimer's Disease

CONTRIBUTOR:

Name: Robert S. Hellman, M.D. and Ronald S. Tikofsky, M.D.
Institution: Medical College of Wisconsin

IMAGING DATA:

Camera: GE 400 AC/T;Star
Isotope: ^{123}I IMP
Collimator: High resolution
Dose: 4.0 mCi

This 69-year-old man was referred for evaluation of progressive signs and symptoms of dementia.

No anatomic imaging studies had been performed.

An N-isopropyl-*p*-iodoamphetamine (IMP) SPECT study (Fig. 6.6), in the transaxial **(A),** coronal **(B),** and sagittal **(C)** planes, revealed decreased radiotracer uptake in the frontal, temporal, and posterior parietal lobes bilaterally, suggesting advanced Alzheimer's disease.

Teaching Point:

Patients with advanced Alzheimer's disease will often show decreased tracer uptake in the frontal lobes bilaterally as well as the typical abnormalities in the temporal and parietal lobes.

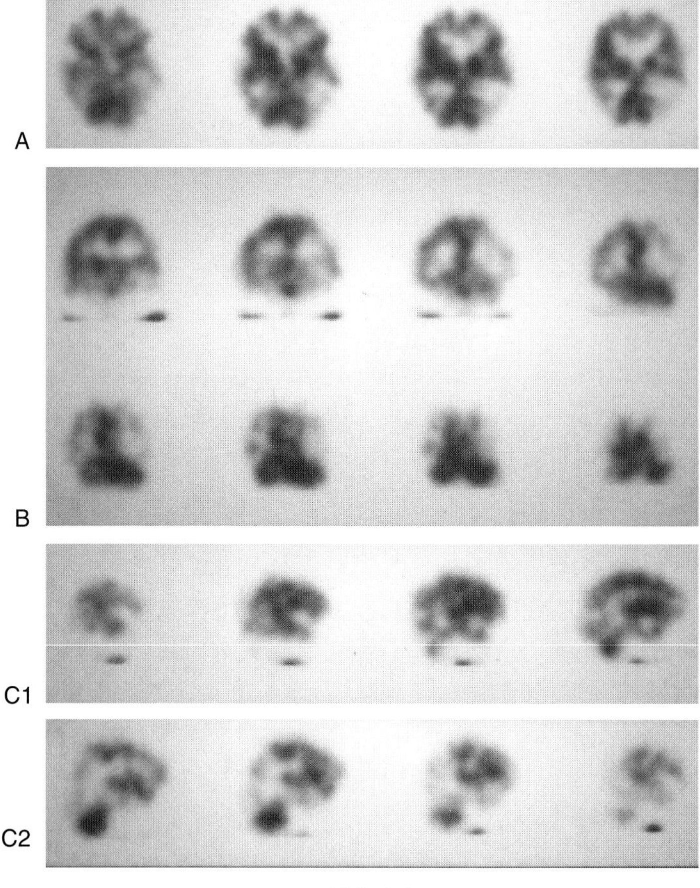

FIG. 6.6

CASE 6-5

Clinical Diagnosis: Possible Alzheimer's Disease

CONTRIBUTOR:	IMAGING DATA:	
Name: Matthew Bloom, M.D. **Institution:** Columbia-Presbyterian Medical Center	**Camera:** Picker Prism 3000 **Isotope:** ^{99m}Tc HMPAO	**Collimator:** Ultra-high resolution, fan bean **Dose:** 20.6 mCi

This 68-year-old woman with an 8-year history of anomia, fluctuating antisocial behavior, and violent outbursts, was referred for evaluation of progressive short-term memory loss.

MRI (T2-weighted) revealed mild generalized atrophy and small lacunas infarct in the right cerebral peduncle.

At the time of the SPECT study, she was quite agitated and uncooperative. As a result a shortened SPECT acquisition was performed. HMPAO SPECT (Fig. 6.7), in the coronal **(A)** and sagittal **(B)** planes, revealed an overall decrease in radiotracer uptake that was most marked in the posterior-parietal-temporal and frontal lobes bilaterally. There is relative sparing of the sensory motor area and the subcortical structures including basal ganglia and thalami.

Teaching Point:

Cerebral SPECT can be very useful in the evaluation of dementia, particularly in patients who are difficult to evaluate with clinical neuropsychological testing such as this patient with anomia. This study further demonstrates the value of shortening the total SPECT acquisition time in agitated or uncooperative patients.

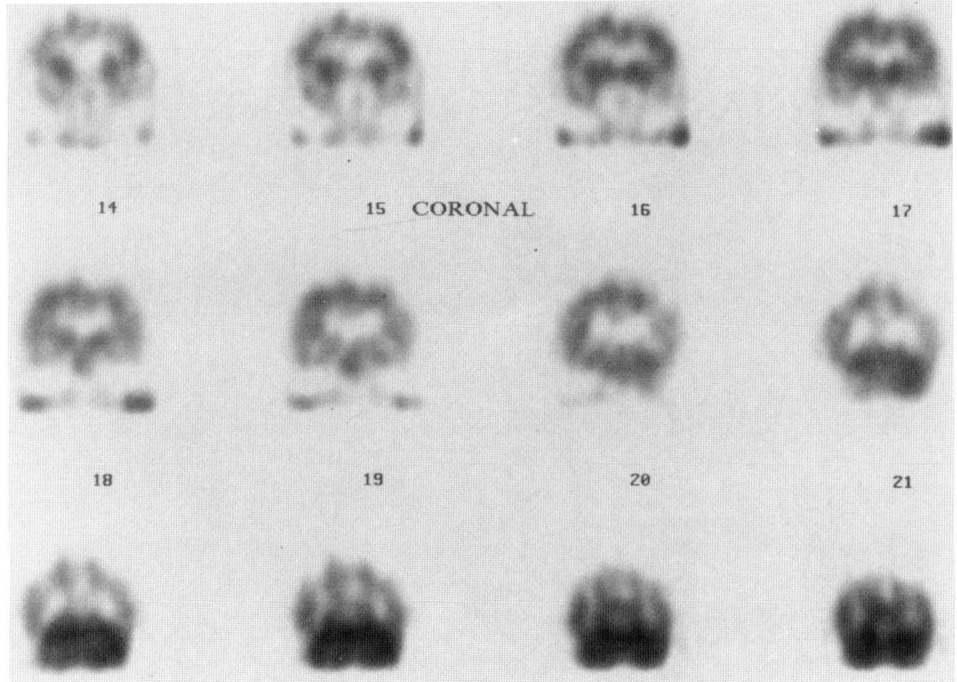

FIG. 6.7A

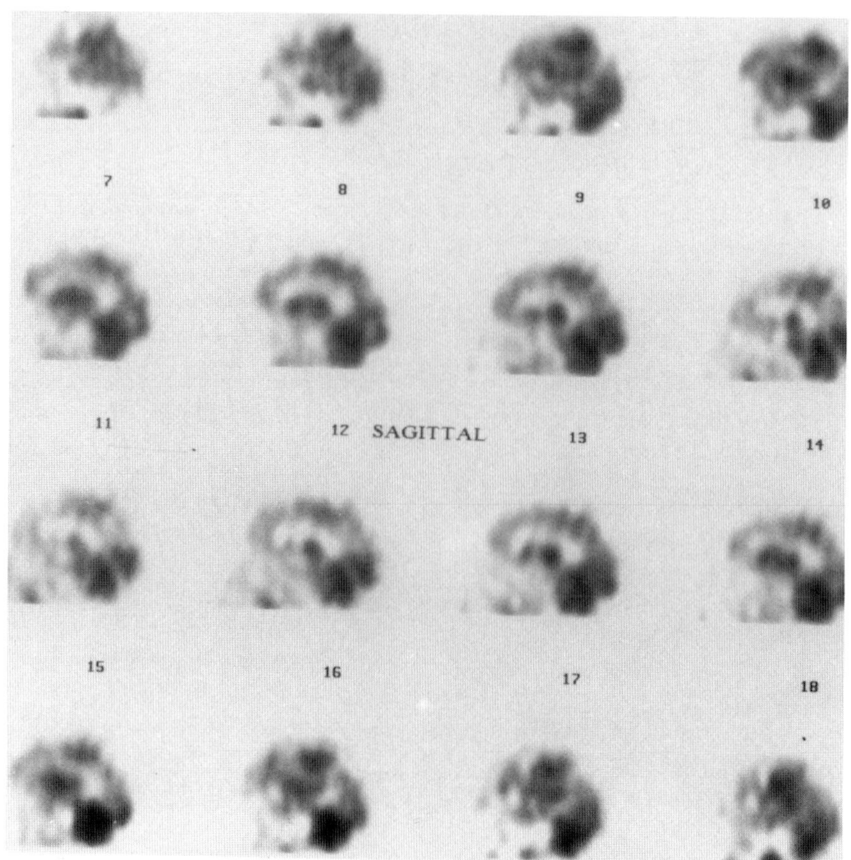

FIG. 6.7B

CASE 6-6

Clinical Diagnosis:
Probable Alzheimer's Disease

CONTRIBUTOR:

Name: Marvin B. Cohen, M.D.
Institution: VA Medical Center

IMAGING DATA:

Camera: Siemens Rota Camera
Isotope: ^{123}I IMP
Collimator: LEAP
Dose: 3.0 mCi

This 65-year-old man was referred for evaluation of probable Alzheimer's disease.

The cerebral SPECT study (Fig. 6.8), in the transaxial **(A)** and sagittal **(B)** planes, revealed a mild bilateral decreased tracer deposition in the posterior parietal region *(arrow)*. The pattern is consistent with the pattern seen in the early stages of Alzheimer's disease.

Teaching Point:

Early in the course of Alzheimer's disease, anatomic studies may reveal atrophic changes in the medial temporal (hippocampus) regions. At about the same time, SPECT studies, even with single detector technology, have frequently been reported to demonstrate early diminished tracer uptake in the posterior parietal-temporal cortical regions.

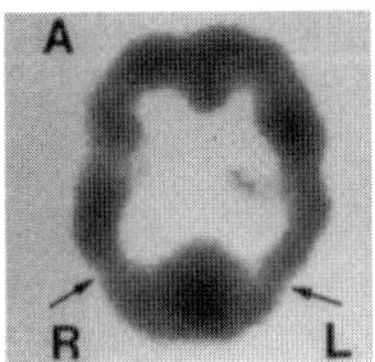

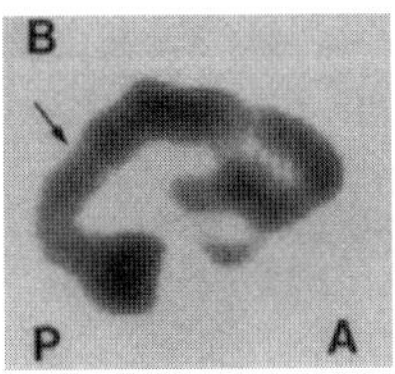

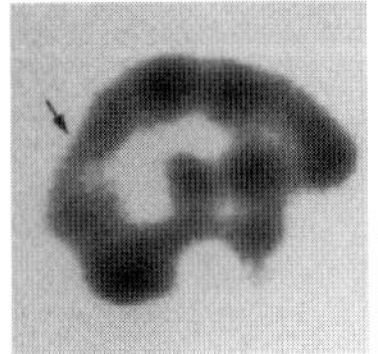

FIG. 6.8

CASE 6-7

Clinical Diagnosis: Amnestic Syndrome, Possible Alzheimer's Disease

CONTRIBUTOR:

Name: Robert S. Hellman, M.D. and Ronald S. Tikofsky, M.D.
Institution: Medical College of Wisconsin

IMAGING DATA:

Camera: GE 400 AC/T;Star
Isotope: ^{123}I IMP
Collimator: High resolution
Dose: 5.0 mCi

This 74-year-old woman with a known prior history of three motor vehicle accidents and alcohol/phenobarbital abuse was referred for evaluation of progressive memory changes. Her memory changes were first noted in 1983 following the third motor vehicle accident. Although her Mini-Mental Status Examination at the present time was within the normal range (29/30), she did show a mild impairment on the Blessed Dementia rating scale (8.5/16). The brief psychiatric rating scale and Hachinski cerebral ischemia score were within normal range. The criteria used for amnestic syndrome were those of the National Institute of Neurological and Communicative Disorders and Stroke/(NINCDS/ADRDA).

An MRI scan showed diffuse cerebral atrophy with mild senescent white matter changes.

An HMPAO SPECT study (Fig. 6.9), in the transaxial plane, revealed decreased radiotracer activity in the mesial anterior temporal and posterior frontal lobes. In addition, mild decreased tracer activity was noted bilaterally, right greater than left, in the posterior parietal lobes.

Teaching Point:

This is an atypical presentation for Alzheimer's disease. However, repeat scans will typically show the progression of the disease over time. Approximately 80 percent of patients with amnestic syndrome progress to Alzheimer's disease within 5 years of onset.

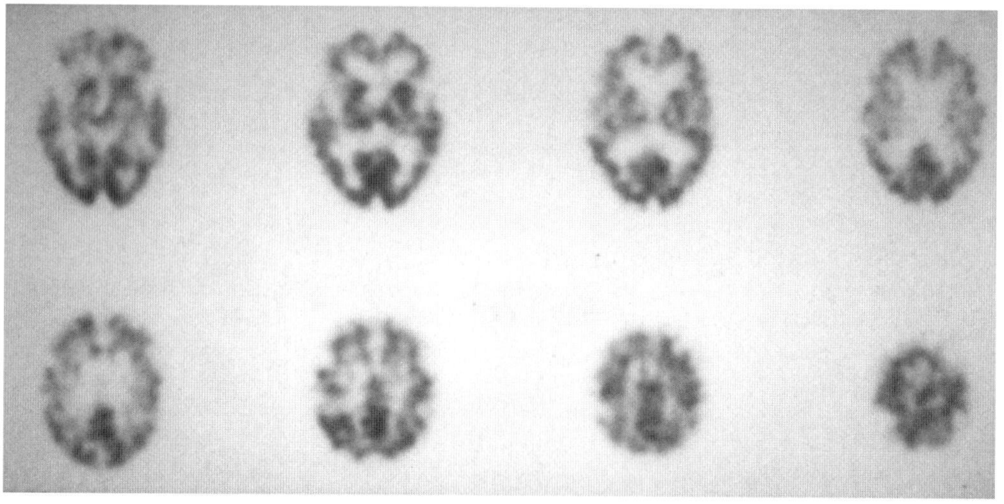

FIG. 6.9

CASE 6-8

Clinical Diagnosis:
Mixed Alzheimer's and Multi-Infarct Dementia

CONTRIBUTOR:

Name: Robert S. Hellman, M.D. and Ronald S. Tikofsky, M.D.
Institution: Medical College of Wisconsin

IMAGING DATA:

Camera: GE 400 AC/T;Star
Isotope: ^{123}I IMP
Collimator: High resolution
Dose: 4.0 mCi

This 77-year-old woman was referred for further evaluation of signs and symptoms of dementia. Her chief complaints were memory loss with associated verbal and physical aggression toward relatives. The Dementia Clinic evaluation was most consistent with a diagnosis of probable Alzheimer's disease (NINCDS/ADRDA criteria); however, the patient also manifested a stepwise progression of symptoms consistent with an evolving multi-infarct dementia.

A CT scan (Fig. 6.10) showed generalized cerebral and cerebellar atrophy. In addition, multiple white matter hypodensities were seen in the centrum ovale region which were felt to be secondary to small vessel disease.

An IMP SPECT study (Fig. 6.11), in the transaxial **(A),** coronal **(B),** and sagittal **(C)** planes, revealed bilateral decreased, but not absent, radiotracer activity in the posterior temporal and parietal regions, greater on the left than right. Decreased radiotracer activity in the posterior frontal lobes was also evident. These findings are consistent with Alzheimer's disease.

Teaching Point:

Patients with Alzheimer's disease will often have asymmetric changes in the posterior regions of the brain along with involvement of the frontal lobes. The SPECT findings of greater reduction of tracer in the left hemisphere typically correlate with the clinical findings of significant language disturbance.

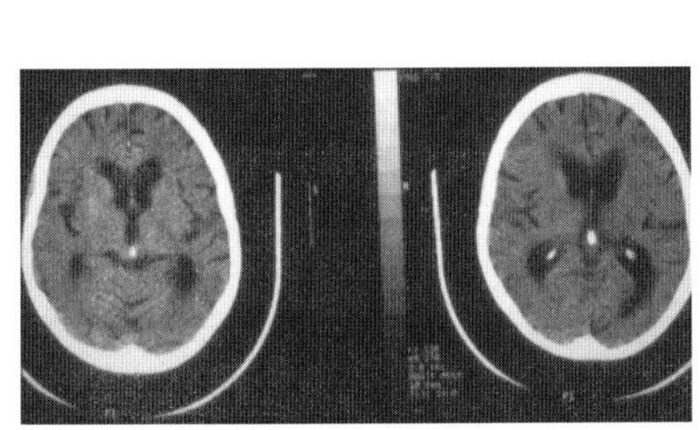

FIG. 6.10

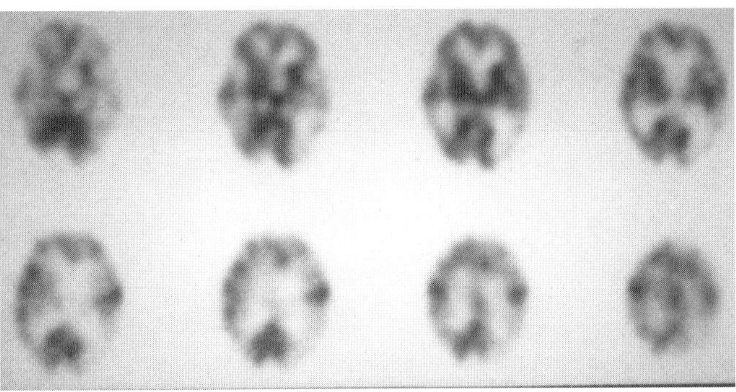

FIG. 6.11A

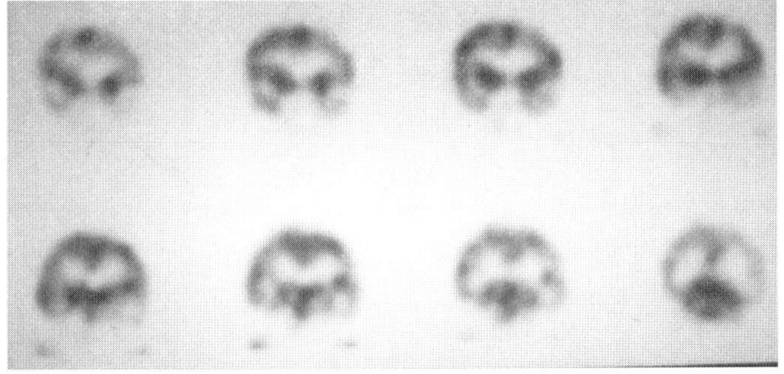

FIG. 6.11B

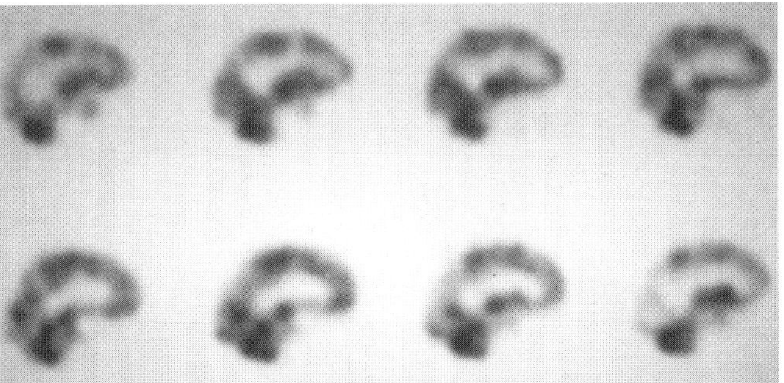

FIG. 6.11C

CASE 6-9

Clinical Diagnosis:

Mixed Dementia—Dementia of the Alzheimer's Type and Vascular Dementia

CONTRIBUTOR:

Name: Robert S. Hellman, M.D. and Ronald S. Tikofsky, M.D.

Institution: Medical College of Wisconsin

IMAGING DATA:

Camera: GE 400 AC/T;Star
Isotope: ^{123}I IMP

Collimator: High resolution
Dose: 4.5 mCi

This 85-year-old woman had been admitted to Geriopsychiatry on an emergency basis after she was found wandering away from her home. The patient was unaware of the reason for her admission. Her relatives noted that she had had increasing confusion, memory impairment, and poor concentration over the 2 years prior to admission. The patient scored 8/28 on the Folstein Mini-Mental State examination. In addition, her insight and judgement were observed to be severely impaired.

A CT scan revealed diffuse cortical atrophy and a hypodensity in the distribution of the right middle cerebral artery consistent with an area of infarction.

An IMP brain SPECT study (Fig. 6.12), in the transaxial plane, showed a large area of absent radiotracer uptake in the right frontal, anterior parietal, and temporal lobes extending down to the basal ganglia. Crossed cerebellar diaschisis was also evident. In addition, reduction of radiotracer in the anterior frontal lobes in the distribution of the anterior cerebral artery was observed. The area of decreased radiotracer activity in the right cerebral hemisphere seen on the SPECT study was larger than the area of infarction seen on the CT examination. Smaller regions of decreased but not absent radiotracer uptake in the posterior parietal-temporal regions, left greater than right, were also evident. The overall findings were most consistent with the diagnosis of a combined multi-infarct dementia and Alzheimer's disease.

Teaching Point:

This case makes the point that patients presenting with dementia-like signs and symptoms may have complex findings that include those of vascular dementia as well as the more typical patterns, associated with Alzheimer's disease. It is also important to recognize that patients who have sustained a stroke may also develop Alzheimer's disease.

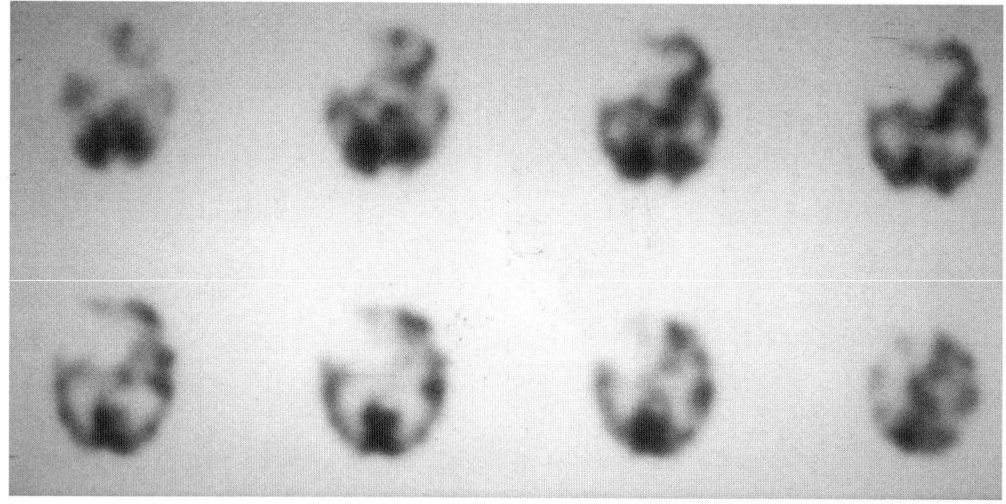

FIG. 6.12

CASE 6-10 Clinical Diagnosis: Vascular Dementia

CONTRIBUTOR:

Name: Robert S. Hellman, M.D. and Ronald S. Tikofsky, M.D.
Institution: Medical College of Wisconsin

IMAGING DATA:

Camera: GE 400 AC/T;Star
Isotope; ^{123}I IMP

Collimator: High resolution
Dose: 5.0 mCi

This 84-year-old, right-handed woman was referred for evaluation of a progressive deterioration in cognitive function.

The CT scan (Fig. 6.13) showed cerebral atrophy with dilation of the lateral ventricles.

The cerebral SPECT study (Fig. 6.14), in the transaxial plane revealed a marked decrease in tracer deposition throughout the periventricular white matter. In addition, a large area of diminished and absent radiotracer deposition was noted in the left hemisphere, particularly in the posterior parietal-temporal and occipital lobes *(arrows)*. The areas of involvement included the cortical territory surrounding the sylvian fissure. Lesions in this area usually result in significant alteration of language production and comprehension. This pattern is not typical of that usually associated with dementia of the Alzheimer's type.

Teaching Point:

This type of pattern may, at times, be very problematic when dementia of the Alzheimer's type (DAT) is a serious clinical consideration. In such situations, a repeat study following acetazolamide (Diamox) or hypercapnic challenge may help to differentiate a vascular dementia from DAT. In addition, serial SPECT studies may also be very helpful.

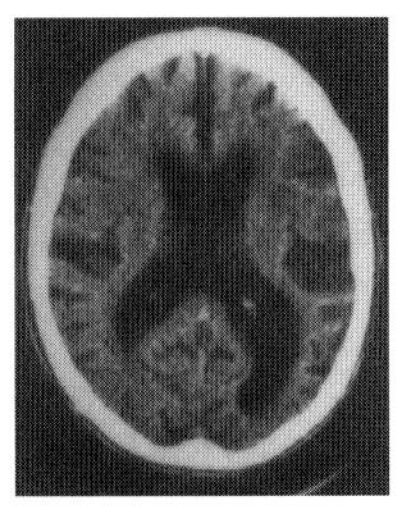

FIG. 6.13

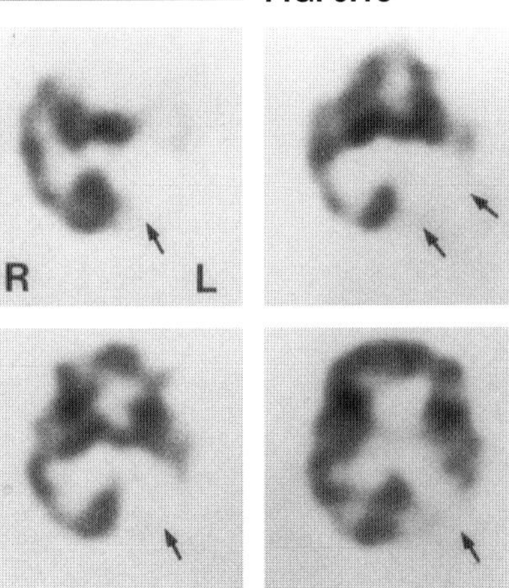

FIG. 6.14

CASE 6-11

Clinical Diagnosis: Multi-Infarct Dementia

CONTRIBUTOR:	IMAGING DATA:	
Name: Ronald L. Van Heertum, M.D.	**Camera:** GE 400 AC/T;Star II	**Collimator:** High resolution
Institution: St. Vincent's Hospital and Medical Center	**Isotope:** ^{123}I IMP	**Dose:** 3.0 mCi

This 64-year-old woman with known multi-infarct dementia was referred for evaluation of the recent onset of hemiplegia.

The CT scan (Fig. 6.15) demonstrated a large area of infarction involving the left occipital lobe. In addition, cortical atrophy and bilateral white matter hypodensity, suggesting microvascular disease, were also noted.

A cerebral SPECT study (Fig. 6.16), in the transaxial **(A),** coronal **(B),** and sagittal **(C)** planes, showed that tracer deposition was absent in the left occipital lobe *(arrows),* left frontal lobe *(arrowheads),* and left basal ganglia.

Teaching Point:

In cases of multi-infarct dementia, the cerebral SPECT study will frequently be more useful than a CT scan and, in some cases MRI, for defining the full extent of disease.

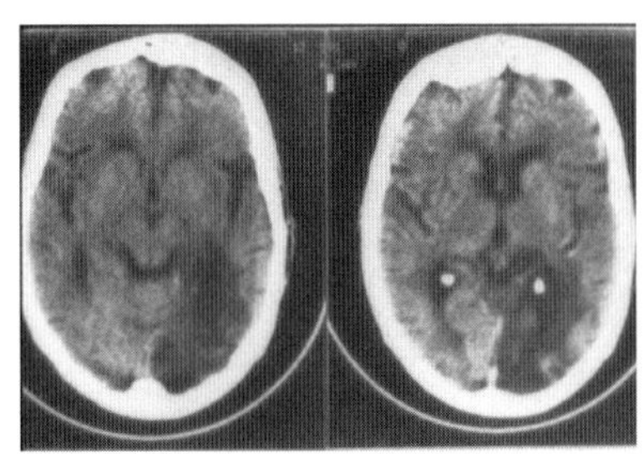

FIG. 6.15

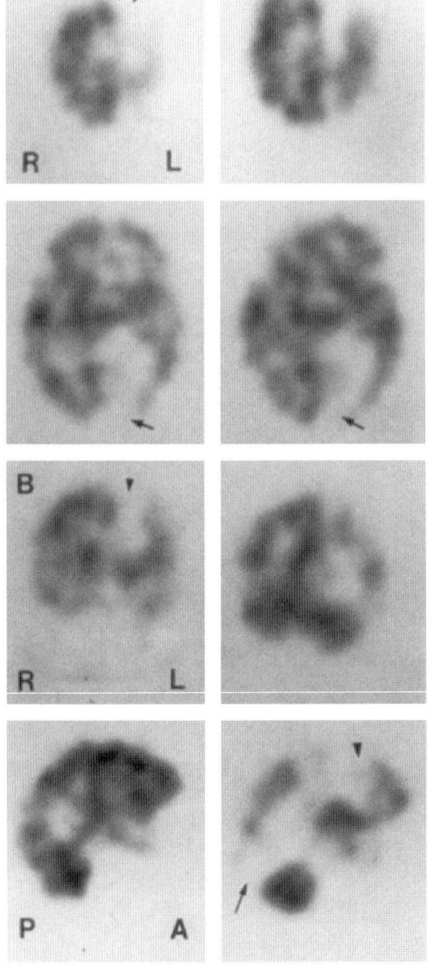

FIG. 6.17

CASE 6-12 Clinical Diagnosis: Vascular Dementia

CONTRIBUTOR:

Name: Robert S. Hellman, M.D. and Ronald S. Tikofsky, M.D.
Institution: Medical College of Wisconsin

IMAGING DATA:

Camera: GE Neurocam
Isotope: ^{123}I IMP
Collimator: High resolution
Dose: 3.2 mCi

This 68-year-old woman was referred by a geriopsychiatrist for a cerebral SPECT scan as part of an Alzheimer's disease workup. No other history was available at the time of the SPECT study. At the time of the SPECT study, no anatomic imaging exams had been performed.

The HMPAO/SPECT study (Fig. 6.17), in the transaxial **(A)** and coronal **(B)** planes, revealed a sharply defined defect in the left occipital and posterior temporal region that was felt to be consistent with an area of infarction involving the posterior circulation. No crossed cerebellar diaschisis was seen. These findings were not consistent with the provisional diagnosis of possible Alzheimer's disease. Correlation with CT or MRI was recommended.

A follow-up CT scan (Fig. 6.18) showed diffuse brain atrophy consistent with the patient's age. In addition, an old left posterior parietal-occipital infarction was observed. No intracranial mass, acute hemorrhage, or acute infarction was reported.

Teaching Point:

When used as an initial screen in patients suspected of Alzheimer's disease, the cerebral SPECT scan may reveal focal deficits compatible with areas of infarction or other abnormalities that do not conform with the original diagnosis. When regions of absent perfusion are observed, CT or MR imaging studies should be requested to clarify the diagnosis further.

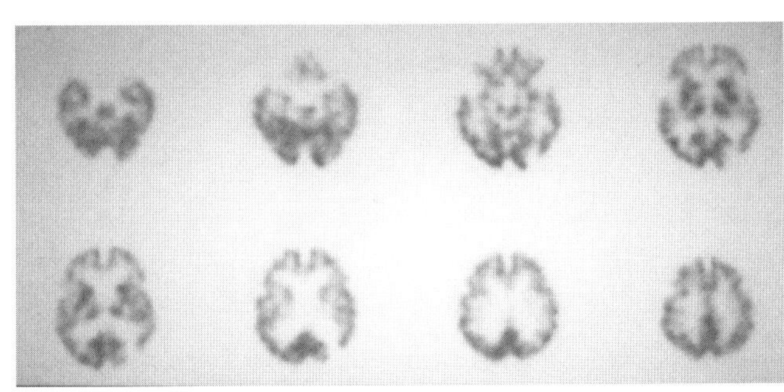

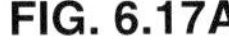

FIG. 6.17A

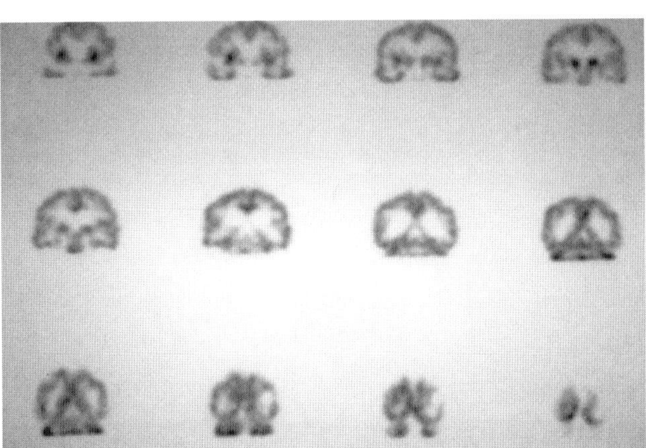

FIG. 6.17B

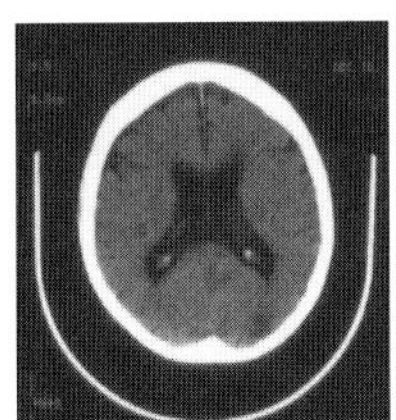

FIG. 6.18

CASE 6-13

Clinical Diagnosis: Bilateral Posterior Parietal-Temporal Infarctions

CONTRIBUTOR:	**IMAGING DATA:**	
Name: Ronald L. Van Heertum, M.D. **Institution:** Columbia-Presbyterian Medical Center	**Camera:** Picker Prism 3000 **Isotope:** ^{99m}Tc HMPAO	**Collimator:** Ultra-high resolution, fan beam **Dose:** 20.0 mCi

This 78-year-old man was referred for further evaluation of progressive memory loss. The patient had a known prior history of cerebrovascular disease.

A CT scan (Fig. 6.19) revealed bilateral temporal parietal hypodensities consistent with infarctions.

An HMPAO SPECT study (Fig. 6.20), in the transaxial **(A),** coronal **(B),** and sagittal **(C)** planes, revealed absent radiotracer activity bilaterally in the areas of infarction seen on the prior CT scan.

Teaching Point:

This case emphasizes the importance of correlating the SPECT scan results with an anatomic study (CT or MRI), as not all bilateral temporal-parietal defects are due to Alzheimer's disease.

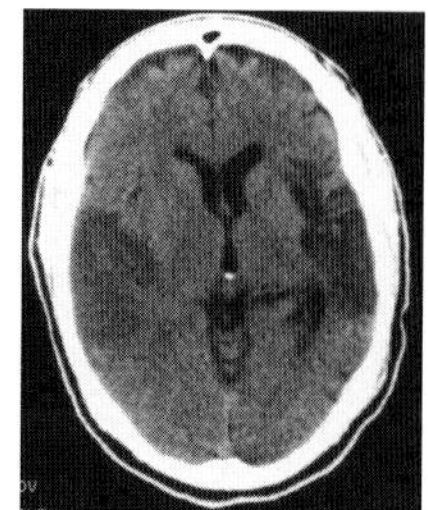
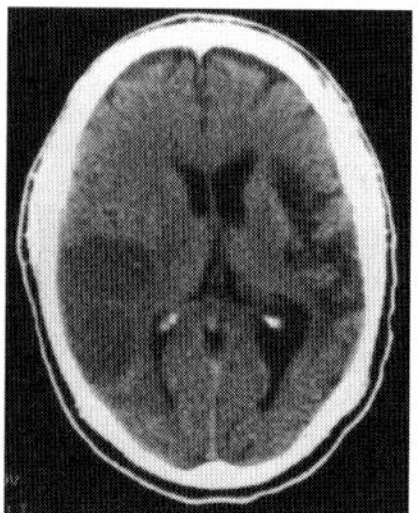

FIG. 6.19

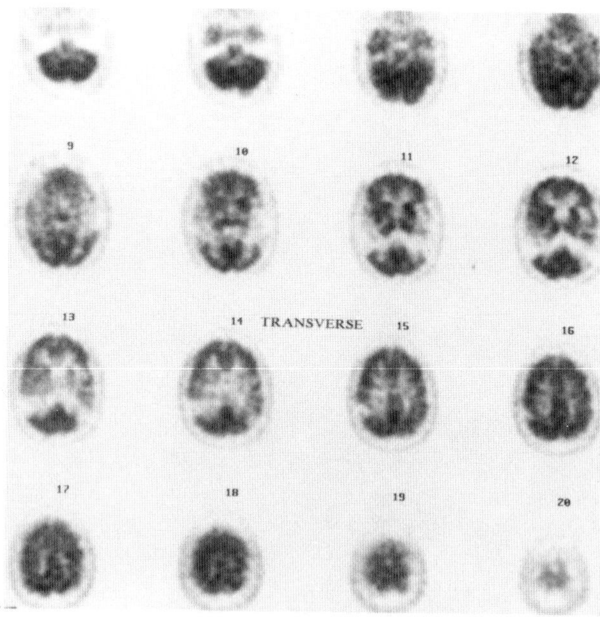

FIG. 6.20A

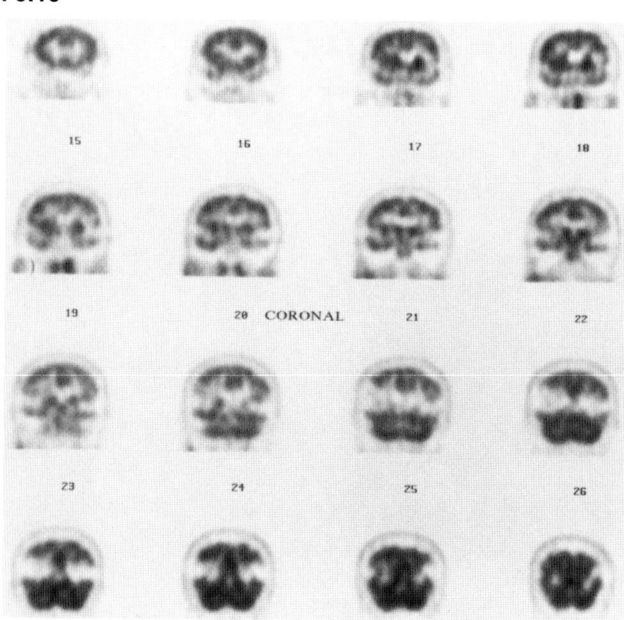

FIG. 6.20B

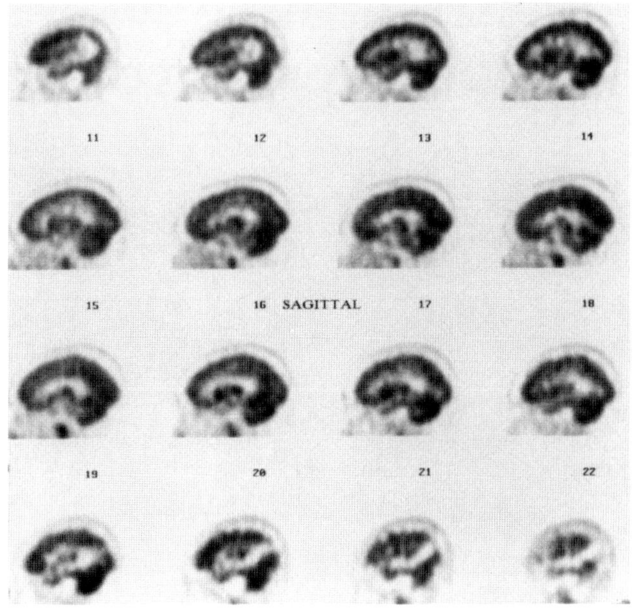

FIG. 6.20C

CASE 6-14

Clinical Diagnosis: Major Depressive Disorder

CONTRIBUTOR:	**IMAGING DATA:**	
Name: Ronald L. Van Heertum, M.D.	**Camera:** GE 400 AC/T;Star II	**Collimator:** High resolution
Institution: St. Vincent's Hospital and Medical Center	**Isotope:** ^{123}I IMP	**Dose:** 3.0 mCi

This 77-year-old man presented with mild dementia and severe depression. An electro encephalogram (EEG) revealed diffuse slow wave activity. The CT scan (Fig. 6.21) revealed moderate cortical atrophy.

A cerebral SPECT study (Fig. 6.22), in the transaxial **(A),** coronal **(B),** and sagittal **(C)** planes, revealed reduced tracer deposition in the frontal and anterior parietal lobes *(arrows)*. This pattern was more pronounced on the left side.

In addition, there was a mild degree of decreased tracer activity in the periventricular white matter corresponding to the cortical atrophy noted on the CT scan.

Teaching Point:

The overall findings on the cerebral SPECT study are consistent with a pattern of severe depression as a cause of the patient's symptoms.

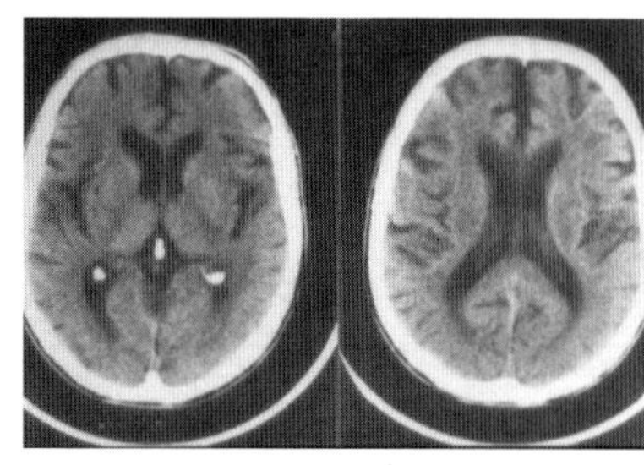

FIG. 6.21

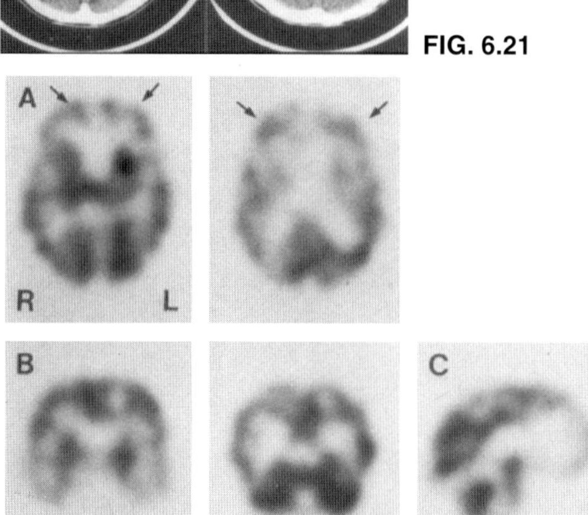

FIG. 6.22

CASE 6-15

Clinical Diagnosis: Pick's Disease

CONTRIBUTOR:

Name: Robert S. Hellman, M.D. and Ronald S. Tikofsky, M.D.
Institution: Medical College of Wisconsin

IMAGING DATA:

Camera: GE Neurocam
Isotope: ^{123}I IMP
Collimator: High resolution
Dose: 3.0 mCi

This 65-year-old man began to manifest progressively more bizarre behavior approximately 6 to 7 years prior to referral for evaluation. His long-term memory was reported to be intact, but recent memory was impaired. The patient had no significant past medical or psychiatric history. Neuropsychological testing, performed 2 years prior to his current evaluation, showed a normal cognitive performance except for the Wisconsin Card Sorting Test, which was suggestive of frontal lobe dysfunction. An EEG study was normal, and clinical examination was suggestive of frontal lobe syndrome, with a high likelihood of Pick's disease. Repeat neuropsychological examination showed a minimal decline from the previous testing with significant impairment noted on the Wisconsin Card Sorting Test with preservation. The overall findings were considered highly suggestive of a frontal lobe syndrome such as Pick's disease.

An MRI study revealed atrophy in the temporal and possibly frontal lobes.

An HMPAO SPECT (Fig. 6.23), in the transaxial plane, showed decreased radiotracer uptake in the frontal lobes bilaterally.

Teaching Point:

Bilateral decreased radiotracer uptake in the frontal lobes is a typical SPECT finding scan in frontal lobe dementias. This finding correlates well with neuropsychological performance deficits indicative of frontal lobe dysfunction. This combination of findings is often indicative of Pick's disease.

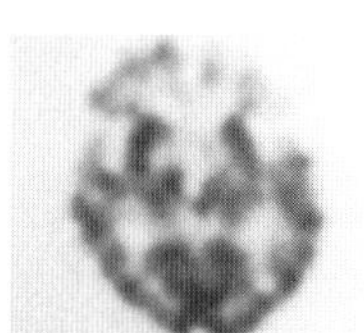
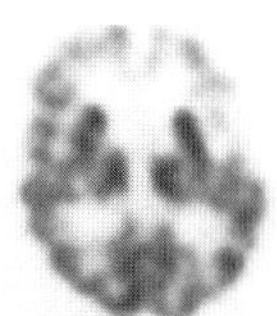
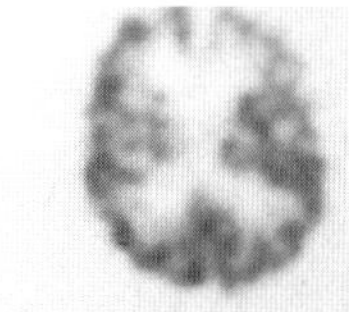

FIG. 6.23

CASE 6-16

Clinical Diagnosis:

Primary Degenerative Dementia: Pick's Disease vs. Frontal Lobe Dementia; Parkinsonism Secondary to Primary Degenerative Dementia

CONTRIBUTOR:

Name: Robert S. Hellman, M.D. and Ronald S. Tikofsky, M.D.

Institution: Medical College of Wisconsin

IMAGING DATA:

Camera: GE Neurocam

Isotope: ^{123}I IMP

Collimator: High resolution

Dose: 8.1 mCi

This 76-year-old woman with a 2-year history of mental deterioration was admitted to the behavioral psychiatry unit for further evaluation. Neuropsychological evaluation was suggestive of senile dementia of the Alzheimer's type (SDAT). At the time of evaluation her speech showed perserveration and echolalia. Rehospitalizations in 1992 and 1993 indicated that Parkinson's disease had developed secondary to the primary dementia and that she was showing further decline in cognitive and motor functions suggestive of frontal lobe dysfunction.

An MRI showed marked atrophy with enlarged ventricles.

An HMPAO SPECT study (Fig. 6.24) in the transaxial **(A)** and saggital **(B)** planes showed a significant decrease in radiotracer uptake in the frontal lobes bilaterally, which was felt to be consistent with frontal lobe dementia, possibly Pick's disease.

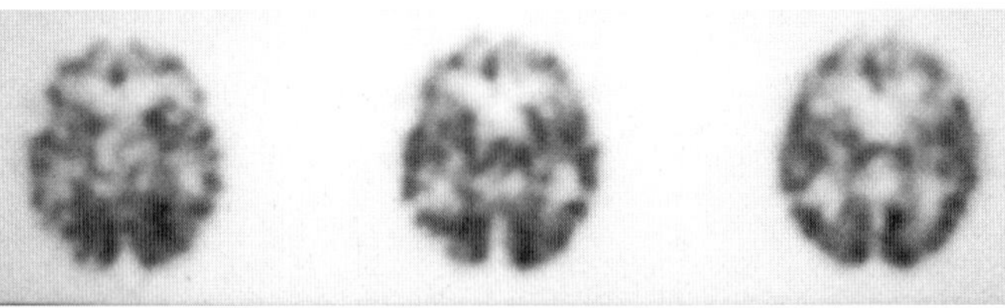

FIG. 6.24A

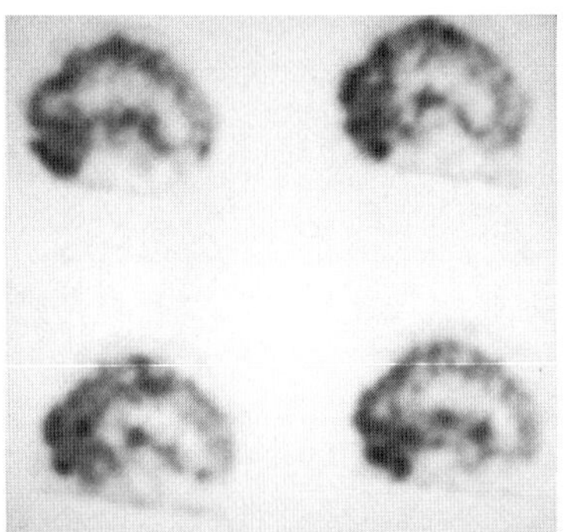

FIG. 6.24B

CASE 6-17

Clinical Diagnosis: Parkinson's Disease with Dementia

CONTRIBUTOR:	**IMAGING DATA:**	
Name: Robert S. Hellman, M.D. and Ronald S. Tikofsky, M.D.	**Camera:** GE 400 AC/T;Star	**Collimator:** High resolution
Institution: Medical College of Wisconsin	**Isotope:** ^{123}I IMP	**Dose:** 4.1 mCi

This 73-year-old man presented as an outpatient to the Dementia Clinic with the chief complaint of a progressive change in memory and cognitive function over 1 1/2 years. During this period the patient's Parkinson's disease had also progressed. The patient was reported to be aggressive, paranoid, increasingly confused, and disoriented. The Mini-Mental Status Examination revealed the patient to be severely impaired (0/30).

An MRI showed senescent cerebral and cerebellar white matter changes consistent with underlying small vessel disease, as well as mild diffuse cortical atrophy.

An HMPAO SPECT study (Fig. 6.25) in the transaxial **(A)** and sagittal **(B)** planes showed diffuse decreased radiotracer activity throughout the entire cortex except for the cerebellum, basal ganglia, motor/sensory, and occipital regions.

The pathologic diagnosis based on autopsy brain examination was that of moderate Alzheimer's disease and Parkinson's disease, an old cerebellar infarct, and slight changes in the thalamus.

Teaching Point:

Cerebral SPECT scans will not always show changes in the basal ganglia in patients with Parkinson's disease. However, cortical changes reflecting the presence of a dementing process associated with Parkinson's disease will frequently be evident.

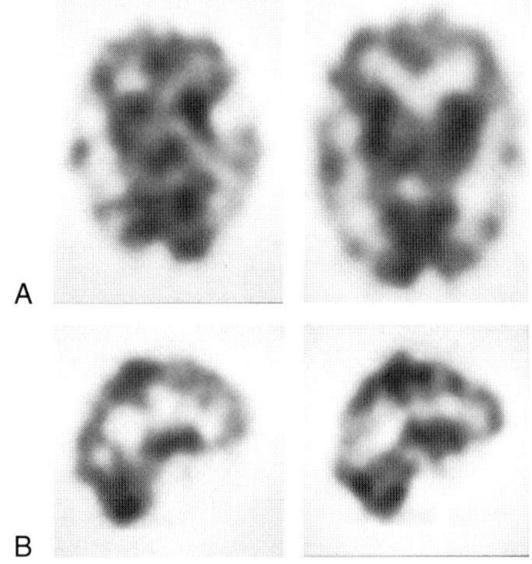

FIG. 6.25

CASE 6-18 Clinical Diagnosis: Normal Pressure Hydrocephalus

CONTRIBUTOR:

Name: Robert S. Hellman, M.D. and Ronald S. Tikofsky, M.D.
Institution: Medical College of Wisconsin

IMAGING DATA:

Camera: GE 400 AC/T;Star
Isotope: ^{123}I IMP
Collimator: High resolution
Dose: 5.0 mCi

This 55-year-old woman was referred for evaluation of a rapid onset of confusion, ataxia, and urinary incontinence.

T2-weighted initial MRI study (Fig. 6.26) showed markedly enlarged lateral and third ventricles and abnormal periventricular high signal.

A cerebral SPECT study (Fig. 6.27) in the transaxial plane showed that tracer activity was reduced in the periventricular white matter, corresponding to the ventricular dilation demonstrated on the MRI scan. In addition, tracer activity was decreased in the right occipital lobe.

A follow-up cerebral SPECT study (Fig. 6.29) performed the next day showed a normal, symmetric distribution of tracer.

Two months after a ventriculoperitoneal shunt procedure, a repeat MRI study (Fig. 6.28) demonstrated a significant decrease in the size of the lateral ventricles, with a VP shunt L tube in place.

Clinically, the patient appeared normal in all physical and mental functions.

Teaching Point:

The pattern in this case is typical of the findings noted in normal pressure hydrocephalus.

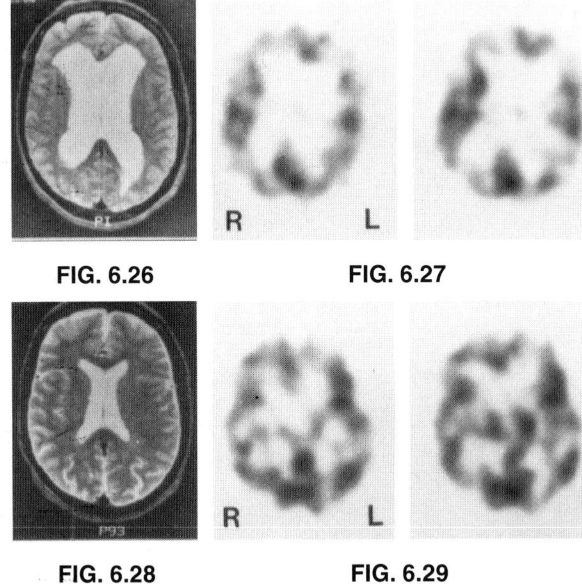

FIG. 6.26 FIG. 6.27

FIG. 6.28 FIG. 6.29

CASE 6-19

Clinical Diagnosis:
Huntington's Disease

CONTRIBUTOR:

Name: Ronald L. Van Heertum, M.D.
Institution: St. Vincent's Hospital and Medical Center

IMAGING DATA:

Camera: GE 400 AC/T;Star II
Isotope: ^{123}I IMP
Collimator: High resolution
Dose: 3.0 mCi

This 55-year-old man was referred for an ongoing evaluation of his known Huntington's disease with mild dementia of 9 years' duration.

A CT scan (Fig. 6.30) showed diffuse atrophy of the cerebral cortex.

The cerebral SPECT study (Fig. 6.31), in the transaxial **(A),** coronal **(B),** and sagittal **(C)** planes, revealed decreased tracer deposition throughout the cerebral cortex and periventricular white matter, corresponding to the cortical atrophy noted on the CT scan. In addition, tracer deposition was absent bilaterally in the caudate nuclei *(arrows).*

Teaching Point:

Absent or markedly diminished tracer activity in the caudate nuclei is a frequent and characteristic pattern observed in patients with Huntington's disease.

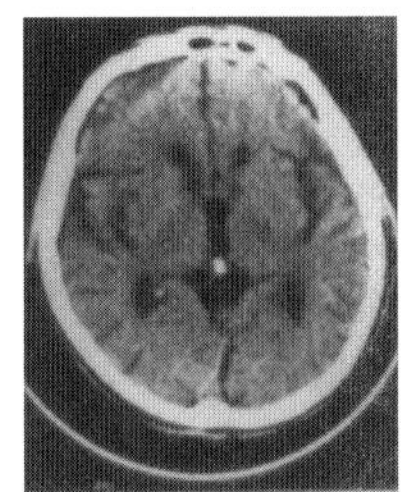

FIG. 6.30

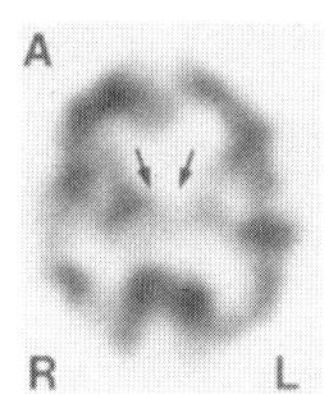

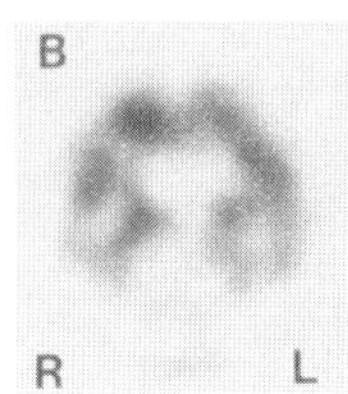

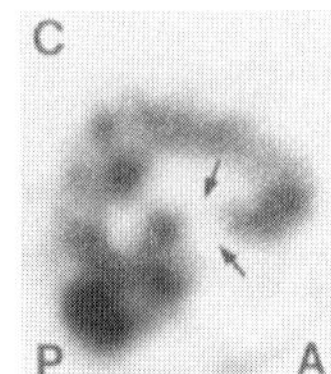

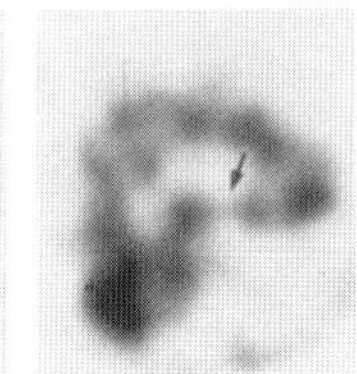

FIG. 6.31

CASE 6-20

Clinical Diagnosis:
Huntington's Disease with Progressive Dementia

CONTRIBUTOR:

Name: Ronald L. Van Heertum, M.D.
Institution: St. Vincent's Hospital and Medical Center

IMAGING DATA:

Camera: GE 400 AC/T;Star II
Isotope: ^{123}I IMP
Collimator: High resolution
Dose: 3.0 mCi

This 45-year-old man was referred for evaluation of progressive dementia and athetosis. The patient's mother had previously been given a diagnosis of Huntington's disease.

A cerebral SPECT study (Fig. 6.32), in the transaxial **(A),** coronal **(B),** and sagittal **(C)** planes, revealed a marked decrease in tracer deposition in the caudate nuclei *(arrows).* The findings were felt to be compatible with Huntington's disease.

Teaching Point:

This case presents an earlier form of Huntington's disease. In this particular case, the cerebral SPECT study was helpful in establishing the final diagnosis.

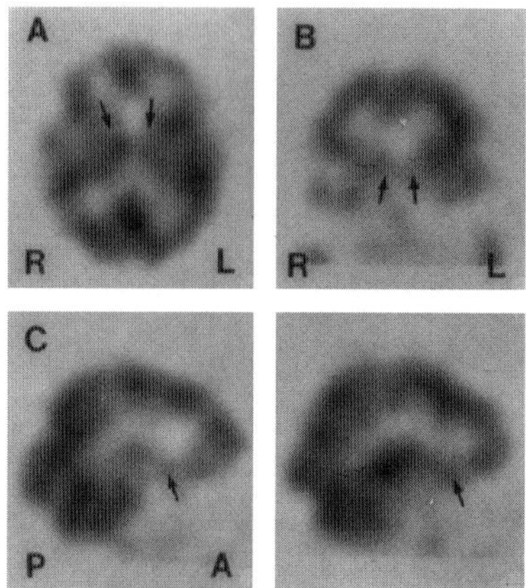

FIG. 6.32

CASE 6-21

Clinical Diagnosis: Huntington's Disease

CONTRIBUTOR:

Name: Robert S. Hellman, M.D. and Ronald S. Tikofsky, M.D.
Institution: Medical College of Wisconsin

IMAGING DATA:

Camera: GE Neurocam
Isotope: ^{123}I IMP
Collimator: High resolution
Dose: 3.0 mCi

This 33-year-old woman with a known history of Huntington's disease was referred for evaluation of an exacerbation of symptoms. At the time of presentation, the patient's symptoms had progressed, with a recent increase in uncontrollable movements and episodes of choking during eating.

An MRI (Fig. 6.33) demonstrated atrophic caudate nuclei bilaterally consistent with the patient's diagnosis of Huntington's disease. There was also a subtle increase in signal intensity in the putamen bilaterally.

An HMPAO SPECT study (Fig. 6.34) in the transaxial plane showed decreased tracer uptake in both caudate nuclei, right greater than left. Decrease in tracer uptake was also observed in the right temporal region. These findings are compatible with the diagnosis of Huntington's disease.

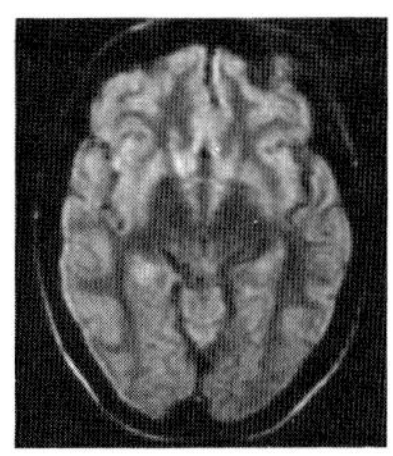

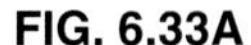

FIG. 6.33A

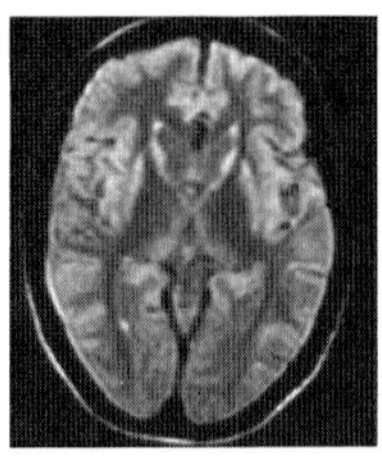

FIG. 6.33B

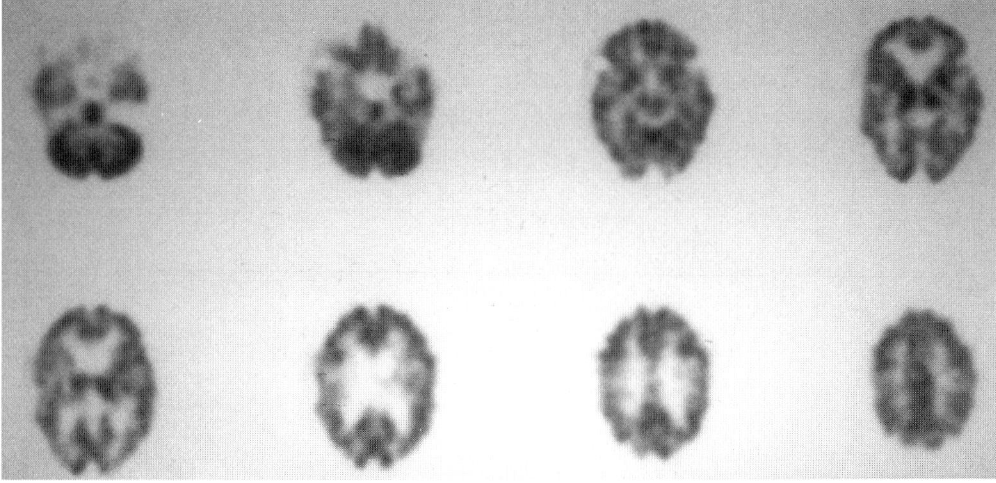

FIG. 6.34

CASE 6-22

Clinical Diagnosis: Huntington's Disease

CONTRIBUTOR:	**IMAGING DATA:**	
Name: Robert S. Hellman, M.D. and Ronald S. Tikofsky, M.D.	**Camera:** GE Neurocam	**Collimator:** High resolution
Institution: Medical College of Wisconsin	**Isotope:** ^{123}I IMP	**Dose:** 3.0 mCi

This 40-year-old woman was referred for further evaluation of a long history of Huntington's disease with progressive dementia.

A CT scan (Fig. 6.35) showed diffuse cerebral atrophy with mild dilation of the lateral and third ventricles. In addition, the caudate nuclei were indistinctly visualized.

An HMPAO study (Fig. 6.36) in the transaxial plane revealed markedly decreased tracer uptake in the caudate nuclei. The decrease in tracer activity was greater on the left. There is also decreased tracer uptake in the right inferior frontal lobe.

Teaching Point:

The caudate nuclei will not be well visualized in Huntington's disease. SPECT images will reflect either absent tracer uptake or various degrees of reduced tracer uptake. These findings may be asymmetric. The presence of decreased tracer uptake in the cortex typically occurs with changes in cognitive function.

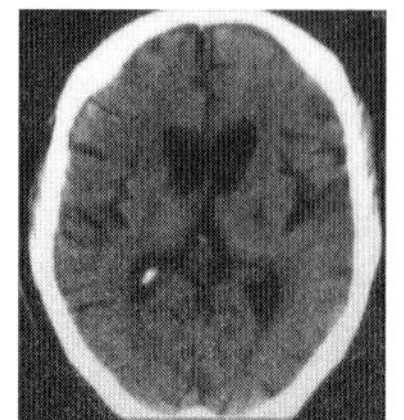

FIG. 6.35A

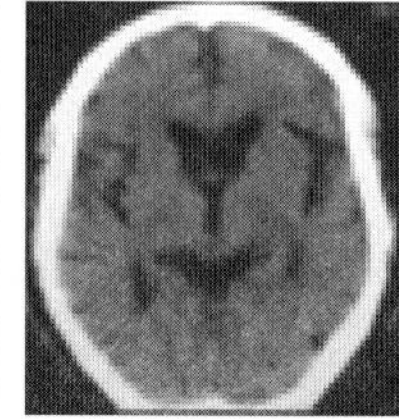

FIG. 6.35B

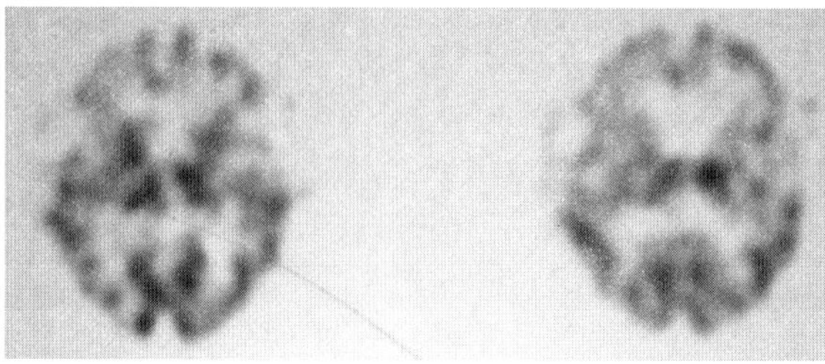

FIG. 6.36

CASE 6-23

Clinical Diagnosis: AIDS-Related Dementia

CONTRIBUTOR:	**IMAGING DATA:**	
Name: Ronald L. Van Heertum, M.D.	**Camera:** GE 400 AC/T;Star II	**Collimator:** High resolution
Institution: St. Vincent's Hospital and Medical Center	**Isotope:** ^{123}I IMP	**Dose:** 3.0 mCi

This 37-year-old bisexual man was referred for evaluation of the acute onset of dementia; he also complained of blurred vision and generalized headaches. His neurological examination revealed a right hemiparesis and an expressive aphasia. Laboratory tests showed him to be seropositive for the HIV antigen.

A CT scan (Fig. 6.37) was negative.

A SPECT study (Fig. 6.38), in the transaxial **(A),** coronal **(B),** and sagittal **(C)** planes, showed a decreased tracer deposition in the left frontal and parietal-occipital lobes *(arrowheads),* with a slight decrease in tracer activity in the right parietal-occipital lobe *(open arrow).* Tracer deposition was also decreased in then thalamus, particularly on the left side *(arrow).*

Teaching Point:

As shown in this case, the cerebral SPECT study may be positive despite a negative CT or MRI scan. The typical pattern in AIDS-related dementia shows random cortical defects combined with subcortical defects.

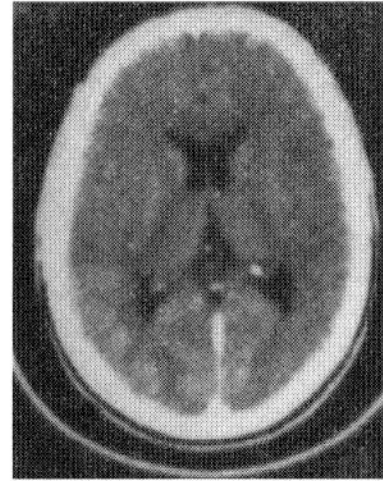

FIG. 6.37

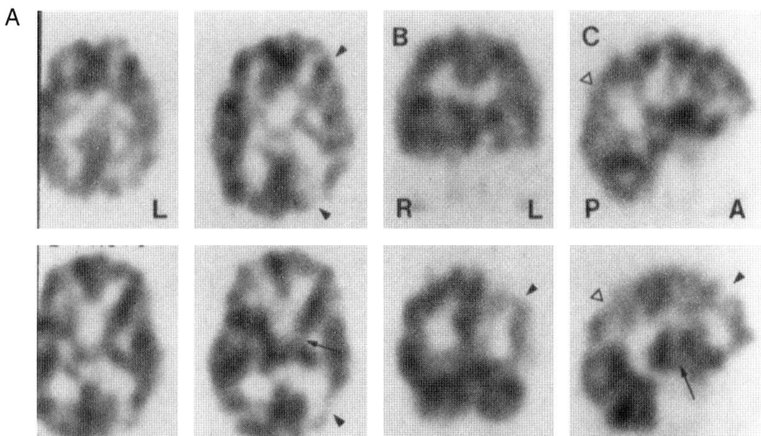

FIG. 6.38

CASE 6-24 Clinical Diagnosis: HIV Encephalopathy

CONTRIBUTOR:

Name: Scott Miller, M.D.
Institution: Columbia-Presbyterian Medical Center

IMAGING DATA:

Camera: GE Neurocam
Isotope: ^{99m}Tc HMPAO
Collimator: Ultra-high resolution
Dose: 21.7 mCi

This 42-year-old woman with known AIDS was referred for evaluation of a progressive alteration in her mental status characterized by increasing apathy, confusion, and progressive memory loss.

An MRI examination revealed mild cortical atrophy.

HMPAO SPECT (Fig. 6.39), in the transaxial **(A),** coronal **(B),** and sagittal **(C)** planes, revealed an overall decrease in radiotracer uptake with a superimposed markedly heterogeneous distribution pattern throughout the cerebral cortex.

Published with permission: ***Radiol Clin North Am* 1993;31:881–907.**

Teaching Point:

Cerebral SPECT is a highly sensitive technique for the detection of HIV encephalopathy.

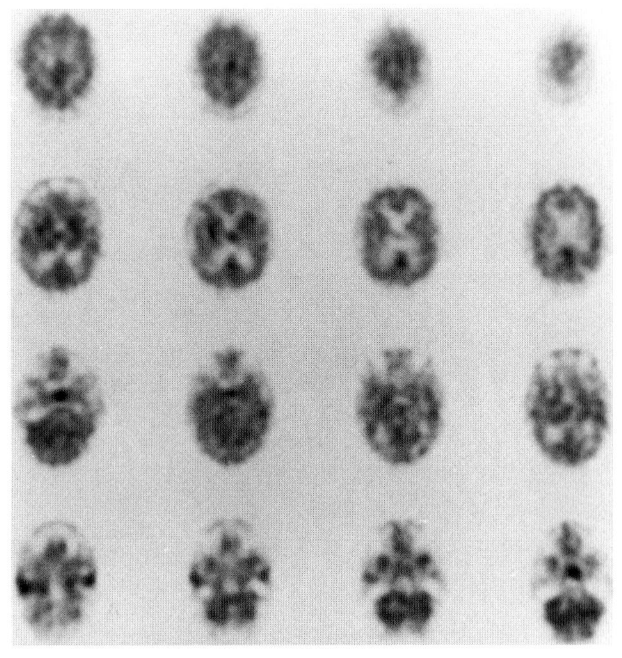

FIG. 6.39A

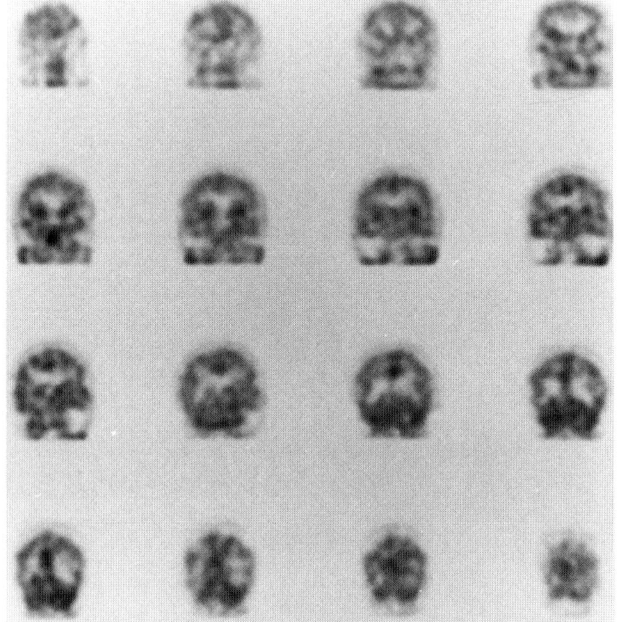

FIG. 6.39B

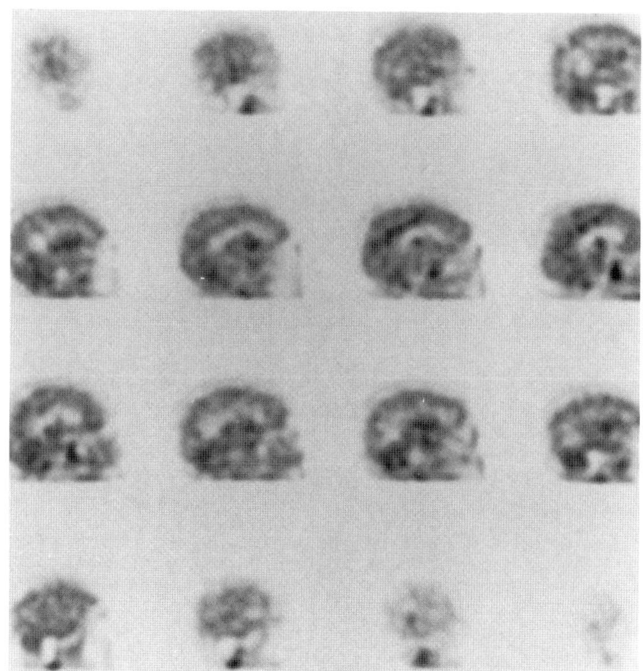

FIG. 6.39C

CASE 6-25 Clinical Diagnosis: Severe HIV Encephalopathy

CONTRIBUTOR:

Name: Ronald L. Van Heertum, M.D.
Institution: Columbia-Presbyterian Medical Center

IMAGING DATA:

Camera: GE 3000 XCT
Isotope: ^{123}I IMP
Collimator: LEAP
Dose: 4.0 mCi

This 42-year-old known HIV-seropositive man presented for evaluation of progressive memory impairment and spasticity of his lower extremities.

CT scan (Fig. 6.40) revealed severe diffuse cortical atrophy.

IMP SPECT (Fig. 6.41) in the coronal **(A)** and sagittal **(B)** planes revealed a diffusely reduced and heterogeneous cortical radiotracer uptake with marked prominence of the periventricular white matter was disproportionately larger than the size of the ventricles noted on CT.

Teaching Point:

This case demonstrates the advanced changes that may be seen in HIV encephalopathy.

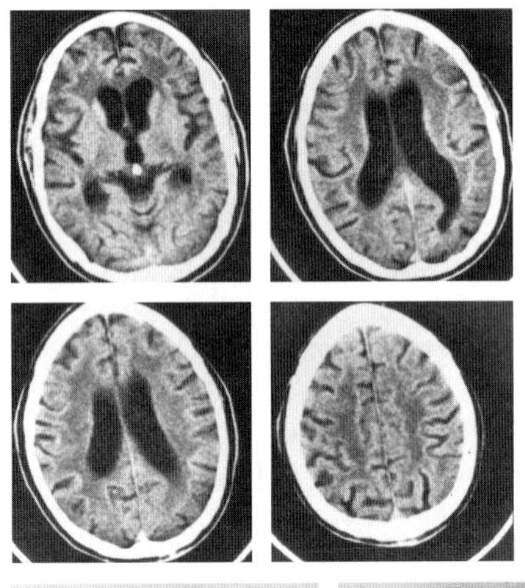

FIG. 6.40

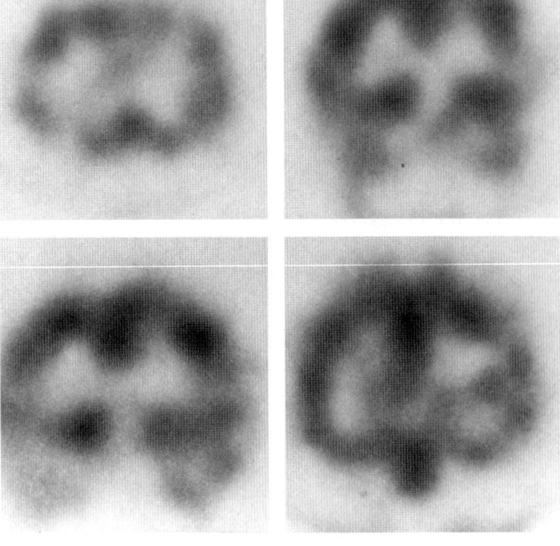

FIG. 6.41A

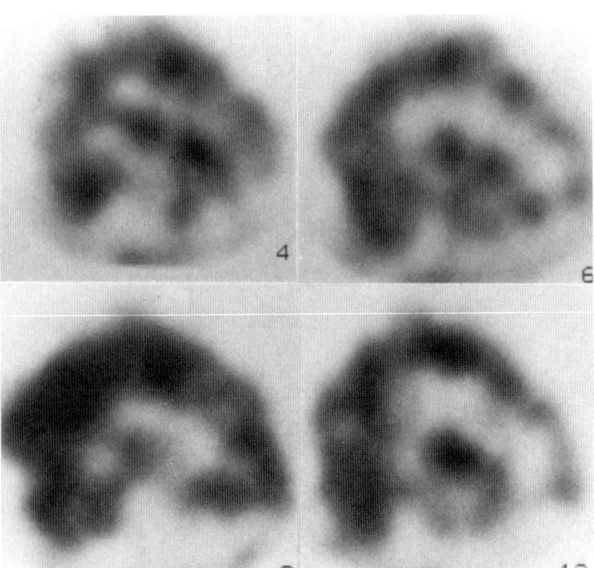

FIG. 6.41B

CASE 6-26

Clinical Diagnosis: HIV Encephalopathy: Pre- and Post Azodithymidine Therapy

CONTRIBUTOR:	**IMAGING DATA:**	
Name: Ronald L. Van Heertum, M.D.	**Camera:** GE 3000 XCT	**Collimator:** Ultra-high resolution
Institution: Columbia-Presbyterian Medical Center	**Isotope:** ^{99m}Tc HMPAO	**Dose:** 1) 21.0 mCi; 2) 20.5 mCi

This 30-year-old known HIV-seropositive man presented for evaluation of progressive memory loss.

CT scan was negative.

The initial HMPAO SPECT (Fig. 6.42), in the coronal **(A)** and sagittal **(B)** planes, revealed a mild overall reduction in radiotracer uptake with a heterogeneous distribution throughout the cortex.

Subsequent to the initial SPECT scan the patient was placed on azodithymidine with significant clinical improvement.

A follow-up HMPAO SPECT study (Fig. 6.43), in the coronal **(A)** and sagittal **(B)** planes, revealed an overall improvement in radiotracer distribution.

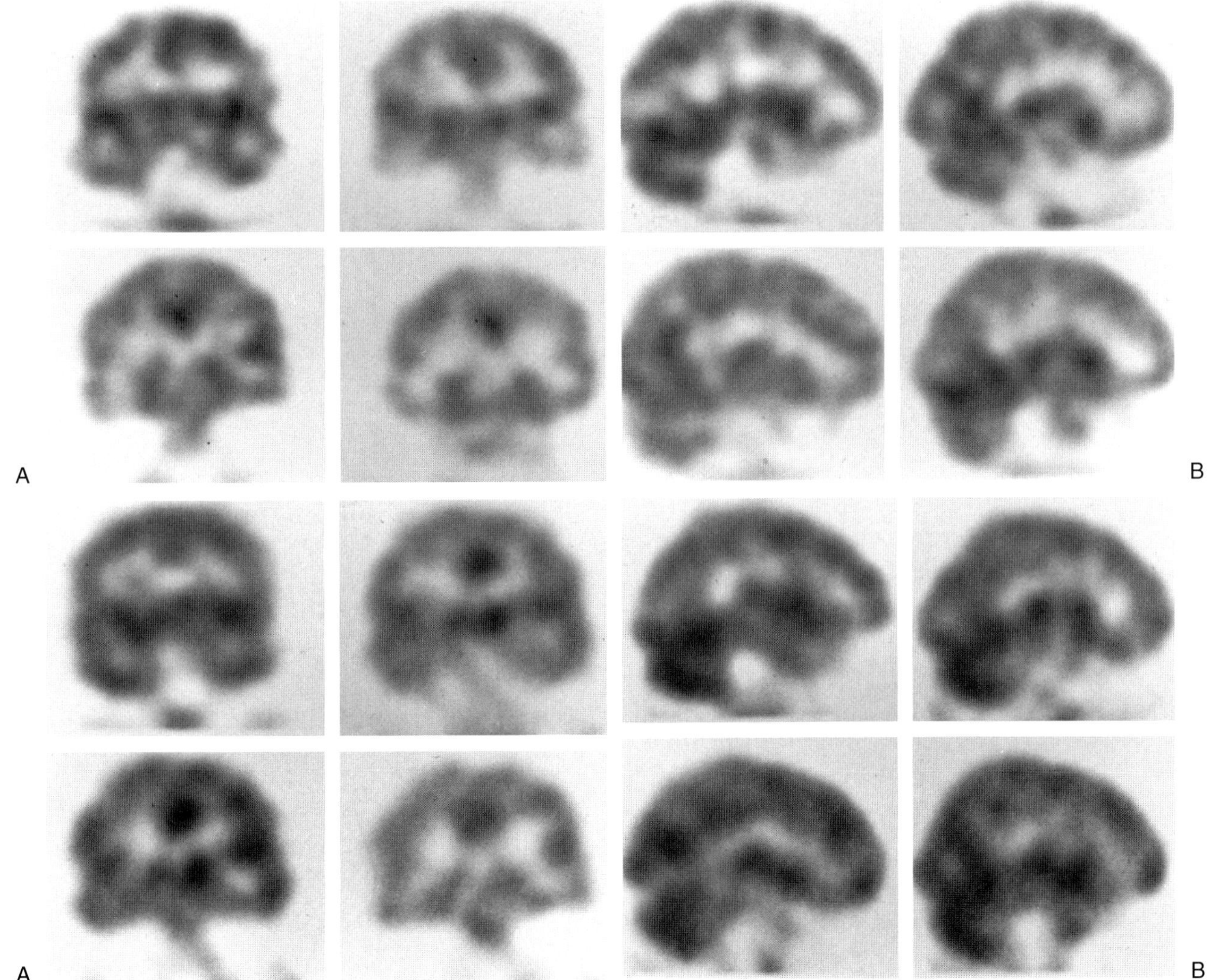

FIG. 6.42 (top) and **FIG. 6.43** (bottom)

CASE 6-27

Clinical Diagnosis:

Left Arachnoid Cyst

CONTRIBUTOR:	IMAGING DATA:	
Name: David L. Kaufman, M.D.	**Camera:** GE 400 ACT.T;Star II	**Collimator:** High resolution
Institution: St. Vincent's Hospital and Medical Center	**Isotope:** ^{123}I IMP	**Dose:** 3.0 mCi

This 40-year-old homosexual man, known to be seropositive for HIV, was referred for evaluation of a progressive loss of concentration over 3 months.

A cerebral SPECT study (Fig. 6.44), in the transaxial **(A),** coronal **(B),** and sagittal **(C)** planes, showed absent tracer deposition in the left frontal lobe laterally. The area of absent activity appeared to be extracerebral.

As a consequence of this finding, a follow-up CT scan (Fig. 6.45) was performed; it demonstrated a large cystic area at the lateral aspect of the left frontal lobe.

Teaching Point:

The findings on cerebral SPECT studies may be lacking in specificity. In such instances, CT or MRI scans should be correlated with the SPECT studies to characterize the abnormality better.

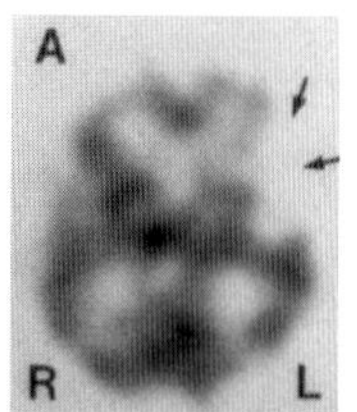

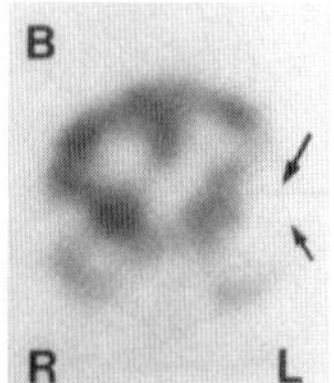

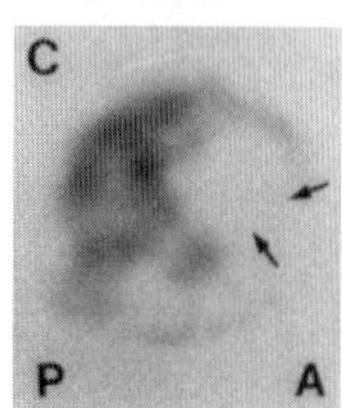

FIG. 6.44

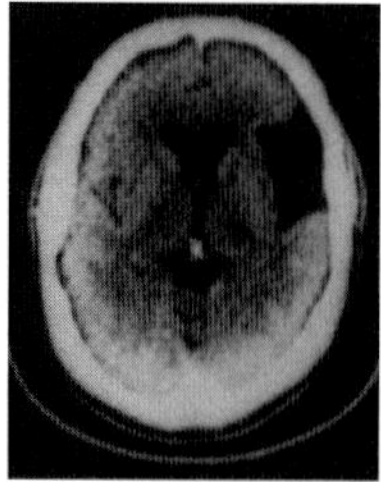

FIG. 6.45

CASE 6-28

Clinical Diagnosis: AIDS with Cerebral Toxoplasmosis

CONTRIBUTOR:

Name: Ronald L. Van Heertum, M.D.
Institution: St. Vincent's Hospital and Medical Center

IMAGING DATA:

Camera: GE 400 AC/T;Star II
Isotope: ^{123}I IMP
Collimator: High resolution
Dose: 3.0 mCi

This 39-year-old homosexual man was referred for evaluation of severe headaches of 1 month's duration. In addition, he reported blurred vision, intermittent chills, and night sweats. Neurological examination revealed a left homonymous hemianopsia.

A CT scan showed a large right parietal-occipital hypodensity with ring enhancement, with a mass effect on the surrounding structures.

A cerebral SPECT study (Fig. 6.46) in the transaxial plane demonstrated absent tracer deposition in the right parietal-occipital and posterior temporal areas *(arrows)*, corresponding to the area of abnormality on the CT scan. The overall findings were compatible with the final diagnosis of cerebral toxoplasmosis.

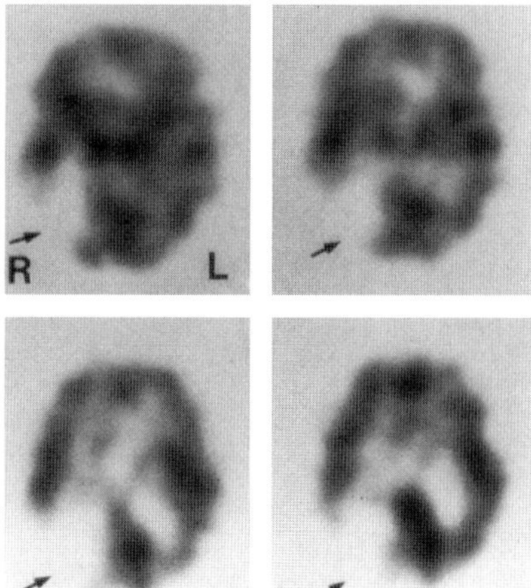

FIG. 6.46

CASE 6-29 Clinical Diagnosis:

Chronic Ethanol Abuse

CONTRIBUTOR:

Name: Ronald L. Van Heertum, M.D.
Institution: St. Vincent's Hospital and Medical Center

IMAGING DATA:

Camera: GE 400 AC/T;Star II
Isotope: ^{123}I IMP
Collimator: High resolution
Dose: 3.0 mCi

This 26-year-old man was referred for evaluation of progressive loss of memory. He had a long history of alcohol abuse, with frequent episodes of violent behavior when intoxicated.

A CT scan (Fig. 6.47) was within normal limits.

A cerebral SPECT study (Fig. 6.48), in the transaxial **(A)**, coronal **(B)**, and sagittal **(C)** planes, showed a highly heterogeneous pattern of tracer distribution throughout the cerebral cortex and cerebellar hemispheres.

Teaching Point:

This pattern of tracer distribution is typical of alcohol and drug abuse patients. This heterogeneous distribution is quite different from the patterns seen in Alzheimer's disease, vascular dementia, and pseudodementia of major depression. The pattern of uptake may, however, be difficult, if not impossible, to differentiate from HIV encephalopathy.

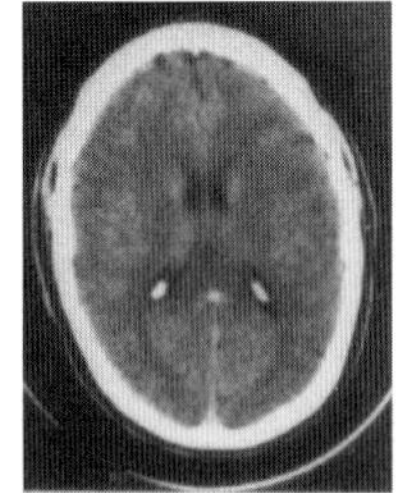

FIG. 6.47

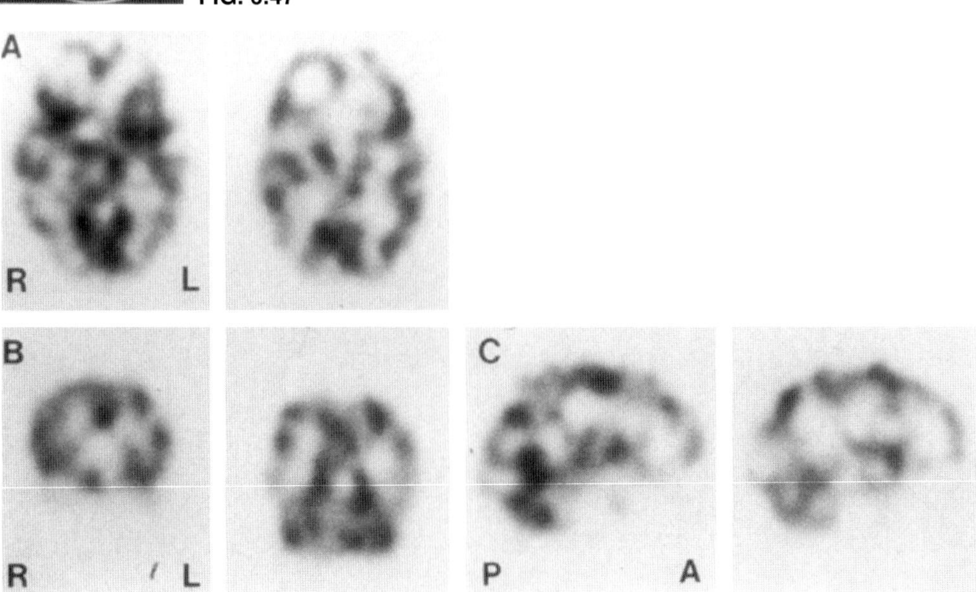

FIG. 6.48

CASE 6-30 Clinical Diagnosis: Chronic Polysubstance Abuse

CONTRIBUTOR:

Name: L.M. Konopka, M.D., J.W. Crayton, M.D., and T.J. Milo, M.D.
Institution: Hines VA Hospital

IMAGING DATA:

Camera: TRIAD
Isotope: ^{99m}Tc HMPAO
Collimator: Ultra-high, fan beam
Dose: 25 mCi

This 32-year-old male presented with a 4-year history of cocaine and alcohol abuse. The patient stated that he free-based approximately 300 to 500 dollars of cocaine weekly. He had last used cocaine 1 week prior to admission. The patient also admitted that he had consumed a pint to a fifth of whiskey each day for the past 2 years. At the time of presentation, the patient noted frequent blackouts and migraine headaches, which were treated with Motrin 600 mg tid. He denied any history of delirium tremens or seizures.

The HMPAO SPECT study (Fig. 6.49) in the transaxial plane revealed multiple small deficits throughout the cortex, consistent with polysubstance abuse.

Teaching Point:

The perfusion brain SPECT pattern seen in known polysubstance abuse patients may be indistinguishable from the pattern of abnormality seen in AIDS-related dementia.

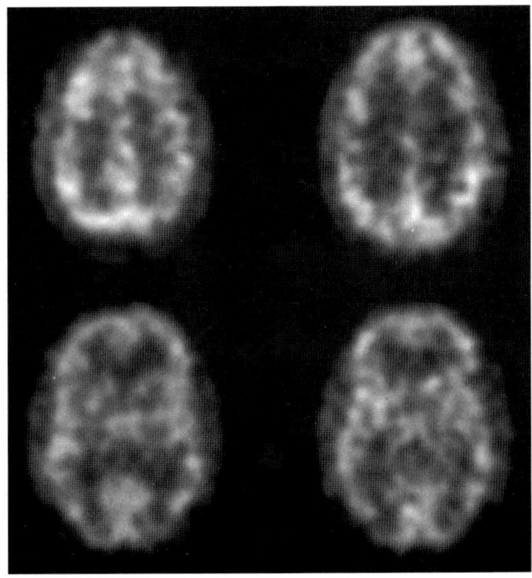

FIG. 6.49

CASE 6-31

Clinical Diagnosis:

Chronic Crack Abuse

CONTRIBUTOR:	IMAGING DATA:	
Name: David A. Weber, Ph.D. and Dinko Franceschi, M.D.	**Camera:** Toshiba-901	**Collimator:** ^{123}I
Institution: Brookhaven National Laboratory	**Isotope:** ^{123}I IMP	**Dose:** 3.0 mCi

This 32-year-old man with a 5-year history of crack use was referred for further evaluation. The patient stated that he had used 10 gs/week of crack for the past 5 years. He denied any other substance abuse and at present was asymptomatic.

The IMP SPECT study (Fig. 6.50) in the transaxial plane revealed multiple focal areas of decreased or absent radiotracer activity throughout the cerebral cortex.

Teaching Point:

IMP SPECT studies may reveal significant alterations in rCBF despite the fact that patients are reported to be clinically asymptomatic. The extent and severity of the SPECT changes correlate well with the degree of impairment noted on neuropsychological testing.

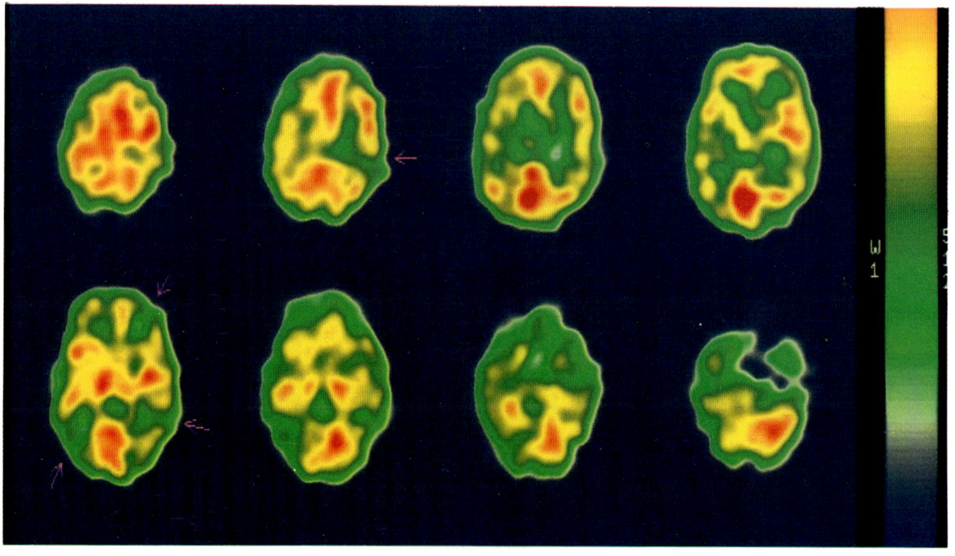

FIG. 6.50

CASE 6-32

Clinical Diagnosis: Chronic Crack Abuse

CONTRIBUTOR:	IMAGING DATA:	
Name: David A. Weber, Ph.D. and Dinko Franceschi, M.D.	**Camera:** Toshiba 901-A	**Collimator:** ^{123}I
Institution: Brookhaven National Laboratory	**Isotope:** ^{123}I IMP	**Dose:** 3.0 mCi

This 32-year-old man with a known 9-year history of crack abuse was referred for further evaluation. This patient stated that he had used 12 gs/week of crack for the past 9 years.

The IMP SPECT study (Fig. 6.51) in the transaxial plane revealed extensive cortical perfusion deficits diffusely throughout both cerebral hemispheres.

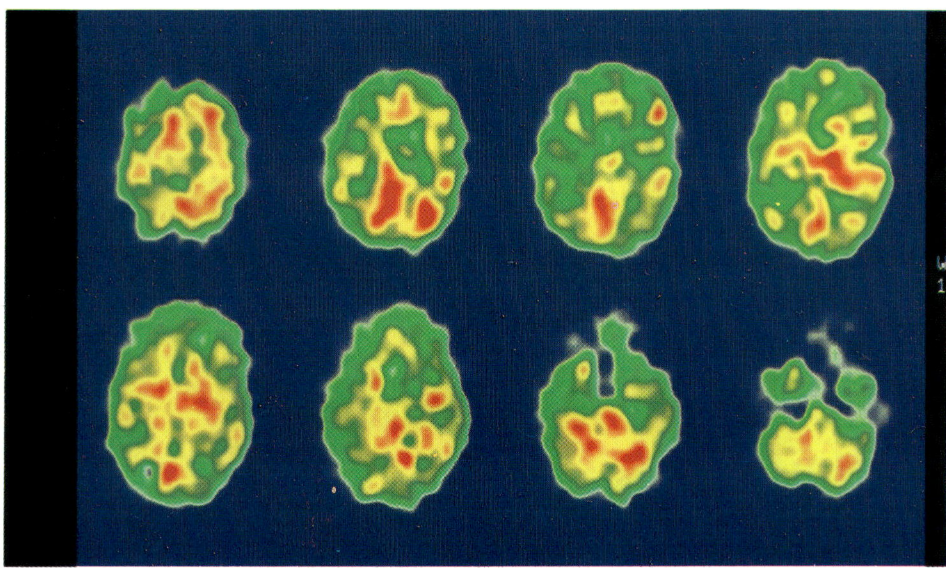

FIG. 6.51

CASE 6-33

Clinical Diagnosis:
Meningioma; Possible Alzheimer's Disease

CONTRIBUTOR:	IMAGING DATA:	
Name: Ramy Nour, M.D.	**Camera:** GE 400 AC/T;Star	**Collimator:** High resolution
Institution: Columbia-Presbyterian Medical Center	**Isotope:** ^{123}I IMP	**Dose:** 21.6 mCi

This 71-year-old woman with a known hypertension and diabetes mellitus, presented with a 1-year history of progressive cognitive decline. In particular, she was noted to have profound short- and long-term memory loss, language dysfunction, and impaired abstract reasoning.

An MRI scan (Fig. 6.52) in the axial **(A)** and coronal **(B)** planes demonstrated a mass lesion consistent with a meningioma adjacent to the left temporal lobe.

The finding of a meningioma was felt to be an incidental finding unrelated to the patient's cognitive decline. As a result, the patient had been given a provisional clinical diagnosis of Alzheimer's disease.

An HMPAO SPECT study (Fig. 6.53) in the transaxial plane revealed a focal area of increased radiotracer activity corresponding to the meningioma seen on the MRI study.

Teaching Point:

This case demonstrates the importance of correlating the SPECT and MRI studies. Other causes of focal increase in radiotracer activity include other tumors, seizure disorders, and luxury perfusion.

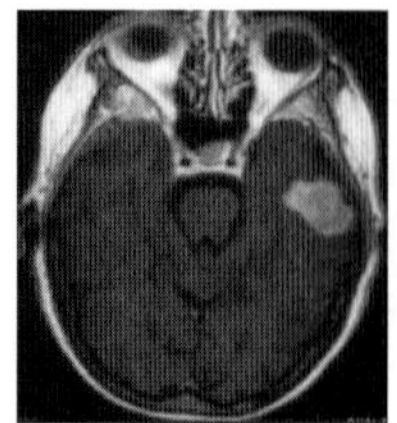

FIG. 6.52A

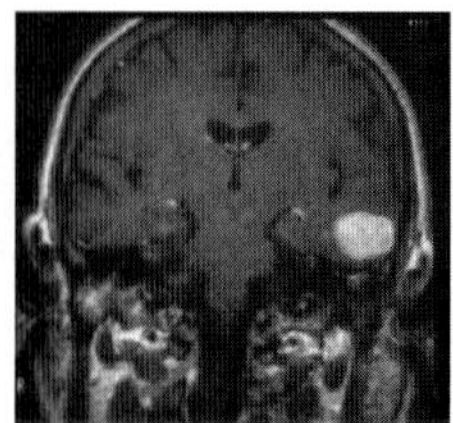

FIG. 6.52B

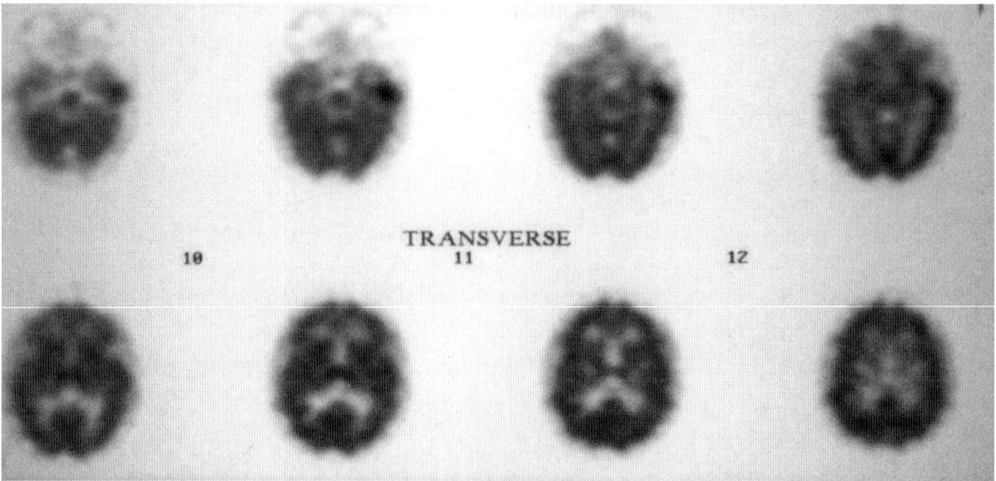

FIG. 6.53

Cerebral SPECT Imaging, Second Edition,
edited by R.L. Van Heertum and R.S. Tikofsky.
Raven Press, Ltd., New York © 1995.

CHAPTER 7

Seizure Disorders

Ronald S. Tikofsky and Ronald L. Van Heertum

Devous (1) notes that approximately 50,000 persons in the United States have medically refractory seizures; of this group, 500 patients a year undergo surgical treatment to eliminate or reduce the seizures. The number of patients undergoing this treatment is expected to increase as techniques for localizing the seizure focus improve.

The clinical application of SPECT imaging in the study of patients with complicated epilepsy is becoming increasingly common in centers for the surgical treatment of complex partial seizures (2,3). Whenever a seizure patient is referred for SPECT imaging, it is important to determine the type of seizure pattern and its localization. This will help in the evaluation of the images. Many epileptic patients present with more than one type of seizure pattern. It is therefore important for the nuclear medicine community to appreciate the variability in seizure disorders. An attempt was made in 1989 to establish a universal classification system for the epilepsies by the International League against Epilepsy (ILAE) (4). At present, this classification system is still most commonly used.

The major classes of epilepsy are divided into two groups. The first separates the epilepsies with generalized seizures from those with focal or partial seizure. The latter are localization-related, partial or focal epilepsies. The second classification type distinguishes epilepsies with a known etiology (termed symptomatic or secondary) from the idiopathic (primary) and cryptogenic (those epilepsies whose etiology is unclear or occult).

The seizure syndromes that will most often be seen in the nuclear medicine laboratory are often called temporal lobe syndromes. The components of the syndrome are: simple partial seizures, complex partial seizures, and sometimes generalized seizures. In some patients there may be a combination. It is important to distinguish between simple partial seizures, whose features are autonomic and/or psychic symptoms and possibly sensory phenomena, and complex partial seizures, which often begin with motor arrest followed by automatisms. These seizures usually last < 1 min. and are followed by postictal confusion, amnesia, and gradual recovery.

Two other types of temporal lobe seizures are frequently seen. One is amygdalohippocampal, sometimes referred to as mesiobasal limbic or rhinencephalic. These are very similar to the temporal lobe group described above, but rarely are there auditory symptoms. They are characterized by epigastric distress, marked autonomic signs, fear, panic, and olfactory-gustatory hallucinations. The other groups are referred to as lateral temporal seizures (LTS). Patients with LTS, simple seizures, will have auditory hallucinations or illusions, dream-like states, and language and visual misperceptions depending on the hemisphere involved. If there is seizure propagation to the mesial temporal or extratemporal structures the simple seizures could become complex partial seizures.

Another major group of seizure patterns requires mention here. They are the frontal lobe epilepsies, which can present as simple, complex partial, secondarily generalized, or any combination of these patterns. Seizures related to the frontal lobes will occur frequently in the course of the day and may even occur during sleep; status epilepticus can be a frequent complication. Frontal lobe seizures tend to be short. In complex partial seizures, postictal confusion is unusual; there are tonic or postural motor manifestations with frequent complex gestural automatisms when the seizures begin. In the case of bilateral discharges, falling is common. Specific patterns of seizures are related to particular regions of seizure activity in the various frontal lobe territories (supplementary motor, cingulate, motor cortex,

R. S. Tikofsky: Department of Radiology, Section of Nuclear Medicine, Medical College of Wisconsin, Milwaukee, Wisconsin 53226.

R. L. Van Heertum: Department of Radiology, Columbia University College of Physicians and Surgeons, and Department of Nuclear Medicine, Columbia Presbyterian Medical Center, New York, New York 10032.

etc.). Less frequently occurring seizure patterns arise from the parietal and occipital lobes.

Numerous research reports (5,6) demonstrate that SPECT imaging can play a major role in the identification of epileptogenic foci in patients with medically intractable complex partial seizures who are being considered for surgery. In addition to performing interictal (baseline) SPECT studies, two other options are possible in studying this patient population. One is to inject the patient during ictus (7), versus in the immediate postictal state (8,9). The choice of options is somewhat dependent on institutional logistics for performing the studies and the stability of the radiopharmaceutical. Unless a stable radiopharmaceutical is available, it is very difficult to prepare the tracer and get it to the seizure unit and still capture a seizure in progress (most seizures are very brief). Stable isotopes (stable up to 6 hr) make it more likely that one can inject during seizure activity. The best situation for injecting during ictus is to have the tracer available in the unit with a member of the epilepsy team trained to prepare the kit if necessary or to inject from a prepared vial of stable tracer. While the ideal situation is to inject during the seizures, thus capturing the brain's perfusion and metabolic activity at a key point in time, postictal injections (within 5 min. after ictus) can yield clinically useful information regarding seizure localization.

The great advantage of the recently developed radiotracers for seizures studies is the fact that they provide a "snapshot" of the activity at the time of injection. Because the newer SPECT radiopharmaceuticals remain fixed in the brain, the patients can be imaged up to several hours after injection without significant changes in tracer deposition occurring. This allows sufficient time for patients to be brought to an imaging area, and it increases the probability of identifying the physiologic changes associated with an active seizure focus. Seizure patterns observed on SPECT imaging parallel those reported with positron emission tomography (PET) (10). During the interictal period, in approximately 50 percent of patients, the seizure focus is identified as an area of reduced perfusion and metabolism, and baseline (interictal) scans will often have a normal appearance; during an active seizure in approximately 80 to 90 percent of patients, an area of increased perfusion and metabolism marks the active seizure focus. In the immediate postictal period the seizure locus is often characterized by a significant reduction of tracer activity, often in the medial temporal lobe, with a spread of decreased perfusion to the remaining temporal lobe. In some instances, changes in perfusion may be seen in the opposite hemisphere or in the entire ipsilateral hemisphere. Therefore SPECT imaging, with its wide clinical availability, is becoming more widely identified as an important method of identifying single and multiple seizure foci and of minimizing the need for invasive electrophysiological studies. Used in conjunction with computed tomography (CT), magnetic resonance imaging (MRI), and electroencephalographic (EEG) studies, SPECT increases the accuracy of lesion identification and improves the rate of surgical success (11).

Another application of SPECT in connection with seizure disorders is to use the procedure in conjunction with mapping the distribution of amobarbital sodium in intracarotid Wada testing. This is a test to localize speech, memory function, and hemispheric dominance in patients being considered for surgical treatment of temporal lobe seizures. One of the critical issues in performing this test is to be certain that the amobarbital sodium is reaching the intended site. By injecting a radiotracer such as ^{99m}Tc hexamethylpropyleneamine-oxime (HMPAO) and performing SPECT imaging, the distribution of the amobarbital distribution can be more accurately traced. Jeffery et al. (12) (1991) reported on 25 patients that were studied with this technique. Their findings and those of Biersack et al. (13) demonstrate that it is possible to determine the distribution of the amobarbital used in the Wada test. Similar findings have also been reported by Hietala et al. (14). While this technique has not been widely incorporated into the routine Wada evaluation, it is likely that those centers performing temporal lobe surgery may find it to be a useful application of SPECT imaging.

Some of the more typical findings associated with regional cerebral blood flow (rCBF)/SPECT scans of patients with seizure disorders are reviewed in Table 7.1.

TABLE 7.1 *General findings in image interpretation associated with seizure disorders*

Interictal (seizure free for approximately 24 hr at time of injection)
Scan may have a normal appearance
In some patients there may be regions of absence or reduced tracer uptake associated with structural abnormalities
Ictal study (injected during the seizure or within 1 to 3 min of the seizure)
There is increased uptake in the region of seizure focus
There may be other focal or global changes in tracer uptake
Postictal study (injected 3 to 20 min after ictus)
Reduction of tracer uptake, usually in the region of the medial temporal lobe (hippocampal area) at site of seizure, is seen
There may be surrounding regions of reduced tracer uptake within hemisphere or in some cases bilateral changes

REFERENCES

1. Devous MD Sr. Comparison of SPECT applications in neurology and psychiatry. *J Clin Psychiatry* 1992;53(Suppl11):13–19.
2. Devous MD Sr, Leroy RF, Homan RW. Single photon emission computed tomography in epilepsy. *Semin Nucl Med* 1990; 20: 325–342.
3. Duncan R, Patterson J, Roberts R, et al. Infra/postictal SPECT in the presurgical localization of complex partial seizures. *J Neurol Neurosurg Psychiatry* 1993;56:141–148.
4. Commission on Classification and Terminology of the International League against Epilepsy. Proposal for revised classification of epilepsies and epileptic syndromes. *Epilepsia* 1989;30:389–399.
5. Rowe CC, Bercovic SF, Sia STB, et al. Localization of epileptic foci with postictal single photon emission computed tomography. *Ann Neurol* 1989;26:660–668.
6. Harvey AS, Hopkins IJ, Bowe JM, et el. Frontal lobe epilepsy: clinical seizure characteristics and localization with ictal 99m Tc-HMPAO SPECT. *Neurology* 1993;43:1966–1980.
7. Newton MR, Austin MC, Chan JG, et al. Ictal SPECT using technetium-99m-HMPAO: methods for rapid preparation and optimal deployment of tracer during spontaneous seizures. *J Nucl Med* 1993; 34:666–670.
8. Newton MR, Berkovic SF, Austin MC, et al. Postictal switch in blood flow distribution and temporal lobe seizures. *J Neurol Neurosurg Psychiatry* 1992;55:891–894.
9 Rowe CC, Barcovic SF, Austin MC, et al. Patterns of postictal cerebral blood flow in temporal lobe epilepsy: quantitative and qualitative findings. *Neurology* 1991;41:1096–1193.
10. Ryvlin P, Philippon B, Cinotti L, et al. Functional neuroimaging strategy in temporal lobe epilepsy: a comparative study of 18 FDG-PET and 99mTc-HMPAO-SPECT. *Ann Neurol* 1992;31:650–656.
11. Tikofsky RS, Morris GL, Hellman RS, et al. rCBF/SPECT seizure evaluation in surgical candidates: reader agreement and relation to surgical site. *Epilepsia* 1993;34 (suppl): 134.
12. Jeffery PJ, Monsieu LH, Szabo Z, et al. Mapping the distribution of amobarbital sodium in the intra caratoid Wada test for use of Tc-99m HMPAO with SPECT. *Radiology* 1991; 178: 847–850.
13. Biersack HJ, Linke D, Brassel F, et al. Technetium-99m-HMPAO brain SPECT in epileptic patients before and during unilateral hemispheric anesthesia (Wada Test): Report of three cases. *J Nucl Med* 1987;28:1763–1767.
14. Hietala S-O, Sivenius H, Aasley J, Olivecrona M, Jonsson L. Brain perfusion with intracarotid injection of 99m-Tc-HMPAO in partial complex epilepsy during amobarbital testing. *Eur J Nucl Med* 1990; 16:683–687.

SUGGESTED READINGS

Biersack HJ, Stefan H, Reichman K. Brain imaging with 99mTc-HMPAO SPECT, CT, and NMR—results in epilepsy. *J Nucl Med* 1986;27:1028–1032.

Duncan R, Patterson J, Hadley DM, et al. CT, MR and SPECT imaging in temporal lobe epilepsy. *J Neurol Neurosurg Psychiatry* 1990;53:11–15.

Duncan R, Patterson J, Bone I, et al. Tc99m HMPAO single photon emission tomography in temporal lobe epilepsy. *Acta Neurol Scand* 1990; 81:287–293.

Homan RW, Paulman RG, Devous MD, Sr, et al. Cognitive function and regional cerebral blood flow in partial seizures. *Arch Neurol* 1989; 46:964–970.

Launes J, Iivanainen M, Salmi T, et al. Interictal brain 99Tc-HM-PAO SPECT hypoperfusion in patients with unstable partial epilepsy and normal CT. *Acta Neurol Scand* 1992;86:558–562.

Rowe CC, Bercovic SF, Austin MC. Visual and quantitative analysis of interictal SPECT with technetium 99m HMPAO in temporal lobe epilepsy. *J Nucl Med* 1991;32:1688–1694.

Stephan H, Bauer J, Feistel H, et al. Regional cerebral blood flow during focal seizures of temporal and frontocentral onset. *Ann Neurol* 1990;27:162–166.

CASE 7-1

Clinical Diagnosis:

Visual Hallucinations Secondary to Right Occipital Lobe Seizure Focus

CONTRIBUTOR:	**IMAGING DATA:**	
Name: Ronald L. Van Heertum, M.D.	**Camera:** GE 400AC/T;STAR II	**Collimator:** High resolution
Institution: St. Vincent's Hospital and Medical Center	**Isotope:** ^{123}I IMP	**Dose:** 3.0 mCi

This 31-year-old man was referred for evaluation of a recent seizure with associated occipital headaches, photophobia, and intermittent flashes of light (visual hallucinations). There was no history of prior seizure activity.

An EEG revealed a right temporal lobe spike focus.

A CT scan (Fig. 7.1) with intravenous contrast and an MRI study were negative. The patient was having visual hallucinations at the time of the CT and MRI scans, and also at the time of the SPECT study.

The SPECT study (Fig 7.2), in the transaxial **(A),** coronal **(B),** and sagittal **(C)** planes, revealed a focus of intense, increased activity in the right occipital and posterior temporal lobes *(arrows)*.

Teaching Point:

A focus of intense, increased tracer deposition is typical of an epileptogenic focus in the ictal phase. The cerebral SPECT study may be highly useful in defining such foci, particularly when both the CT and MRI scans are negative.

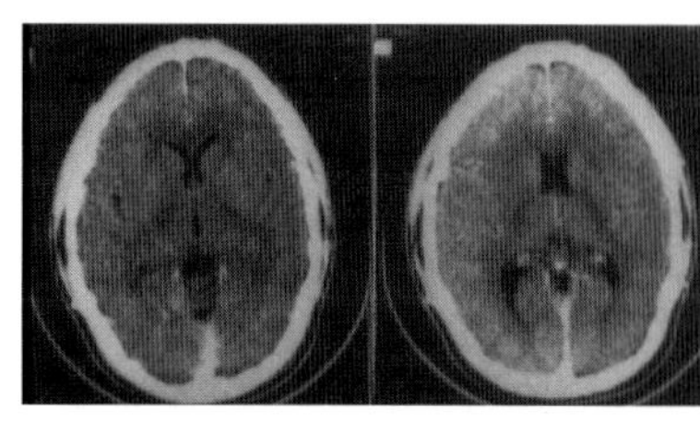

FIG. 7.1

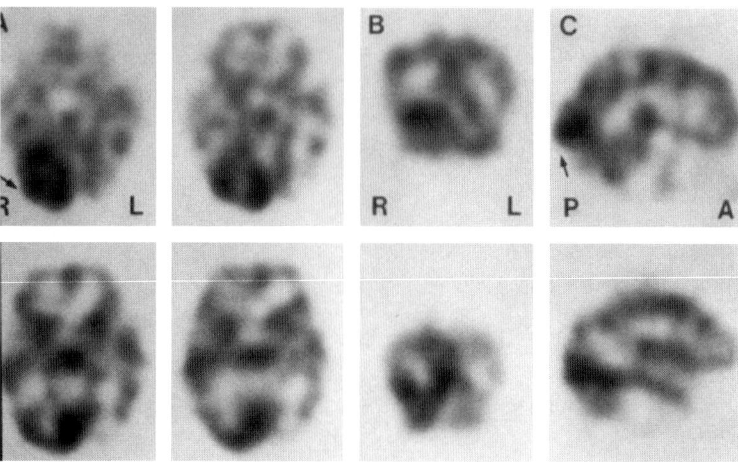

FIG. 7.2

CASE 7-2

Clinical Diagnosis: Status Epilepticus

CONTRIBUTOR:	**IMAGING DATA:**	
Name: Thomas C. Hill, M.D.	**Camera:** Strichman SME-810	**Collimator:** High resolution
Institution: New England Deaconess Hospital	**Isotope:** ^{123}I IMP	**Dose:** 3.0 mCi

This 94-year-old woman was referred for evaluation of status epilepticus. Her seizure activity began 8 hr before her hospital admission. There was no history of a prior seizure disorder.

An EEG showed continuous bursts of left frontal temporal seizure activity. At the time of admission the patient was started on intravenous phenytoin, which was continued over the next 2 days; she slowly became more responsive but was still disoriented.

An emergency CT scan (Fig. 7.3) was unremarkable except for a benign calcification in the left temporal lobe.

Four days after admission, a cerebral SPECT study (Fig. 7.4) in the transaxial plane showed an intense focus of increased tracer deposition in the left frontal lobe *(arrowhead)*. As a result, the patient's medication was adjusted, and she became more oriented and alert.

Teaching Point:

In this case, the cerebral SPECT study was very helpful in determining the presence of persistent seizure activity despite what was thought to be adequate dosage levels of anticonvulsant medication.

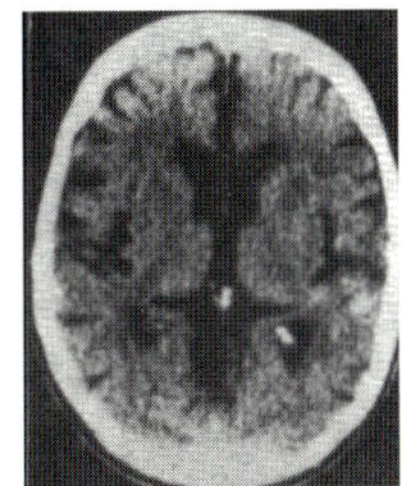

FIG. 7.3

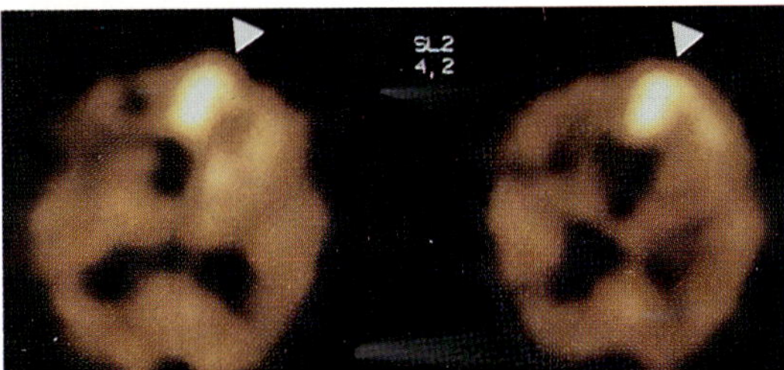

FIG. 7.4

CASE 7-3

Clinical Diagnosis:
Recurrent Complex Partial Seizure Disorder

CONTRIBUTOR:

Name: Robert S. Hellman, M.D. and Ronald S. Tikofsky, Ph.D.
Institution: Medical College of Wisconsin

IMAGING DATA:

Camera:	GE 400AC/ T;STAR	Studies 1 and 2	**Collimator:** High resolution
	GE Neurocam	Studies 3 and 4	**Collimator:** Ultra-high resolution
Isotope:	^{123}I IMP	Studies 1 and 2	**Dose:** 30. mCi
	Tc^{99m} HMPAO	Studies 3 and 4	**Dose:** 30. mCi

This 45-year-old right-handed woman, with a long history of migraine headaches, was referred for evaluation of a recurrence of complex partial seizures. The patient first experienced seizure activity approximately 5 years prior to her current presentation. At that time a CT scan was normal.

An initial N-isopropyl-P-iodoamphetamine (IMP) cerebral SPECT study (Fig. 7.5), in the transaxial **(A),** coronal **(B),** and sagittal **(C)** planes, done in the immediate postictal period while the patient was still complaining of generalized headaches, showed a significant increase in tracer deposition in the right temporal, posterior frontal, and anterior parietal lobes and in the adjacent subcortical areas *(arrows).*

A subsequent MRI study (Fig. 7.6) showed increased signal intensity in the medial aspect of the right temporal lobe, without associated edema or mass effect.

An EEG was abnormal with a significant slow wave in the right temporal lobe.

A follow-up cerebral SPECT study (Fig. 7.7) performed interictally 8 days after the first study, showed a normal pattern of tracer distribution. For approximately the next 5 years, the patient was successfully treated with anticonvulsant medication. The patient currently presented for assessment of a recurrence of the seizure activity that was uncontrolled with medication.

A repeat MRI scan showed a focus of abnormal increased signal intensity in the medial aspect of the right temporal lobe most likely secondary to sclerosis of the mesial temporal lobe.

An HMPAO SPECT study (Fig. 7.8), in the transaxial **(A)** and coronal **(B)** planes, revealed a focus of increased radiotracer activity in the medial aspect of the right temporal lobe. The patient subsequently underwent partial resection of the right temporal lobe.

A follow-up HMPAO SPECT study (Fig. 7.9), in the transaxial **(A)** and coronal **(B)** planes, revealed an area of absent radiotracer activity in the right temporal lobe in the area of surgical resection. However, seizure activity recurred.

Teaching Point:

The cerebral SPECT study, with IMP or HMPAO, may be useful in localizing and monitoring the seizure activity of epileptogenic foci, as this case demonstrates.

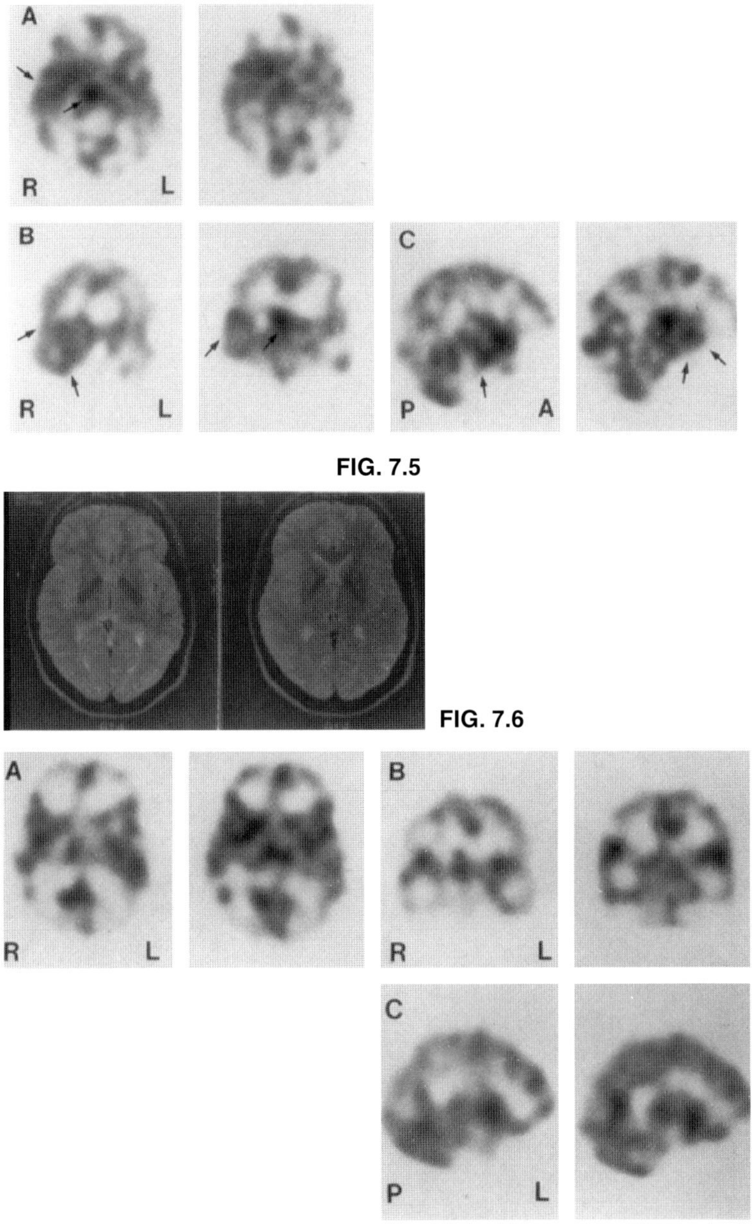

FIG. 7.5

FIG. 7.6

FIG. 7.7

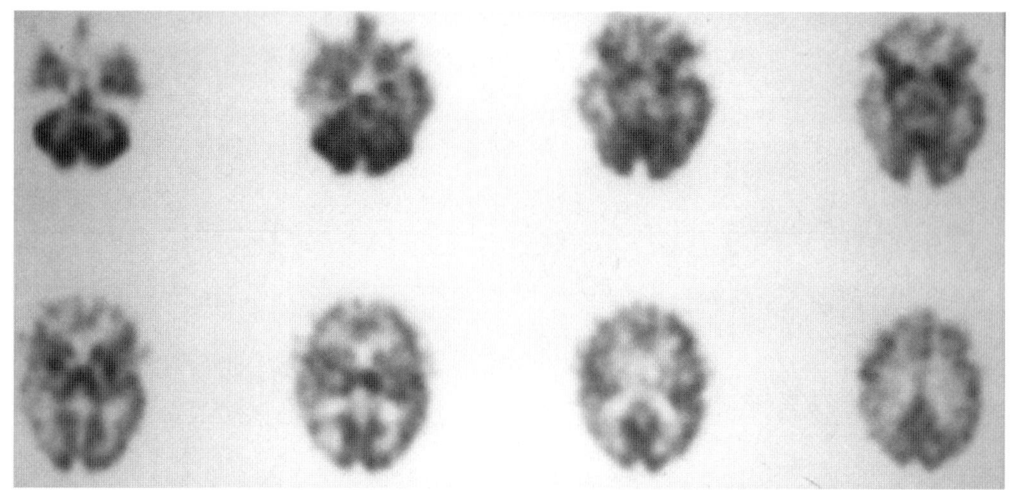

FIG. 7.8A

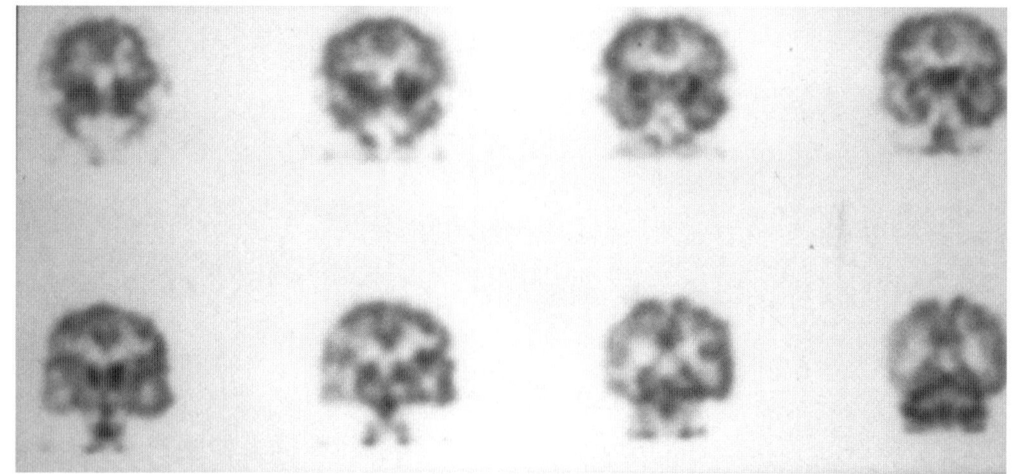

FIG. 7.8B

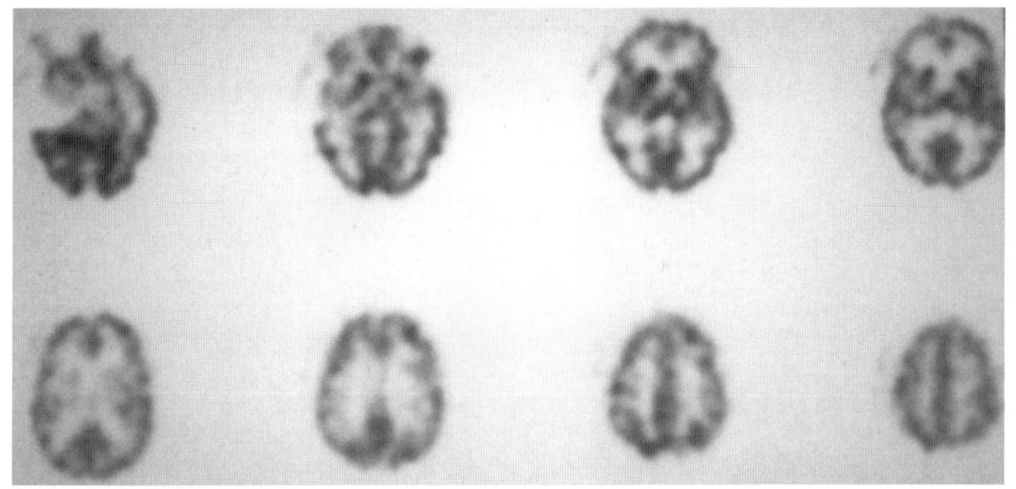

FIG. 7.9A

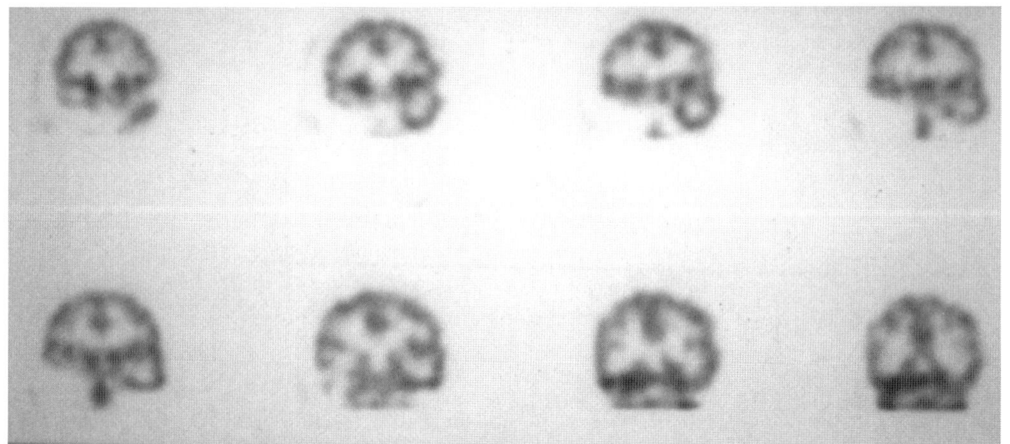

FIG. 7.9B

CASE 7-4 Clinical Diagnosis: Atypical Seizure Disorder

CONTRIBUTOR:

Name: S. Askienazy, M. D., and M.O. Habert, M.D.
Institution: C.H. Sainte-Anne/Service Medicine Nucleaire Paris, France

IMAGING DATA:

Camera: SOPHY
Isotope: ^{99m}Tc HMPAO
Collimator: Ultra-high resolution
Dose: 25 mCi

This 56-year-old woman presented with a history of recurrent episodes of left-hand hemiparesis. Three years prior to her current presentation, she had sustained a traumatic right temporal lobe contusion. At present, neurological examination revealed a left lateral homonymous hemianopsia. Scalp EEG demonstrated the presence of permanent lateralized epileptiform discharge (PLEDS). After 1 week of antiepileptic therapy, a follow-up scalp EEG demonstrated the disappearance of PLEDS.

CT scan (Fig. 7.10) revealed a hypodensity in the right temporal lobe consistent with prior trauma to the temporal lobe.

The initial HMPAO SPECT study (Fig. 7.11), in the transaxial **(A)** and coronal **(B)** planes, revealed increased radiotracer activity in the right posterior temporal lobe. A follow-up HMPAO SPECT scan (Fig. 7.12), in the transaxial **(A)** and coronal **(B)** planes, showed a decrease in radiotracer activity in the right temporal lobe following treatment with anticonvulsants.

Teaching Point:

Cerebral SPECT imaging can be a useful tool in the assessment of epilepsy patients not only for the localization of the seizure focus, but also for establishing the diagnosis of epilepsy, when the patient's clinical presentation is atypical.

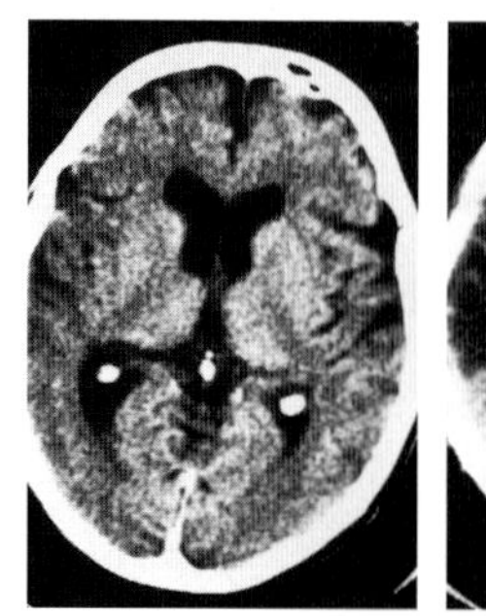
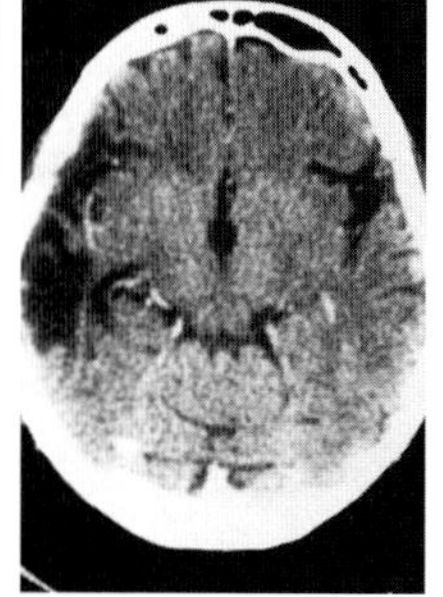

FIG. 7.10

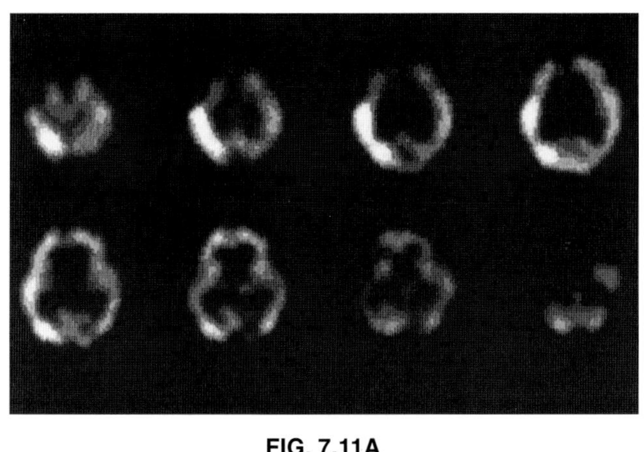

FIG. 7.11A

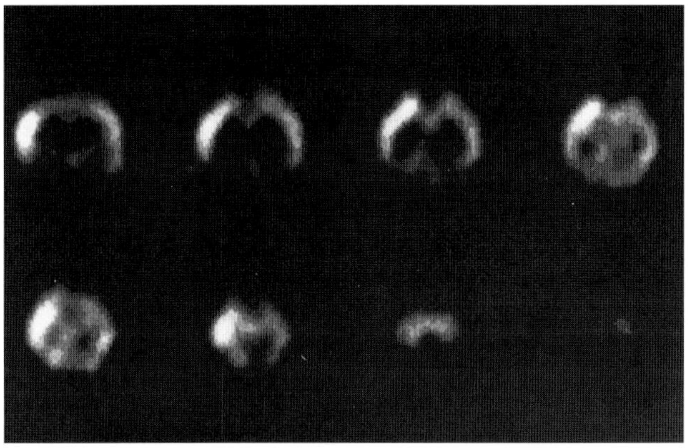

FIG. 7.11B

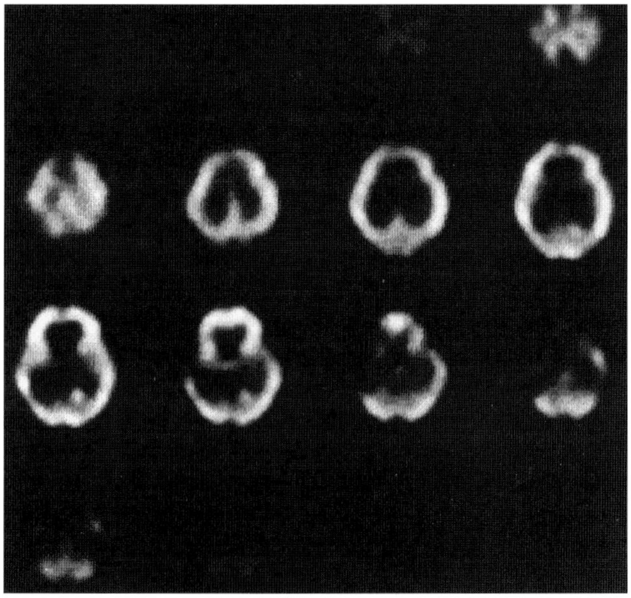

FIG. 7.12A

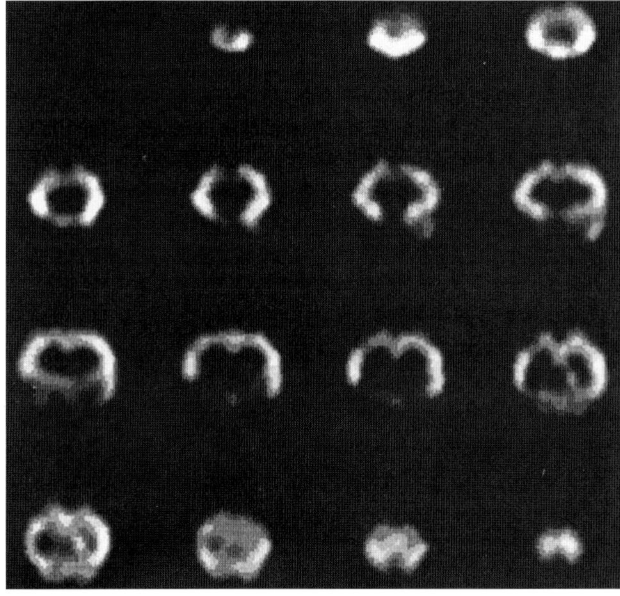

FIG. 7.12B

CASE 7-5

Clinical Diagnosis: Medically Intractable Seizure Disorder

CONTRIBUTOR:	IMAGING DATA:	
Name: James Mountz, M.D., Ph.D.	**Camera:** ADAC dual-headed Genesys	**Collimator:** High resolution
Institution: University of Alabama Hospital	**Isotope:** ^{99m}Tc HMPAO	**Dose:** 15 mCi

This 10-year-old boy with known seizures since age 2 1/2 years, was referred for evaluation of progressively increasing seizure activity uncontrolled by medication. At the time of referral the patient averaged 30 to 40 seizures/day. The seizures were characterized by tonic extension of the left arm and nonpurposeful movement of the arm with preservation of consciousness. Repeat EEGs showed mild background slowing with occasional sharp discharges and slow wave activity in the right frontocentroparietal region interictally.

Multiple CT and MRI examinations were performed, and all were negative (Fig. 7.13).

An HMPAO SPECT study (Fig. 7.14) in the transaxial plane obtained during ictus revealed a focus of increased radiotracer activity in the right premotor cortex. This finding was felt to represent the site of the seizure focus. This region was surgically excised, and pathologic tissue examination revealed cortical dysplasia.

Teaching Point:

As with ^{123}I IMP SPECT, ^{99m}Tc HMPAO SPECT studies will frequently demonstrate foci of increased radiotracer deposition at the site of the seizure focus at the time of ictus.

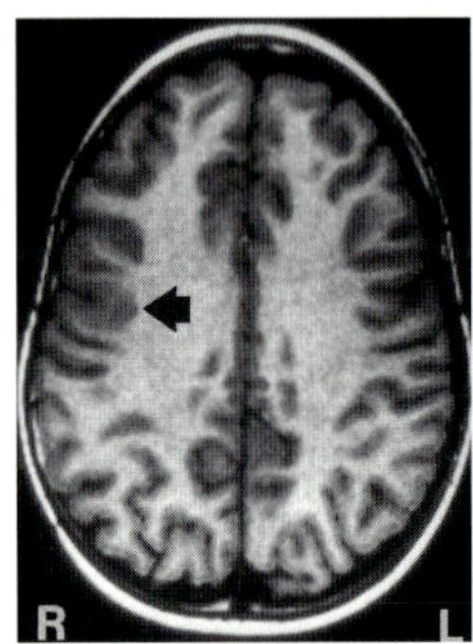

FIG. 7.13

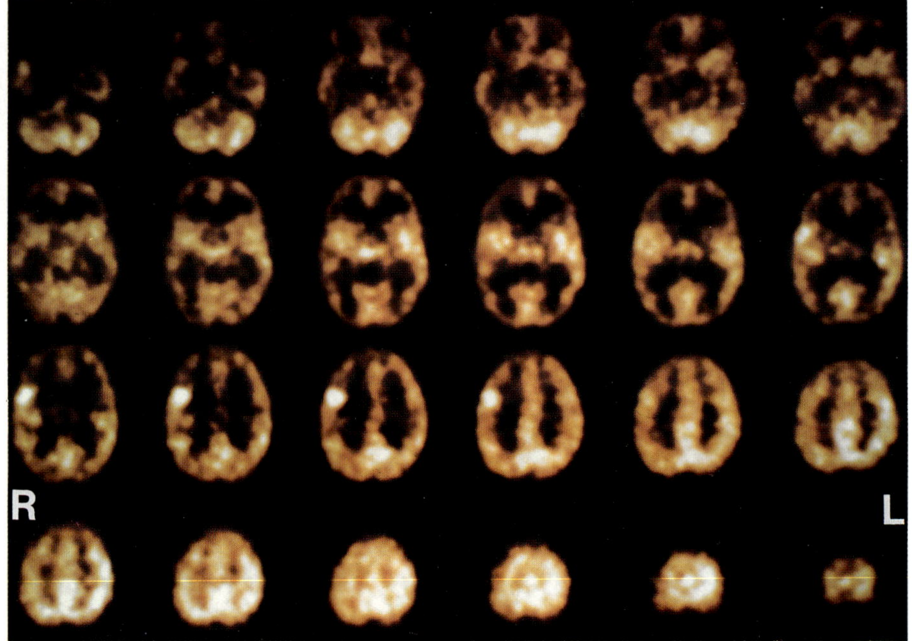

FIG. 7.14

CASE 7-6

Clinical Diagnosis: Intractable Seizure Disorder

CONTRIBUTOR:	IMAGING DATA:	
Name: Amjad Ali, M.D.	**Camera:** Siemens 7500 ZLC; VAX	**Collimator:** LEAP
Institution: Rush Presbyterian/St. Luke's Medical Center	**Isotope:** ^{123}I IMP	**Dose:** 3.0 mCi

This 19-year-old woman had had a known seizure disorder since she was 9 months old. She was referred for an evaluation before surgical removal of the ictal focus.

The CT and MRI scans (Fig. 7.15) were normal.

An IMP cerebral SPECT study (Fig. 7.16) in the transaxial **(A)** and coronal **(B)** planes showed a marked decrease in tracer deposition in the right temporal lobe *(arrows)*, corresponding to the abnormality found on the PET scan and the EEG.

Prolonged EEG monitoring showed prominent epileptiform activity in the right anterior temporal region.

PET scanning with ^{18}F 2-deoxyglucose showed hypometabolic activity in the right temporal lobe.

The patient underwent a resection of the right temporal lobe and was reported to be doing well at a 6-month postsurgical follow-up.

Teaching Point:

As this case illustrates, a cerebral SPECT study done during the interictal phase may be useful for the accurate presurgical localization of an epileptogenic focus.

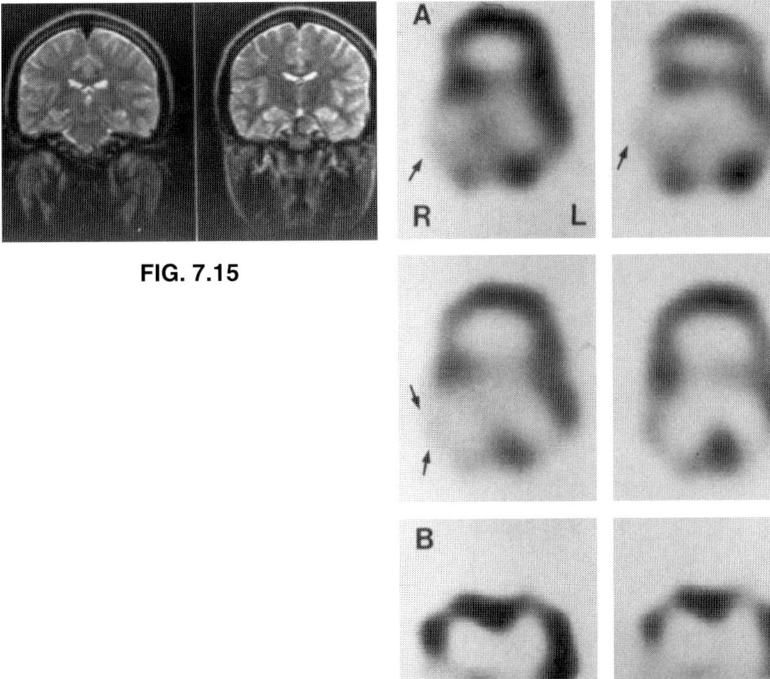

FIG. 7.15

FIG. 7.16

CASE 7-7

Clinical Diagnosis: Intractable Seizure Disorder

CONTRIBUTOR:	**IMAGING DATA:**	
Name: Amjad Ali, M.D.	**Camera:** Siemens 7500 ZLC; VAX	**Collimator:** LEAP
Institution: Rush Presbyterian/St. Luke's Medical Center	**Isotope:** ^{123}I IMP	**Dose:** 3.0 mCi

A 22-year-old man with a history of epilepsy since the age of 9 years was referred for the presurgical evaluation of an epileptogenic focus.

A cerebral SPECT study in the transaxial plane (Fig. 7.17) revealed a decreased tracer deposition in the left temporal lobe and adjacent posterior parietal region *(arrows).*

A follow-up MRI showed increased signal activity in the left posterior temporal-parietal region.

A PET scan with ^{18}F 2-deoxyglucose demonstrated hypometabolism in the left posterior temporal and inferior parietal lobes.

Surface EEG showed frequent bursts of epileptiform activity in both posterior frontal regions, with slightly greater predominance of activity on the right side.

A subsequent EEG done during a Wada test showed similar findings. A methohexitol test demonstrated epileptiform foci in the left frontal anguli gyrus and the left temporal lobe.

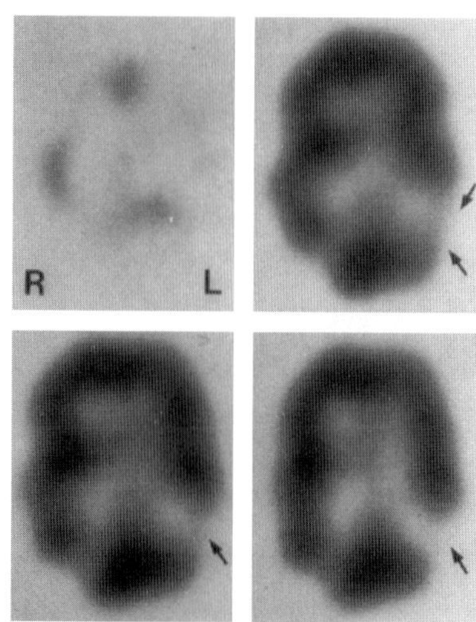

FIG. 7.17

CASE 7-8

Clinical Diagnosis: Seizure Disorder: Interictal Phase

CONTRIBUTOR:

Name: David Moon, M.D. and Paul Hoffer, M.D.
Institution: Yale University School of Medicine

IMAGING DATA:

Camera: Picker Prism 3000
Isotope: ^{99m}Tc HMPAO
Collimator: High resolution, fan beam
Dose: 20 mCi

This 33-year-old man was referred for further evaluation of his seizure disorder.

An HMPAO SPECT study (Fig. 7.18), in the transaxial **(A)** and coronal **(B)** planes, revealed asymmetric tracer activity in the temporal lobes with a relative increase of radiotracer uptake in the right temporal lobe compared with the left side. No other perfusion abnormalities were noted.

Teaching Point:

In an interictal setting, this asymmetrical SPECT finding is more suggestive of a seizure focus in the left temporal lobe. Frequently the area of the seizure focus will appear as a site of diminished tracer uptake (photopenic focus) on either IMP or HMPAO interictal SPECT scans. It is essential that care should be taken to compare the tracer activity in the suspected temporal lobe with comparable regions in the contralateral temporal lobe and surrounding cortical structures when attempting to localize the site of the seizure focus. Serial SPECT studies performed ictally and interictally will often be more helpful for accurately defining the seizure focus.

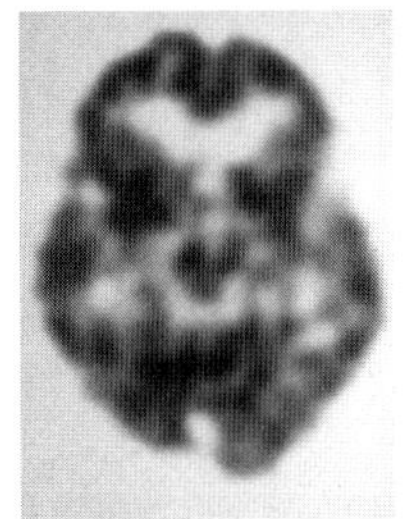

FIG. 7.18A

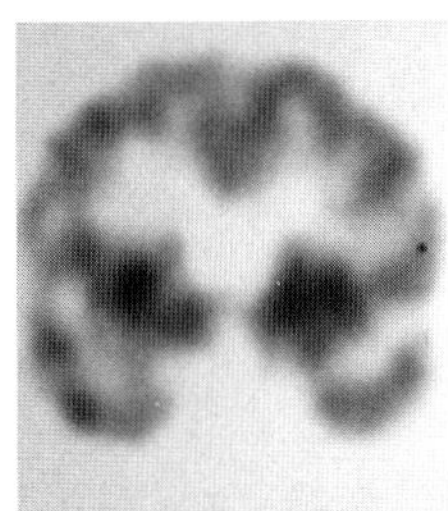

FIG. 7.18B

CASE 7-9

Clinical Diagnosis:
Complex Partial Seizure Disorder

CONTRIBUTOR:

Name: Kastytis Karvelis, M.D.
Institution: Henry Ford Hospital

IMAGING DATA:

Camera: ADAC Genesys
Isotope: ^{99m}Tc HMPAO
Collimator: High resolution
Dose: 20 mCi

This 35-year-old man with known complex partial seizures of uncertain etiology, was referred for further evaluation. Specifically, the patient was referred to determine if the seizures were temporal lobe in origin.

An MRI scan (Fig. 7.19) demonstrated a subarachnoid cyst in the superior aspect of the right parietal occipital lobe.

An HMPAO SPECT study (Fig. 7.20) in the transaxial plane revealed a focus of absent radiotracer activity corresponding to the subarachnoid cyst seen on MRI.

Teaching Point:

In this case, without an accompanying MRI study, the region of absent tracer activity could easily have been interpreted as evidence of an area of infarction. When there is no history of cerebrovascular disease or hemorrhage, anatomic imaging such as CT or MRI is essential in order to establish a correct diagnosis. This case demonstrates a good correlation between SPECT and MRI with respect to lesion locus.

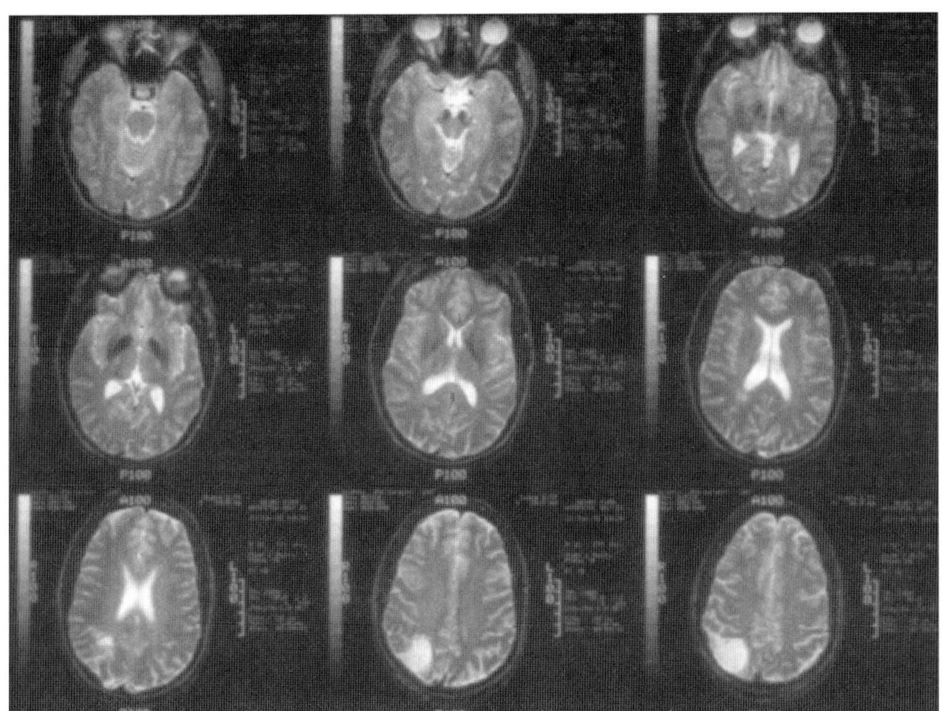

FIG. 7.19

HMPAO
HENRY HOSP
04/01/93
17
18
19
20
21
22
23
24
25
26
27
28
TRANSVERSE
29
30
31
32

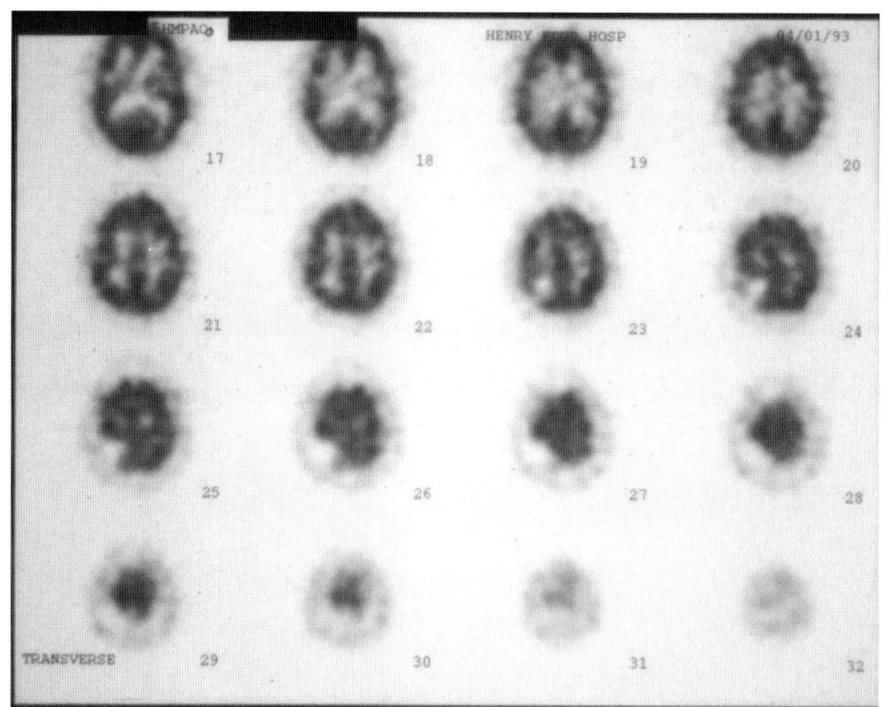

FIG. 7.20

CASE 7-10

Clinical Diagnosis: Schizencephaly

CONTRIBUTOR:	**IMAGING DATA:**	
Name: Ronald L. Van Heertum, M.D.	**Camera:** GE 3000 XCT	**Collimator:** Ultra-high resolution
Institution: Columbia-Presbyterian Medical Center	**Isotope:** ^{99m}Tc HMPAO	**Dose:** 20.4 mCi

This 81-year-old Caucasian man was referred for evaluation of a change in mental status. At the time of initial presentation, he was found to be dysarthric and aphasic (expressive). While in the hospital the patient developed a generalized tonic clonic seizure.

CT (Fig. 7.21) revealed a cleft, lined by cortical gray matter, in the right posterior frontal area that extended to the right lateral ventricle. In addition, dilation of the lateral ventricles is evident.

HMPAO SPECT (Fig. 7.22) in the transaxial plane demonstrated a photopenic cleft defect extending from the cortex of the right frontal lobe to the level of the right lateral ventricle. The cortical gray matter was visually intact through the effect.

Teaching Point:

HMPAO SPECT may be helpful for distinguishing a developmental cleft due to schizencephaly from other etiologies including infarction and localized head trauma.

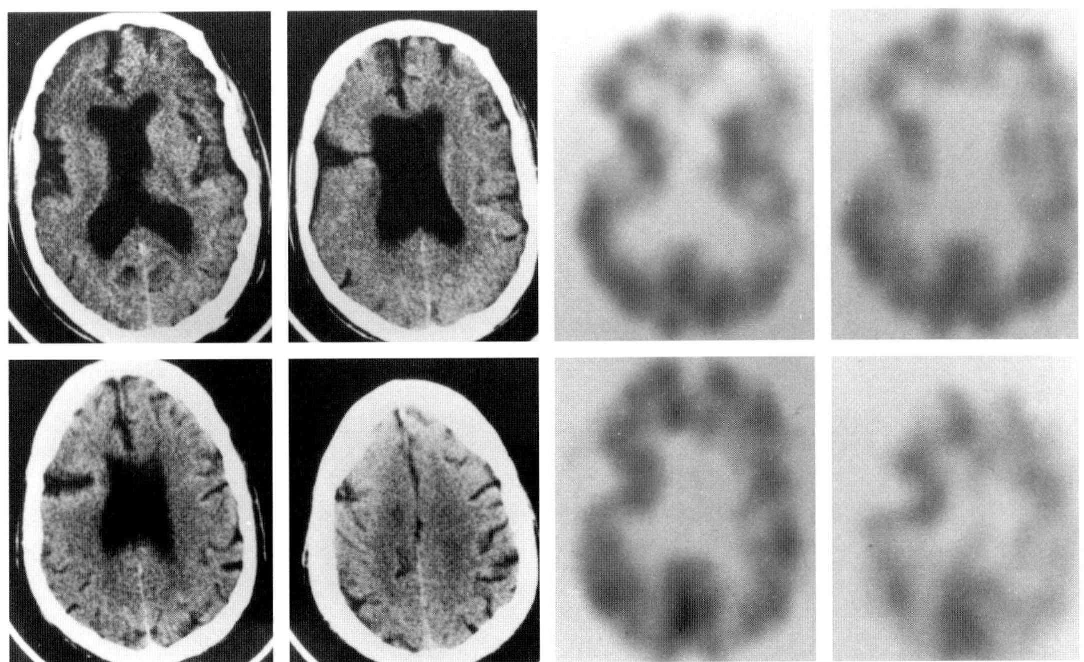

FIG. 7.21 FIG. 7.22

Cerebral SPECT Imaging, Second Edition,
edited by R.L. Van Heertum and R.S. Tikofsky.
Raven Press, Ltd., New York © 1995.

CHAPTER 8

Trauma

Ronald S. Tikofsky and Ronald L. Van Heertum

Head injury is a major medical management problem in the United States. According to Julien Dilks, President of the JMA Foundation, Inc./National Brain Injury Research Group, Inc. (personal communication) there is one head injury each minute each day. According to the National Head Injury Foundation, over 1,190,000 individuals of the 2 million yearly with head injuries survive. There are approximately 300,000 hospitalizations a year for minor head injury, and 34 percent of this group is unable to return to work after 3 months. These epidemiological data confirm that head trauma is a major cause of disability in the United States. Structural brain imaging, particularly computed tomography (CT) and magnetic resonance imaging (MR) is extremely useful in the evaluation of acute and chronic head trauma. Unfortunately, structural imaging techniques, particularly in minor head trauma, do not always correlate with the clinical deficits that these patients manifest.

Regional cerebral blood flow (rCBF)/SPECT imaging in patients with closed cranial trauma is becoming recognized as a clinically useful evaluation procedure (1–4). There is a growing body of literature describing SPECT findings associated with various types of clinical sequelae resulting from closed cranial and other trauma to the brain. SPECT imaging does not replace CT or MRI for the identification of major structural lesions or the presence of hemorrhage, subdural hematomas (SDH), or edema; it does play a role in evaluating cortical, basal ganglia and thalamic changes in perfusion as a consequence of trauma (13,14).

While most of the attention in functional brain imaging has been on closed cranial trauma and its sequalae, SPECT also has a role in evaluating other types of brain injury. Penetrating wounds to the head and brain typically produce focal lesions. These lesions are often the result of missiles penetrating the skull and entering the brain. The CT and MRI modalities can often track the path of the missiles through the brain. However, SPECT may be useful in detecting perfusion deficits secondary to the primary lesion. Neuropsychological changes resulting from, for example, gunshot wounds to the head may be related to both the structural damage detected by CT/MRI and the surrounding perfusion defects seen with SPECT. Penetrating lesions to the brain tend to be focal in nature. On the other hand, closed head injuries resulting from vehicular accidents, falls, or other blows to the head are frequently more diffuse. In many cases of closed head injury the resulting brain damage is a combination of focal and diffuse brain damage. Even when there is diffuse injury, the frontal, temporal, and basomesial areas appear to be the most vulnerable to damage (15). Thus SPECT studies in this patient population can be expected to reveal regions of absent tracer uptake that will, in part, correlate with sites of structural damage seen on anatomic imaging. In addition, SPECT studies may also show the effects of diffuse nonstructural lesions in the form of regional decreases in tracer uptake.

Wilson (16) notes that abnormalities seen using neuroimaging techniques may be classified as follows: by type, locus, extent, and persistence after injury. Hematomas are commonly seen after closed cranial trauma. Hematomas, which may be extradural, subdural, or intracerebral, may produce secondary changes in the brain including contusion, compression, necrosis, and edema. In some cases evacuation of the hematoma will be followed by cortical atrophy. A CT study is an excellent tool for the detection of hematomas. SPECT brain imaging, on the other hand, may be more useful in identifying perfusion deficits following evacuation of the hematoma. Oder el al. (11) suggested that SPECT imaging may be useful in

R. S. Tikofsky: Department of Radiology, Section of Nuclear Medicine, Medical College of Wisconsin, Milwaukee, Wisconsin 53226.

R. L. Van Heertum: Department of Radiology, Columbia University College of Physicians and Surgeons, and Department of Nuclear Medicine, Columbia Presbyterian Medical Center, New York, New York 10032.

predicting outcome in severely injured and comatose patients.

Because SPECT scans can detect alterations in perfusions, the technique is particularly useful in identifying regions of contrecoup injury. These alterations in perfusion, suggesting impaired neural function, can often account for the patient's clinical presentation when no structural lesions are found with CT or MRI. This is of particular importance in evaluating patients with "minor" head trauma who may only experience brief periods of unconsciousness and leave the emergency room with no overt neurological impairment, and who later return with complaints of visual, cognitive, or behavioral changes.

With the availability of stable radiopharmaceuticals, it is possible to inject patients in the emergency room. Comatose patients can then be imaged after they have been stabilized, or in the case of minor trauma after all the other examinations including CT and MRI have been completed.

It is interesting to note that Wilson in 1990 (16) noted that the "new functional tomographic" methods (PET, SPECT) "present exciting, as yet largely untapped, opportunities for the future." The research alluded to earlier in this section and the case material shown in this chapter attest to the potential role that SPECT can play in the clinical evaluation of patients with traumatic brain injury.

The cases presented in this section represent the range of images that are associated with various types of head trauma. Table 8.1 presents the perfusion patterns associated with brain trauma that are most often observed.

TABLE 8.1. General rCBF/SPECT patterns associated with head trauma

Regions of absent tracer uptake
Found at site of trauma (subsequent infarction)
Site of surgical intervention
Regions of reduced tracer uptake
May reflect contrecoup effect
May reflect deafferentation
May reflect axonal shearing
Disorganized patterns of tracer uptake
Seen in prolonged and severe coma
Associated with profound cognitive impairment
Distortion of the cortical rim
Result of pressure from hematomas
Result of persistent edema
Reflect depression of the skull at site of impact

REFERENCES

1. Abdel-Dayem HM, Sadek SA, Kouris K, et al. Changes in cerebral perfusion after acute head injury: comparison of CT with Tc-99m HMPAO SPECT. *Radiology* 1987;165:221–226.
2. Goncalves JM, Vaz R, Cerejo A, et al. HMPAO SPECT in head trauma. *Acta Neurochir* 1992;[Suppl55]:11–13.
3. Reid RH, Gulenchyn KY, Ballinger JR, Ventureyra ECG. Cerebral perfusion imaging with technetium-99m-HMPAO following cerebral trauma. Initial experience. *Clin Nucl Med* 1990;15:383–388.
4. Yamakami I, Yamaura A, Isobe K. Types of traumatic brain injury and regional cerebral blood flow assessed by 99mTc-HMPAO SPECT. *Neurol Med Chir (Tokyo)* 1993;33:7–12.
5. Bullock R, Sakes D, Patterson J, et al. Early post-traumatic cerebral blood flow mapping: correlation with structural damage after focal injury. *Acta Neurochir* 1992;[Suppl]55:286–288.
6. Choksey MS, Costa DC, Patterson J, et al. 1992.
7. Choksey MS, Costa DC, Iannoti F, et al. 99Tcm-HMPAO SPECT studies in traumatic intracerebral hematoma. *J Neurol Neurosurg Psychiatry* 1991;54:6–11.
8. Gray BG, Ichise M, Chung DG, et al. Technetium-99m-HMPAO SPECT in the evaluation of patients with a remote history of traumatic brain injury: a comparison with x-ray computed tomography. *J Nucl Med* 1992;33:52–58.
9. Ichise M, Dae-Gyun C, Wang P, et al. Technetium-99m-HMPAO SPECT, CT, and MRI in the evaluation of patients with chronic traumatic brain injury: a correlation with neuropsychological performance. *J Nucl Med* [in press]
10. Oder W, Goldenberg G, Spatt J, et al. Behavioral and psychosocial sequelae of severe closed head injury and regional cerebral blood flow: a SPECT study. *J Neurol Neurosurg Psychiatry* 1992;55:475–480.
11. Oder W, Goldenberg G, Podreka I, Deecke L. HMPAO SPECT studies in persistent vegetative state after head injury: prognostic indicator of the likelihood of recovery? *Intensive Care Med* 1991;17:149–153.
12. Wilson JTL, Wyper D. Neuroimaging and neuropsychological functioning following closed head injury: CT, MRI, and SPECT. *J Head Trauma Rehabil* 1992;7:29–39.
13. Roper WN, Mena I, King WA, et al. An analysis of cerebral blood flow in acute closed-head injury using technetium-99m-HMPAO SPECT and computed tomography. *J Nucl Med.* 1991;34:1684–1687.
14. Newton MR, Greenwood RJ, Britton KE, et al. A study comparing SPECT with CT and MRI after closed head injury. *J Neurol Neurosurg Psychiatry* 1992;55:92–94.
15. Adams JH. Head injury. In: Adams JH, Corsellis JAN, Duchen LW, eds. *Greenfield's neuropathology,* 4th ed. London: Edward Arnold; 1984;85–124.
16. Wilson JTL. Review: the relationship between neuropsychological function and brain damage detected by neuroimaging after closed head injury. Brain Injury 1990;4:349–363.

SUGGESTED READING

Goldenberg G, Oder W, Spatt J, Podraka I. Cerebral correlates of disturbed executive function and memory in survivors of severe closed head injury: a SPECT study. *J Neurol Neurosurg Psychiatry* 1992;55:362–368.

CASE 8-1 Clinical Diagnosis: Intracranial Gunshot Injury

CONTRIBUTOR:

Name: Robert S. Hellman, M.D. and Ronald S. Tikofsky, M.D.
Institution: Medical College of Wisconsin

IMAGING DATA:

Camera: GE 400 AC/T;STAR
Isotope: ^{123}I IMP
Collimator: High resolution
Dose: 5.0 mCi

This 23-year-old man was referred for evaluation of a left hemiparesis and loss of cognitive function after sustaining a gunshot wound to the head.

An initial CT scan showed hyperdense hematomas in the right frontal and deep right parietal lobes, which appeared hyperdense on a follow-up CT scan.

A cerebral SPECT study (Fig. 8.1) in the transaxial **(A),** coronal **(B),** and sagittal **(C)** planes revealed a marked decrease in tracer deposition throughout the right cerebral hemisphere, plus an absence of tracer activity in the right basal ganglia and the frontal lobes; tracer activity was less reduced in the right parietal lobe. The defect shown by SPECT study was of a larger area than that noted on the CT scan. The pattern of abnormal tracer deposition appreciated by the SPECT study clearly delineated the trajectory of the bullet.

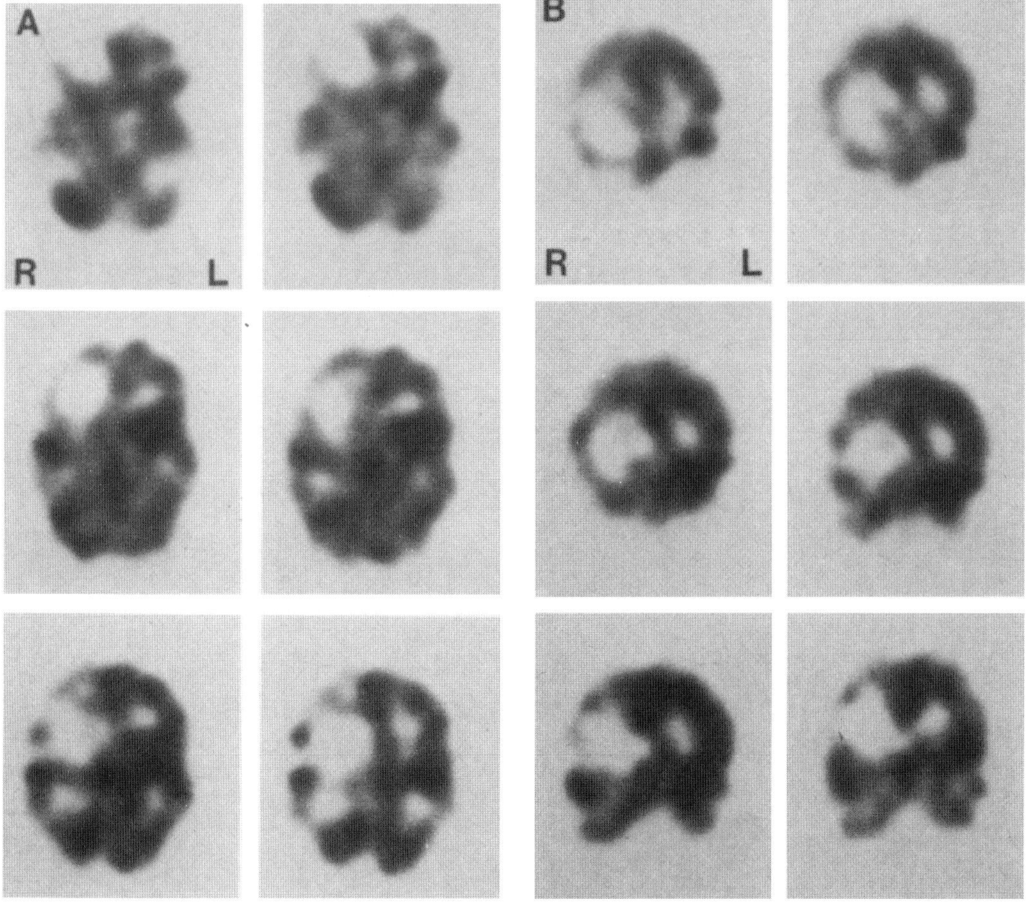

FIG. 8.1A **FIG. 8.1B**

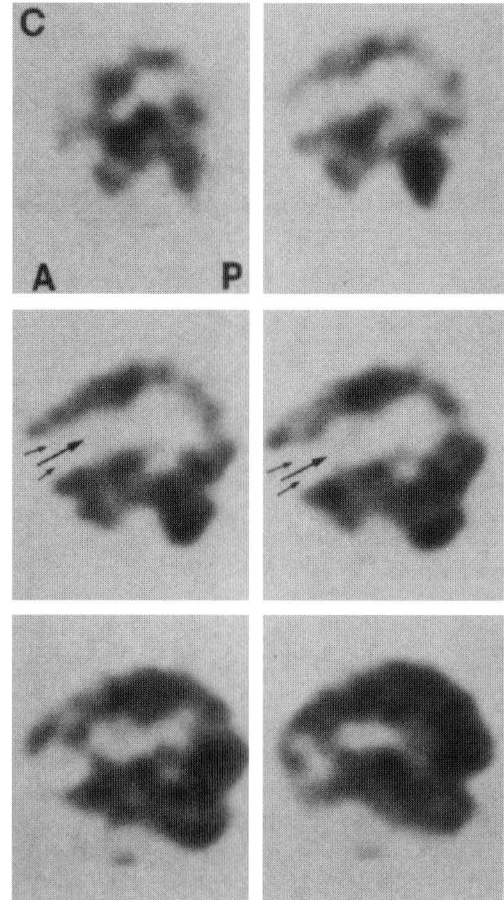

FIG. 8.1C

CASE 8-2

Clinical Diagnosis: Severe Closed Intracranial Trauma

CONTRIBUTOR:

Name: Robert S. Hellman, M.D. and Ronald S. Tikofsky, M.D.
Institution: Medical College of Wisconsin

IMAGING DATA:

Camera: GE 400 AC/T;STAR
Isotope: ^{123}I IMP
Collimator: High resolution
Dose: 5.0 mCi

This 23-year-old man was referred for the evaluation of closed intracranial trauma sustained during an auto-train collision. At the time of evaluation, the patient was in a Grade II coma.

An initial CT scan (Fig. 8.2) revealed a small left temporoparietal epidural hematoma, a small midline hemorrhage in the third ventricle, and a large extracranial scalp hematoma overlying the left frontal temporoparietal calvarium. A follow-up CT scan (Fig. 8.3) 1 month later showed resolution of the areas of hemorrhage, a low-density area in the upper mesencephalon, and some enlargement of the ventricles and sulci (the result of resolution of the cerebral edema).

A cerebral SPECT study (Fig. 8.4) in the transaxial plane showed an overall heterogeneous pattern of tracer distribution, with a lack of normal delineation between the cortical gray and white matter. This was particularly pronounced in the frontal, temporal, and parietal cortex. There was also very poor delineation of subcortical structures.

These findings suggest a gross disorganization of rCBF and metabolism.

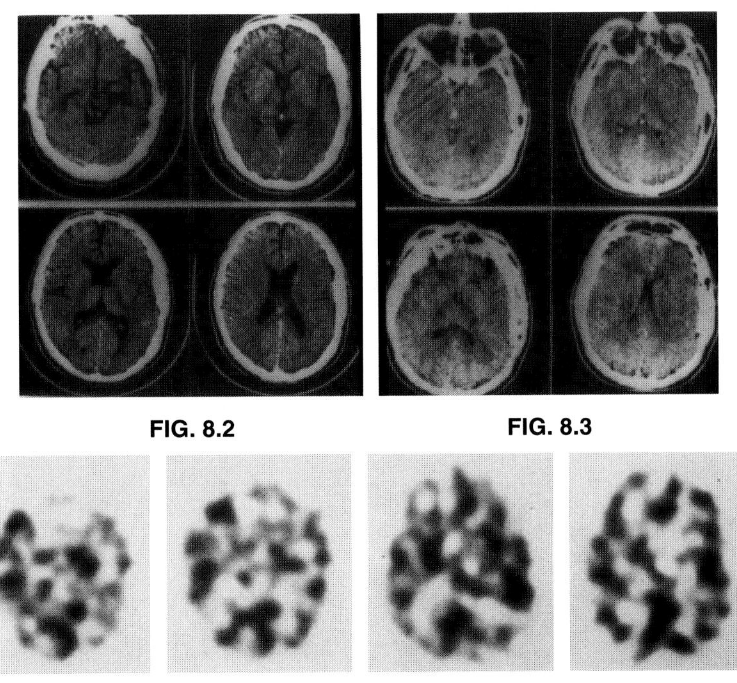

FIG. 8.2

FIG. 8.3

FIG. 8.4

CASE 8-3

Clinical Diagnosis:
Large Right Subdural Hematoma

CONTRIBUTOR:	**IMAGING DATA:**	
Name: Joji Nagawara, M.D.	**Camera:** Shimadzu Headtome Set-031	**Collimator:** High resolution
Institution: Nakamura Memorial Hospital	**Isotope:** ^{123}I IMP	**Dose:**

This 65-year-old man was referred for evaluation of right-sided headaches and a left hemiparesis. Two months previously, he had sustained head trauma.

On a CT scan, a subdural hematoma was noted on the right side.

An initial cerebral SPECT study (Fig. 8.5A) in the transaxial plane revealed decreased peripheral tracer deposition in the right cerebral hemisphere *(arrows)*. In addition, crossed cerebellar diaschisis was observed *(arrowhead)*.

A week after the subdural hematoma was drained, a follow-up cerebral SPECT study (Fig. 8.5B) showed significantly improved tracer deposition in the periphery of the right cerebral hemisphere.

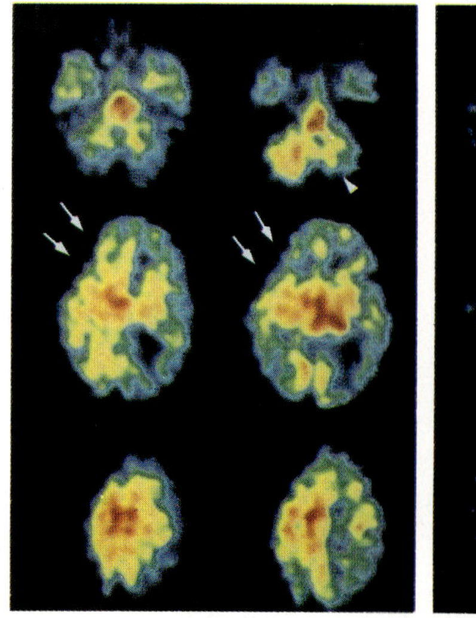

FIG. 8.5A

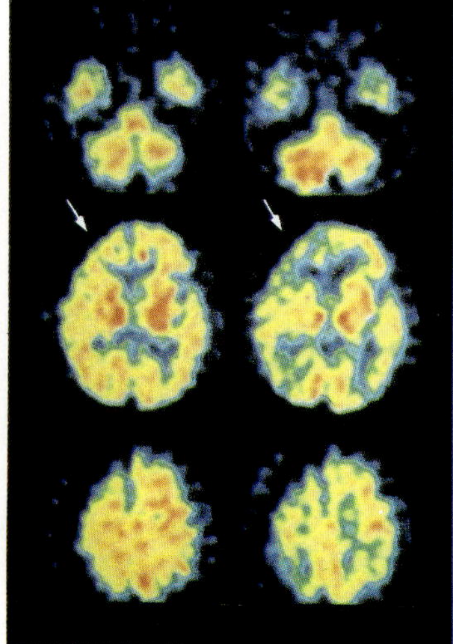

FIG. 8.5B

CASE 8-4

Clinical Diagnosis: Closed Cranial Trauma, Increasing Seizure Activity

CONTRIBUTOR:

Name: Robert S. Hellman, M.D. and Ronald S. Tikofsky, M.D.
Institution: Medical College of Wisconsin

IMAGING DATA:

Camera: GE 400 AC/T;STAR
Isotope: ^{99m}Tc HMPAO
Collimator: High resolution
Dose: 30 mCi

This 31-year-old man with a prior history of seizures and alcohol abuse of 5 years duration, presented to the emergency room after having sustained a basilar skull fracture in a fight.

An admission CT scan revealed bilateral subdural hematomas and an intracerebral hemorrhage in the left temporal lobe. At the time of admission he showed a Glasgow Coma Scale Score of 13 and an alcohol level of 0.288. The patient was subsequently transferred to the Rehabilitation Service for further treatment of his post-traumatic cognitive and language deficits. An EEG revealed a generalized, moderate slowing of brain activity.

A follow-up CT scan of the head (Fig. 8.6), showed areas of hemorrhage and surrounding low density in the left temporal and parietal lobes that were less dense than on the previous study. However, a mass effect with effacement of cortical sulci on the left was still present.

An HMPAO SPECT study (Fig. 8.7), in the transaxial plane, showed a large area of reduced radiotracer deposition in the left temporal lobe and a slightly smaller area of decreased uptake in the superior left parietal region corresponding to the areas of abnormality on CT. Small areas of decreased tracer were also seen in the right posterior parietal-temporal lobes. This latter finding was felt to be secondary to a contrecoup injury.

Teaching Point:

In this case, a large perfusion deficit in the left cerebral hemisphere language region correlated with the patient's severe mixed aphasia. The decreased activity in the right posterior parietal lobe is an example of a contrecoup injury that may be detected with SPECT in spite of a negative CT or MRI study.

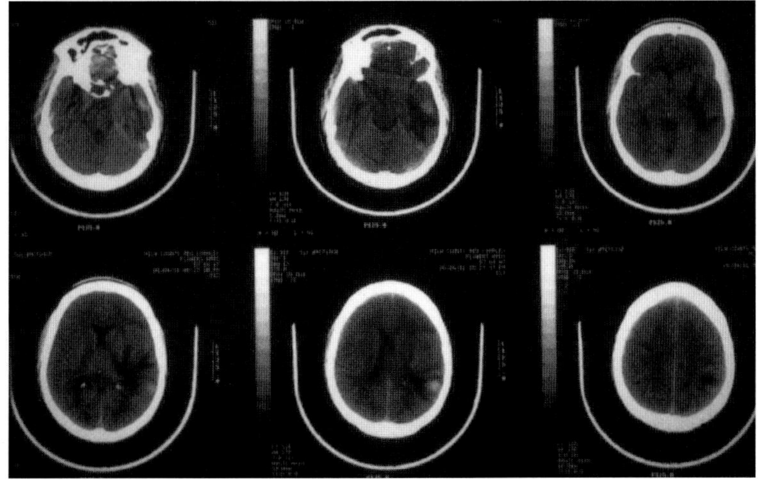

FIG. 8.6

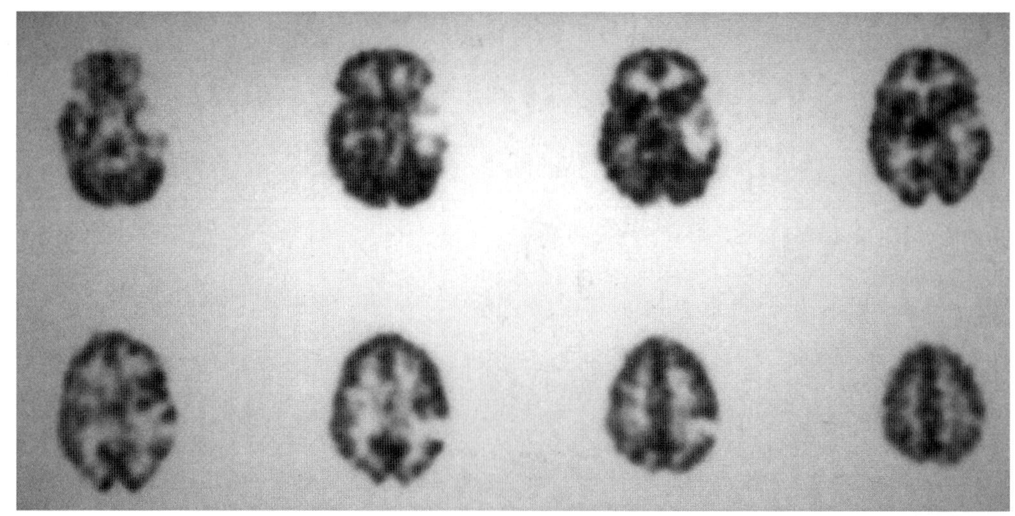

FIG. 8.7

CASE 8-5

Clinical Diagnosis: Traumatic Subarachnoid Hemorrhage

CONTRIBUTOR:	IMAGING DATA:	
Name: Stefanie Jacobs, M.D.	**Camera:** GE Neurocam	**Collimator:** Ultra-high resolution
Institution: Columbia-Presbyterian Medical Center	**Isotope:** ^{99m}Tc HMPAO	**Dose:** 21.3 mCi

This 64-year-old woman with a known history of hypertension was admitted for further assessment and treatment of a depressed level of consciousness and aphasia following a generalized seizure. At the time of the seizures, the patient sustained an injury to the left side of her head. An EEG revealed a diffuse slowing of brain activity with a focus in the left temporal lobe.

An initial CT scan (Fig. 8.8) revealed a localized subarachnoid hemorrhage primarily confined to the left posterior parietal-temporal lobe.

HMPAO SPECT (Fig. 8.9) in the transaxial **(A),** coronal **(B),** and sagittal **(C)** planes revealed decreased radiotracer uptake throughout the left temporal lobe that was felt to be most consistent with an area of contusion.

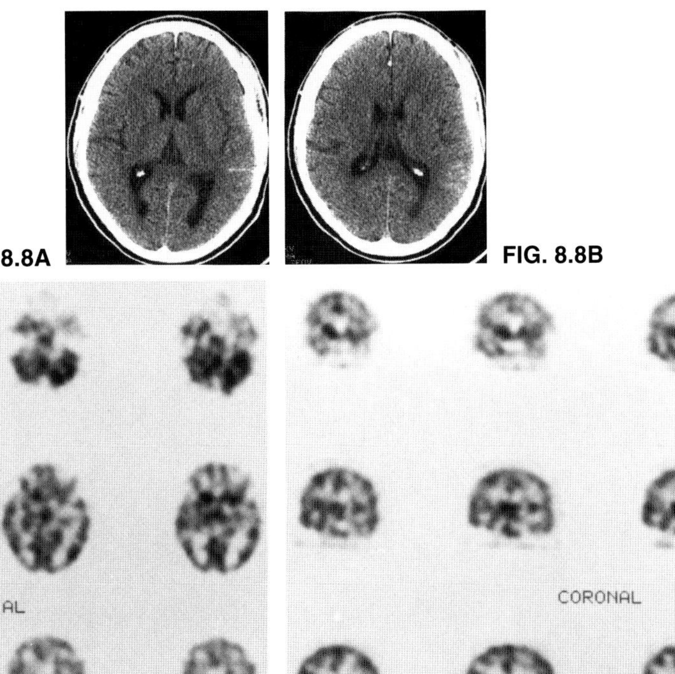

FIG. 8.8A

FIG. 8.8B

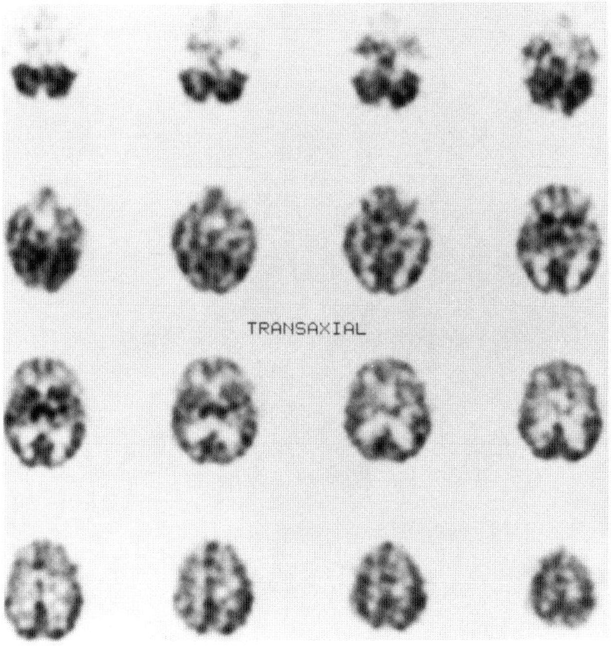

FIG. 8.9A

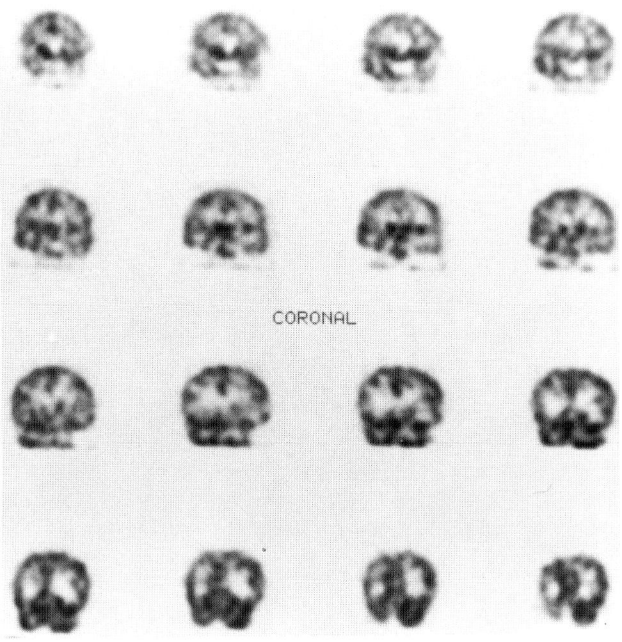

FIG. 8.9B

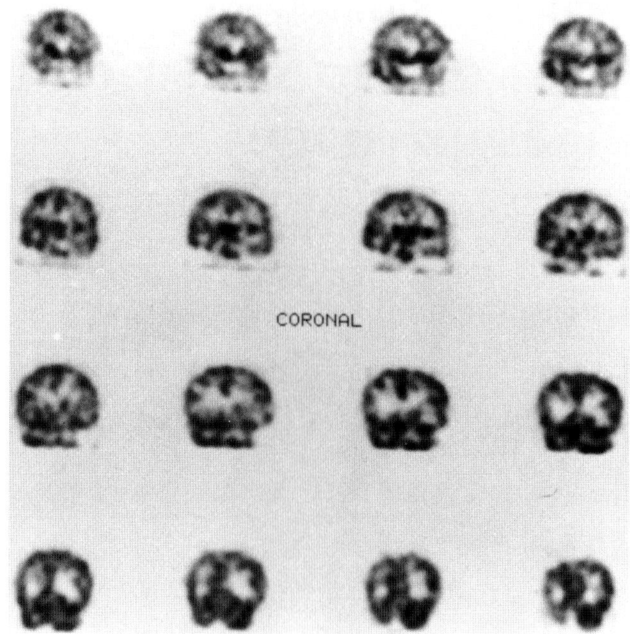

FIG. 8.9C

CASE 8-6 Clinical Diagnosis: Childhood Head Trauma

CONTRIBUTOR:	IMAGING DATA:	
Name: Ronald L. Van Heertum, M.D.	**Camera:** GE-3000 XCT	**Collimator:** Ultra-high resolution
Institution: Columbia-Presbyterian Medical Center	**Isotope:** ^{99m}Tc HMPAO	**Dose:** 20.5 mCi

This 35-year-old woman (transexual), with a long history of polysubstance abuse was referred for evaluation and treatment of pseudoseizures, paranoid ideations, and auditory hallucinations. The patient stated that she thought she had sustained head trauma (left frontal parietal) in early childhood.

A CT scan (Fig. 8.10) revealed an area of localized atrophy and hypodensity in the left frontal and anterior temporal lobes that was felt to be secondary to head trauma in childhood.

An HMPAO SPECT (Fig. 8.11) in the transaxial plane revealed relative decreased radiotracer deposition in the left frontal-temporal lobes corresponding to the area of abnormality on CT.

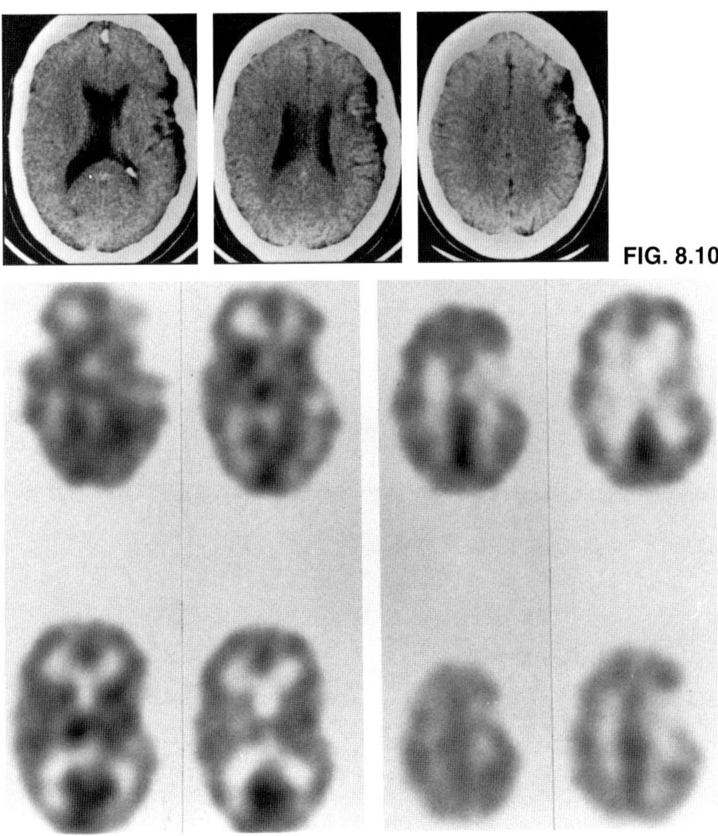

FIG. 8.10

FIG. 8.11

CASE 8-7

Clinical Diagnosis: Chronic Subdural Hematoma

CONTRIBUTOR:

Name: Ronald L. Van Heertum, M.D.
Institution: Columbia-Presbyterian Medical Center

IMAGING DATA:

Camera: Picker Prism 3000
Isotope: ^{99m}Tc HMPAO
Collimator: Ultra-high resolution, fan beam
Dose: 20.4 mCi

This 74-year-old man was referred for evaluation of progressive confusion. The patient stated that he had in the past sustained head trauma without loss of consciousness, which he said was minor and without obvious sequelae.

A CT scan (Fig. 8.12) revealed diffuse cerebral atrophy and bilateral subdural hematoma that were predominately frontal in location.

An HMPAO SPECT study (Fig. 8.13) in the transaxial plane revealed an extrinsic conical deformity in the contour of the cerebral cortex (predominantly frontal) secondary to the bilateral subdural hematomas seen on the CT scan. In addition, bilateral focal areas of absent radiotracer were seen in the occipital lobes. This latter finding was felt to be due to an associated contrecoup intraparenchymal brain injury.

Published with permission: ***Radiol Clin North Am* 1993;31:881–907.**

Teaching Point:

Cerebral SPECT imaging, as shown in this case, may be complementary to CT and MRI in the evaluation of acute and remote head trauma.

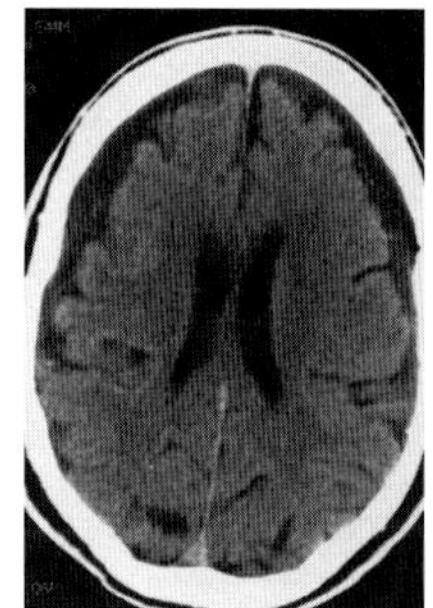

FIG. 8.12

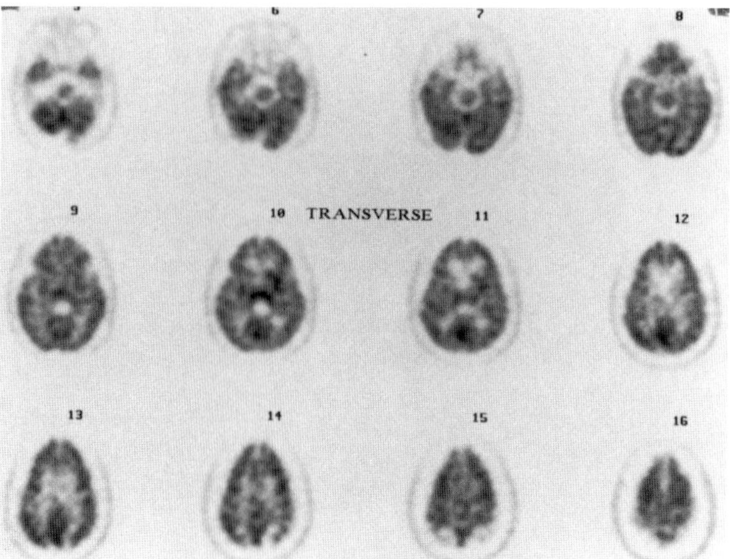

FIG. 8.13

CASE 8-8

Clinical Diagnosis:
Trauma; Motor Vehicle Accident

CONTRIBUTOR:

Name: Robert S. Hellman, M.D. and Ronald S. Tikofsky, M.D.
Institution: Medical College of Wisconsin

IMAGING DATA:

Camera: Neurocam
Isotope: ^{99m}Tc HMPAO
Collimator: High resolution
Dose: 30.7 mCi

This 44-year-old man, who was involved in a motor vehicle accident 3 weeks prior to admission, presented with the chief complaints of recurrent headaches and lethargy. His past history was significant for substance abuse.

An admission CT showed a large space-occupying lesion in the left frontal lobe with a hyperdense rim, which was thought to be due to a large subacute hematoma with surrounding edema or a cerebral abscess (Fig. 8.14). There was also a moderate midline shift from left to right with asymmetric compression of the left lateral ventricles and impending transtentorial herniation on the left as well as subarachnoid hemorrhage.

An MRI study (Fig. 8.15) revealed a large left frontal intracerebral abscess secondary to acute frontal sinusitis. In addition, an apparent defect in the posterior wall of the left frontal sinus was evident.

An HMPAO SPECT study (Fig. 8.16), in the transaxial plane, showed a large zone of absent perfusion in the left frontal region extending across the midline that correlated with the MRI and CT findings. A smaller zone of decreased perfusion in the right posterior parietal region was felt to be due to contrecoupe injury.

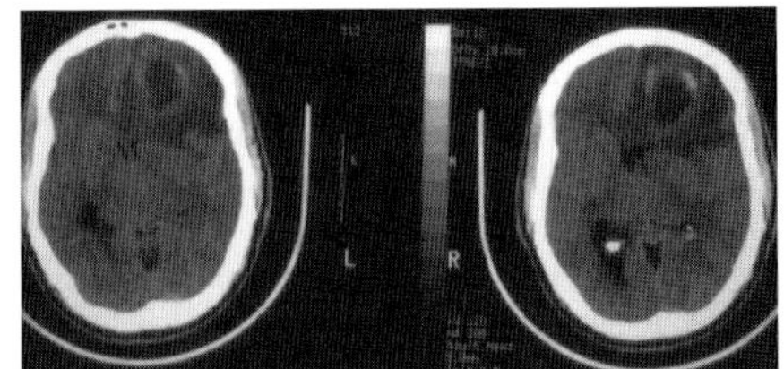

FIG. 8.14

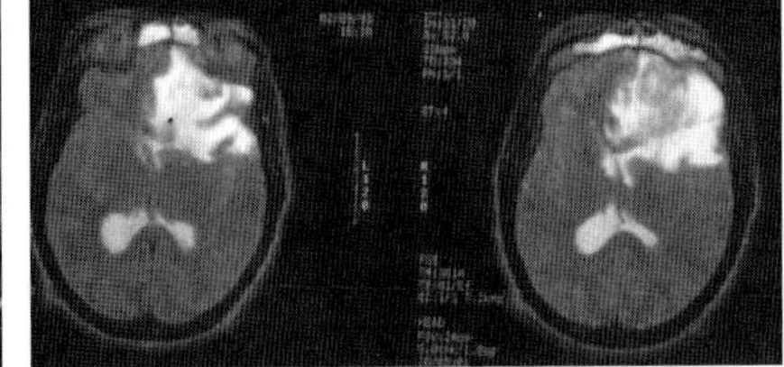

FIG. 8.15

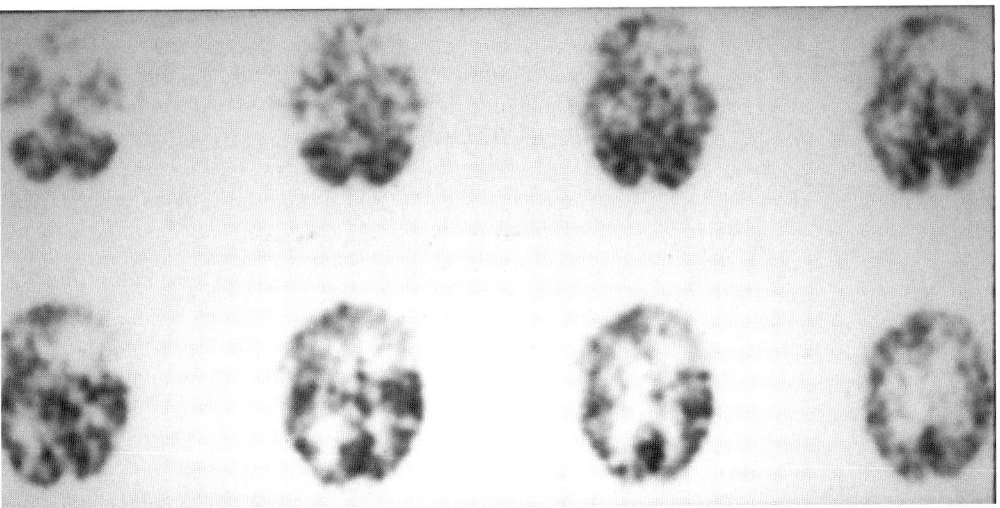

FIG. 8.16

CASE 8-9

Clinical Diagnosis: Trauma

CONTRIBUTOR:

Name: Robert S. Hellman, M.D. and Ronald S. Tikofsky, M.D.
Institution: Medical College of Wisconsin

IMAGING DATA:

Camera: GE Neurocam
Isotope: ^{99m}Tc HMPAO
Collimator: High resolution
Dose: 33 mCi

This 57-year-old left-handed woman presented to the emergency room after having sustained severe head trauma at the time of a motor vehicle accident. Upon presentation to the emergency room, the patient was observed to be unresponsive. The initial workup revealed that she had sustained a right temporal skull fracture with an associated pneumocephalus.

An admission CT showed a large subarachnoid hemorrhage and a right intracerebral frontal-temporal-parietal hematoma with marked midline (right to left) shift. In addition, intraventricular hemorrhage was evident.

An emergency craniotomy was performed to evacuate the intracerebral hematomas. Following surgery, the patient remained comatose for 16 days. In the postcoma period the patient was found to be severely aphasic. In addition, the patient manifested multiple episodes of inappropriate behavior.

A follow-up CT scan (Fig. 8.17) after surgery showed a decrease in the size of the hematomas, an evolving right temporal lobe cerebral contusion, persistent mass effect, and a decrease in the subarachnoid hemorrhage.

An HMPAO SPECT study (Fig. 8.18) in the transaxial plane, performed following evacuation of the subdural hematoma, revealed a large area of absent tracer activity in the posterior and mid-right frontal lobe extending deep into the right basal ganglia. In addition, decreased tracer uptake in the right temporal lobe, corresponding to the area of contusion seen on CT, was observed.

Teaching Point:

This patient illustrates the importance of ascertaining handedness. In this case of a left-handed patient, with right hemisphere dominance, a right-sided lesion was associated with significant aphasia.

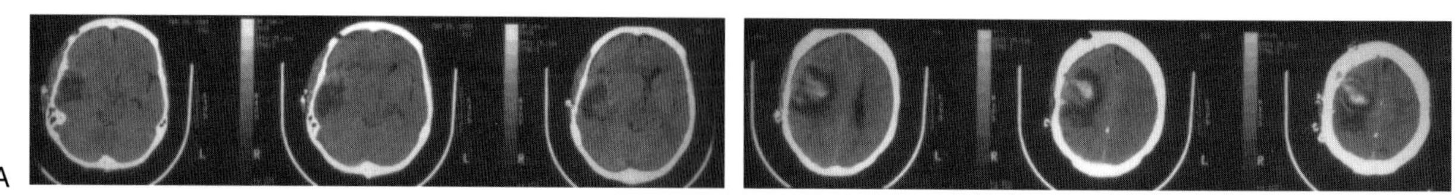

FIG. 8.17A **FIG. 8.17B**

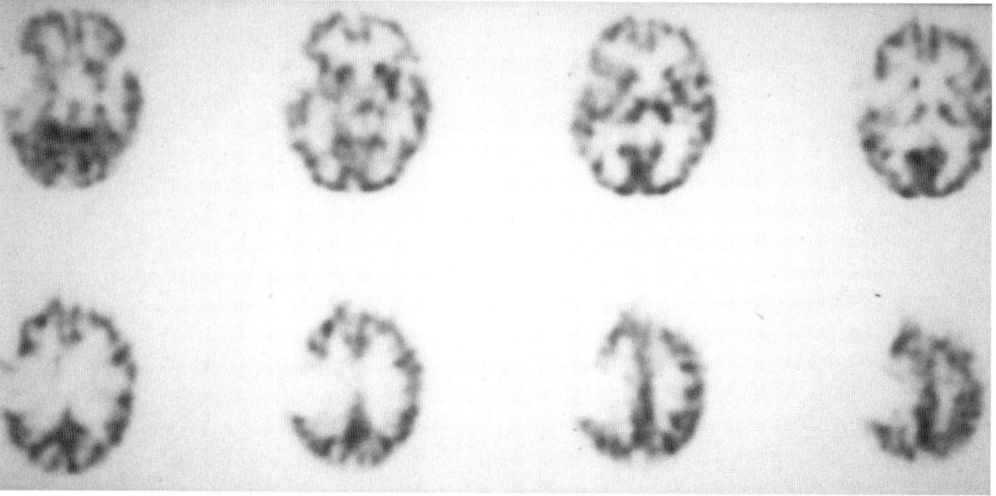

FIG. 8.18

Cerebral SPECT Imaging, Second Edition,
edited by R.L. Van Heertum and R.S. Tikofsky.
Raven Press, Ltd., New York © 1995.

CHAPTER 9

Psychiatric Disorders

R. Anthony O'Connell

The major psychiatric disorders—the schizophrenias and the affective disorders—certainly involve alterations of normal brain mechanisms. This has always been accepted, but the pathophysiology of these disorders has not been determined. The term *functional*, as opposed to *organic*, in describing schizophrenia and manic-depression, was originally used to indicate pathology of function in the absence of gross or microscopic evidence of brain disease. Over the past few years, several methods have been introduced that show great promise for studying the neurobiologic mechanisms related to psychiatric disorders. These new methods include computed tomography (CT), magnetic resonance imaging (MRI), techniques of molecular genetics, tomographic brain mapping, functional brain imaging using positron emission tomography (PET), and SPECT. SPECT imaging shows great potential for helping to understand the pathophysiology of these disorders (1–3).

Psychiatric diagnosis remains essentially a product of the history and mental examination of the patient. There are as yet no specific biological markers for psychiatric diagnoses. The mental status examination is the psychiatric equivalent of the physical examination and requires the collecting of signs and symptoms in a systematic manner. The introduction of the *Diagnostic and Statistical Manual of Mental Disorders* (DSM III, more recently DSM IIIR, and soon DSM IV) has significantly increased the reliability of psychiatric diagnosis by introducing operationalized diagnostic criteria. However, basic questions remain about the validity of many psychiatric diagnostic categories. Most clinicians and researchers today agree that the major diagnostic categories are heterogeneous: they present with similar clinical pictures, but are composed of different subtypes. A nonpsychiatric medical analogy would be the current recognition of at least two subtypes of diabetes mellitus. New methods for looking at brain mechanisms, such as SPECT, may reveal differences within diagnostic categories and possibly give leads to treatment response and prognosis.

In addition to the problems of heterogeneity within diagnostic categories, there are problems of differential diagnosis in psychiatry. In general, psychopathologic signs and symptoms are not specific to a particular diagnosis. For instance, hallucinations are found in schizophrenia, mania, and organic brain syndromes; cognitive impairment is common in dementia and severe depression (the so-called pseudodementia). Techniques such as PET and SPECT may be of help in the differential diagnosis.

SCHIZOPHRENIAS

Studies using CT have shown ventricular enlargements in schizophrenic patients when compared with matched controls. These findings are not specific for schizophrenia: they have also been noted in manic and depressed patients, and they are not found in all schizophrenics.

Studies using MRI, which provide greater resolution and detail than CT, also show ventricular enlargement and changes in frontal and temporal lobes in some schizophrenics. More recently, asymmetric volumetric changes in the left temporal lobe have been described (4). Hypofrontality in schizophrenics, which is correlated with negative symptoms, has also been demonstrated with PET. Studies of basal ganglia metabolism in schizophrenics using PET have been contradictory, with some studies showing a decrease and some an increase. This is a complex and expensive method, so that, while the resolution with SPECT is not quite as good as with PET, SPECT is a more feasible procedure in most clinical settings. SPECT studies using ^{123}I *N*-isopropyl-*P*-iodoamphetamine (IMP) and ^{99m}Tc Hexamethylpropyl-eneamine-opime (HMPAO) are being reported with increasing frequency in the literature (5–11).

R. A. O'Connell: Department of Clinical Psychiatry, New York Medical College, Valhalla, New York; and Department of Psychiatry, St. Vincent's Hospital and Medical Center, New York, New York 10011.

AFFECTIVE DISORDERS

Brain imaging studies in the affective disorders have been less extensive to date. Ventricular enlargement has been noted in bipolar depressions: PET studies have shown overall increased cortical metabolism when patients are in the manic state and decreased cortical metabolism in the same patient in the depressed state. Studies using ^{123}I IMP SPECT in patients with major depressive disorders show an overall decrease in regional cerebral blood flow (rCBF), especially in the frontal lobes, and temporal lobe asymmetries (12,13). This pattern is different from that seen in the dementias, and it may provide a method for the differential diagnosis of dementia and the pseudodementia of depression. The decreased rCBF seen in depressed patients appears to normalize as the patient improves clinically. However, the findings regarding the role of SPECT imaging in the affective disorders is not without controversy. Maes et al. (14), using ^{99m}Tc HMPAO, found no significant differences between normal control subjects and unipolar depressed patients. However, studies reported by Bolwig (15), Ebert et al. (16), and Austin et al. (17), suggest that there are rCBF differences attributable to depression. Final resolution with respect to the role SPECT imaging can play in the evaluation of patients with depression requires more research. However, when taken with other clinical information, SPECT does have the potential to contribute to the diagnosis and evaluation of treatment effectiveness in depression.

More recently, interest in the role of SPECT in evaluating patients with panic disorder has been shown. De Cristofaro et al. (18), in a recent study of panic disorder patients, have reported findings that suggest right-left asymmetric perfusion in the inferior frontal cortex associated with a significant decrease in the hippocampus bilaterally. Much still remains to be done to establish the role of rCBF/SPECT studies in clinical psychiatry. However, the data to date suggest that with further research SPECT imaging has the potential to make a significant contribution to the understanding, diagnosis, and treatment of psychiatric disease.

REFERENCES

1. Schuckit MA. An introduction and overview to clinical applications of neuroSPECT in psychiatry. *J Clin Psychiatry* 1991;Suppl 53:3–6.
2. Wood SW. Regional cerebral blood flow imaging with SPECT in psychiatric disease: focus on schizophrenia, anxiety disorders, and substance abuse. *J Clin psychiatry* 1992;Suppl 53:20–25.
3. Van Heertum RL, O'Connell RA. Functional brain imaging in the evaluation of psychiatric illness. *Semin Nucl Med* 1991;21:24–39.
4. Shenton ME, Kikinis S, Jolesz FA, et al. Left-lateralized temporal lobe abnormalities in schizophrenia and their relationship to thought disorder: a computerized quantitative MRI study. *N Engl J Med* 1992; 327:604–612.
5. Ebmeier KP, Blackwood DH, Murray C, et al. Single-photon emission computed tomography with 99mTc-exametazime in unmedicated schizophrenic patients. *Biol Psychiatry* 1993;33:487–495.
6. Suzuki M, Yuasa S, Minabe Y, Murata M, Kurachi M. Left superior temporal blood flow increases in schizophrenic and schizophreniform patients with auditory hallucination: a longitudinal case study using ^{123}I-IMP SPECT. *Eur Arch Psychiatry Clini Neurosci* 1993; 242:257–261.
7. Syed GM, Barrett JJ, Toone BK. What does rCBF-SPECT offer in schizophrenia? *Nucl Med Commun* 1992;13:879–884.
8. Budinger TF. Critical review of PET, SPECT and neuroreceptor studies in schizophrenia. *J Neural Trans* 1992;Suppl 36:3–12.
9. Sieg KG, Willsie DA, Preston DF, Gaffney GR. Brain imaging: evoked potential, quantitative EEG and SPECT abnormalities in schizophrenia. *J Psychiatry Neurosci* 1991;16:41–44.
10. Erbas B, Kumbasar H, Erbengi G, Bekdik C. Tc-99m HMPAO/SPECT determination of regional cerebral blood flow changes in schizophrenia. *Clin Nucl Med* 1990;15:904–907.
11. Bajc M, Medved V, Basic M, Topuzovic N, Babic D. Cerebral perfusion inhomogeneities in schizophrenia demonstrated with single photon emission computed tomography and Tc99m-hexamethylpropyleneamineoxim. *Acta Psychiatr Scand* 1989;80:427–433.
12. Kumar A, Mozley PD, Dunham C, et al. Semiquantitative I-123 IMP SPECT studies in late onset depression before and after treatment. *Int J Geriatr Psychiatry* 1991;6:775–777.
13. Amsterdam JD, Mozley PD. Temporal lobe asymmetry with iofetamine (IMP) SPECT imaging in patients with major depression. *J Affect Disord* 1992;24:43–53.
14. Maes M, Dierckx R, Meltzer HY, et al. Regional cerebral blood flow in unipolar depression measured with Tc-99m-HMPAO single photon emission computed tomography. *Psychiatry Res* 1993;50:77–88.
15. Bolwig TG. Regional cerebral blood flow in affective disorder. *Acta Psychiatr Scand* 1993;Suppl 371:48–53.
16. Ebert D, Feistel H, Baroca A, Kaschka W, Mokrusch T. A test-retest study of cerebral blood flow during somatosensory stimulation in depressed patients with schizophrenia and major depression. *Eur Arch Psychiatry Clin Neurosci* 1993;242:250–254.
17. Austin MP, Dougall N, Ross M, et al. Single photon emission tomography with 99mTc-exametazime in major depression and the pattern of brain activity underlying the psychotic/neurotic continuum. *J Affect Disord* 1992;26:31–43.
18. De Cristofaro MT, Sessarego A, Pupi A, Biondi F, Faravelli C. Brain perfusion abnormalities in drug-naive, lactate-sensitive panic patients. *Biol Psychiatry* 1993;33:505–512.

CASE 9-1 Clinical Diagnosis: Acute Paranoid Schizophrenia

CONTRIBUTOR:

Name: Ronald L. Van Heertum, M.D.
Institution: St. Vincent's Hospital and Medical Center

IMAGING DATA:

Camera: GE 400AC/T;STAR II
Isotope: ^{123}I IMP
Collimator: High resolution
Dose: 3.0 mCi

This 34-year-old homeless woman was referred for evaluation while having auditory hallucinations and paranoid delusions. The clinical diagnosis was paranoid schizophrenia, which was being treated with fluphenazine, 10 mg bid.

The cerebral SPECT study (Fig. 9.1) in the transaxial **(A),** coronal **(B),** and sagittal **(C)** planes, showed increased tracer deposition in the caudate nuclei *(arrowheads)* and the right posterior temporal region *(regions).*

Published with permission: ***J Neuropsychiatry Clin Neurosci*** **1989;1:145–153.**

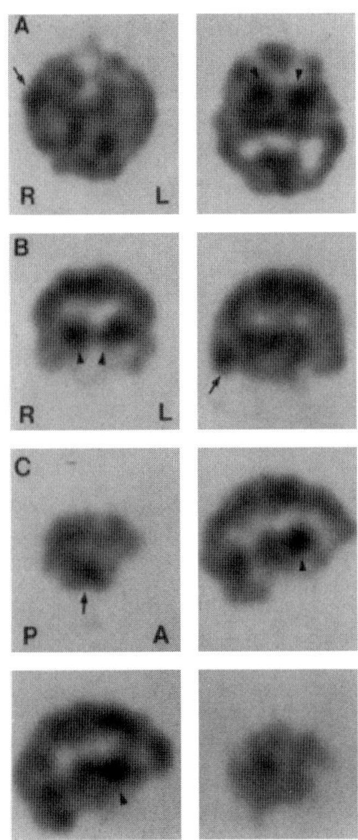

FIG. 9.1

CASE 9-2

Clinical Diagnosis: Acute Paranoid Schizophrenia

CONTRIBUTOR:

Name: Ronald L. Van Heertum, M.D.
Institution: St. Vincent's Hospital and Medical Center

IMAGING DATA:

Camera: GE400AC/T;STAR II
Isotope: ^{123}I IMP
Collimator: High resolution
Dose: 3.0 mCi

This 35-year-old man, a known paranoid schizophrenic, was referred for evaluation of his progressive paranoid delusions and auditory hallucinations. The patient had stopped taking his medication 1 month before admission to the hospital.

A CT scan (Fig. 9.2) was negative.

Before the cerebral SPECT, the patient had been started on fluphenazine, 10 mg bid, and benztropine, 1 mg bid.

The cerebral SPECT study (Fig. 9.3) in the transaxial **(A),** coronal **(B),** and sagittal **(C)** planes revealed increased tracer deposition in the caudate nuclei and slightly increased tracer activity in the right supratemporal region.

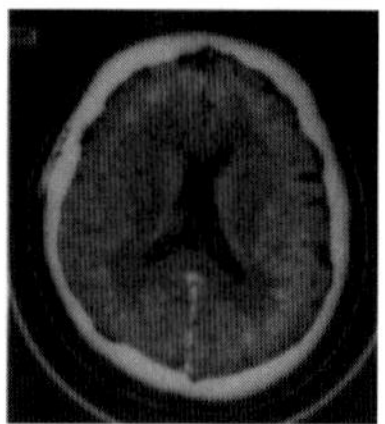

FIG. 9.2

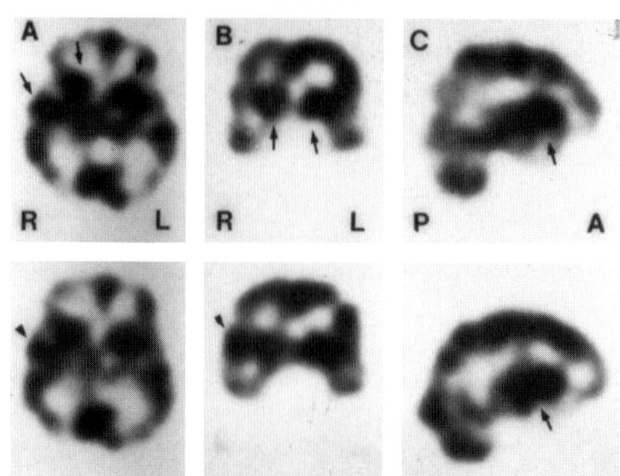

FIG. 9.3

CASE 9-3

Clinical Diagnosis:
Schizoaffective Disorder

CONTRIBUTOR:	IMAGING DATA:	
Name: Professor Hans Biersack and E. Klemm, M.D.	**Camera:** ADAC-Genesys	**Collimator:** Ultra-high resolution
Institution: University of Bonn	**Isotope:** ^{99m}TC	**Dose:** 20 mCi

This 49-year-old patient with a known schizoaffective disorder was referred for further evaluation. At the time of the SPECT study, he was on an antidepressant and a benzodiazepine.

An HMPAO-SPECT study (Fig. 9.4), in the transaxial *(upper row),* coronal *(middle row),* and sagittal *(lower row)* planes, revealed decreased radiotracer in the left temporal region.

Teaching Point:

This is another example of the types of temporal lobe asymmetries that may be seen in psychosis.

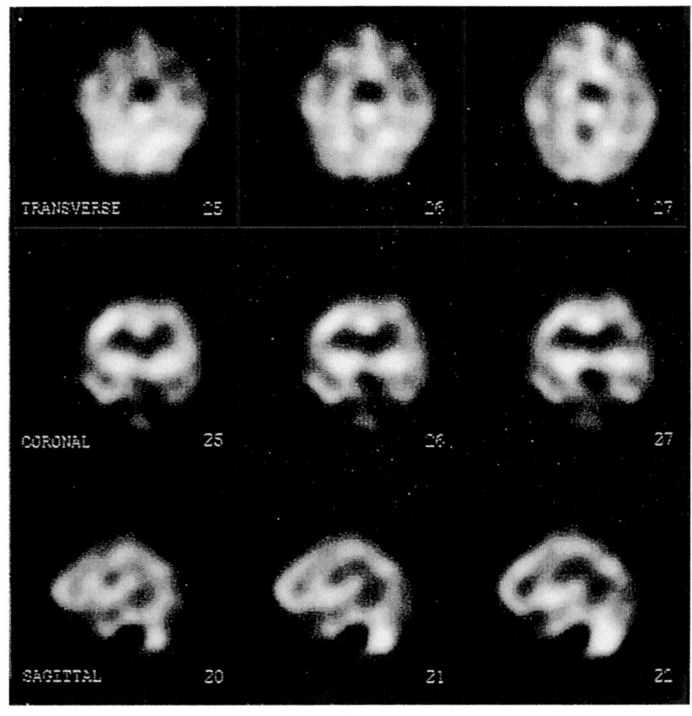

FIG. 9.4

CASE 9-4 Clinical Diagnosis: Autistic Behavior

CONTRIBUTOR:	IMAGING DATA:	
Name: Jane Mountz, M.D., Ph.D.	**Camera:** ADAC Genesys	**Collimator:** Ultra-high resolution
Institution: University of Alabama Hospital	**Isotope:** ^{99m}TC HMPAO	**Dose:** 13 mCi

This 10-year-old boy was referred for further evaluation of a very low IQ and a high level of autistic behavior. At the time of the SPECT study, the patient displayed unpredictable behavior and demonstrated no effectual reactions: language was limited to occasional use of gestures and signs and continuous noncommunicative vocalization.

A CT scan (Fig. 9.5) was normal.

An HMPAO SPECT study (Fig. 9.6), in the transaxial plane, revealed significant reduction of radiotracer uptake in the right hemisphere.

Teaching Point:

Although the patient was injected while in the fully alert autistic state, general anesthesia was administered for scanning. This demonstrates the value of using anesthesia or sedation to image severely noncompliant patients.

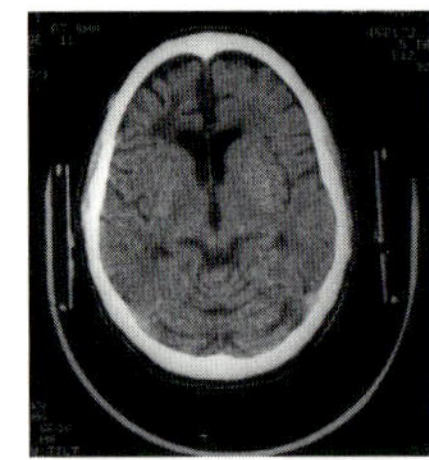

FIG. 9.5

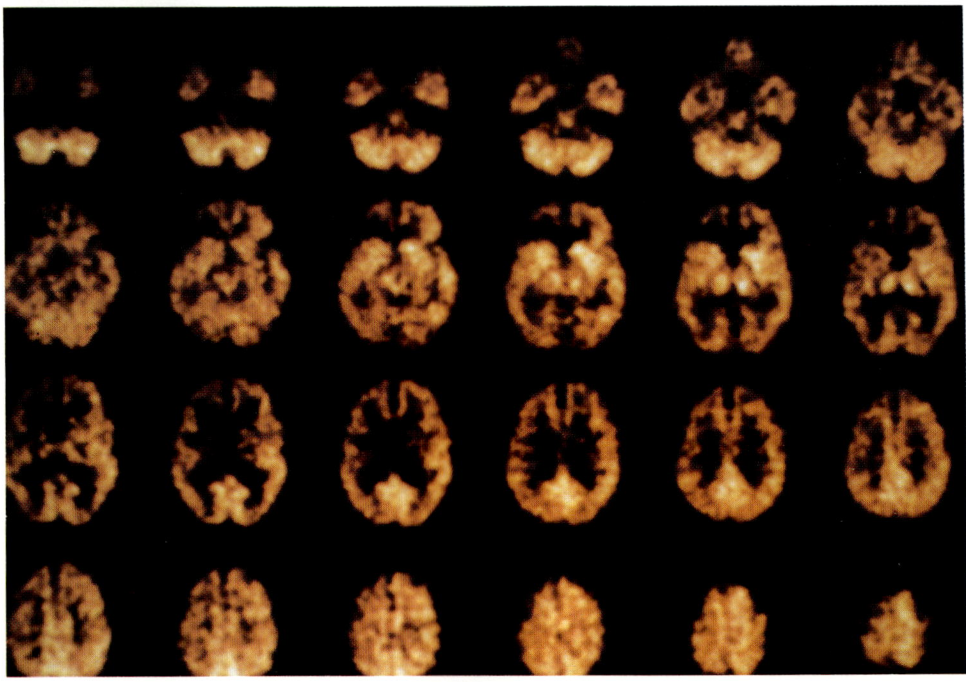

FIG. 9.6

CASE 9-5

Clinical Diagnosis:

Acute Paranoid Schizophrenia: Follow-Up During Treatment

CONTRIBUTOR:

Name: Ronald L. Van Heertum, M.D.
Institution: St. Vincent's Hospital and Medical Center

IMAGING DATA:

Camera: GE 400AC/T;STAR II
Isotope: ^{123}I IMP
Collimator: High resolution
Dose: 3.0 mCi

This 30-year-old man was referred for evaluation of an acute psychosis characterized by paranoid delusions, auditory hallucinations, and destructive behavior that had become progressively worse over the preceding 2 years. An EEG and a CT scan were normal. The clinical diagnosis was acute paranoid schizophrenia.

At the time of the initial SPECT study, the patient was receiving a total daily dose of 100 mg of Ioxapine (an antipsychotic medication). The initial cerebral SPECT study (Fig. 9.7) in the transaxial **(A),** coronal **(B),** and sagittal **(C)** planes revealed an increased tracer deposition in the caudate nuclei, along with a mild decrease of tracer activity in the cortex of the frontal lobes. Two weeks later a follow-up cerebral SPECT study was performed. At that time, the patient was much improved clinically. The follow-up study (Fig. 9.8) demonstrated a significant but partial decrease of tracer activity in the caudate nuclei. A slight focal increase in tracer deposition was noted in the right temporal lobe. This later finding may have been related to the patient's medication lowering the seizure threshold.

Published with permission: ***Adv Functional Neuroimaging*** **1988;1:4–11.**

Teaching Point:

As the preceding three cases illustrate, the pattern of increased tracer activity in the caudate nuclei (with or without decreased tracer uptake in the frontal lobe) may be seen in patients with acute psychoses.

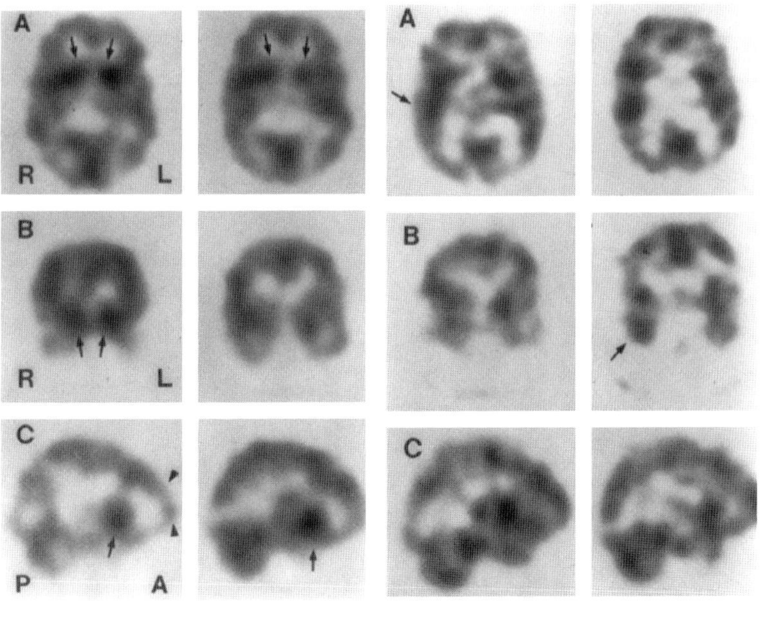

FIG. 9.7 **FIG. 9.8**

CASE 9-6

Clinical Diagnosis: Acute Paranoid Schizophrenia: Change in Treatment

CONTRIBUTOR:

Name: Ronald L. Van Heertum, M.D.
Institution: St. Vincent's Hospital and Medical Center

IMAGING DATA:

Camera: GE 400AC/T;STAR II
Isotope: ^{123}I IMP
Collimator: High resolution
Dose: 3.0 mCi

This 41-year-old woman, known to be paranoid schizophrenic, was referred for evaluation of threatening auditory hallucinations. An EEG and a CT scan (Fig. 9.9) were normal. At the time of the cerebral SPECT examination, she had been receiving trifluoperazine, 50 mg daily, and benztropine, 1 mg daily.

The cerebral SPECT study (Fig. 9.10) in the transaxial(**A**) and sagittal (**B**) planes revealed increased tracer activity in the caudate nuclei, with focal increased uptake of tracer in the right temporal lobe. As a result of her continuing hallucinations and the cerebral SPECT finding of increased temporal lobe activity, the patient's medication was modified to include an anticonvulsant (carbamazepine.)

Following modification of her medication, the patient showed a dramatic improvement, with a marked decrease in the frequency of auditory hallucinations.

Published with permission: ***Clin Nucl Med* 1989;14:319–322.**

Teaching Point:

As this case demonstrates, the cerebral SPECT study may reveal useful information that is not demonstrable on other studies such as the EEG or CT scan.

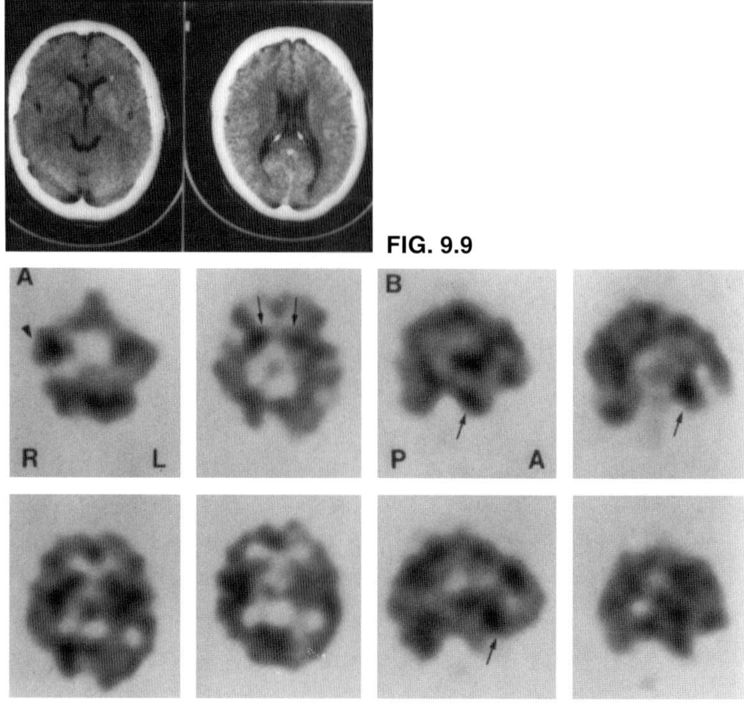

FIG. 9.9

FIG. 9.10

CASE 9-7 Clinical Diagnosis: Severe Depression

CONTRIBUTOR:	IMAGING DATA:	
Name: Ronald L. Van Heertum, M.D.	**Camera:** GE 400AC/T;STAR II	**Collimator:** High resolution
Institution: St. Vincent's Hospital and Medical Center	**Isotope:** ^{123}I IMP	**Dose:** 3.0 mCi

This 32-year-old man was referred for evaluation of severe depression. An EEG and a CT scan (Fig. 9.11) were normal. At the time of the cerebral SPECT study, the patient was not on medication.

The cerebral SPECT study (Fig. 9.12) in the transaxial **(A),** coronal **(B),** and sagittal **(C)** planes revealed an overall decrease in tracer deposition throughout the cerebral cortex. This pattern was most marked in the frontal lobes.

Published with permission: ***J Neuropsychiatry and Clin Neurosci*** **1989;1:145–153.**

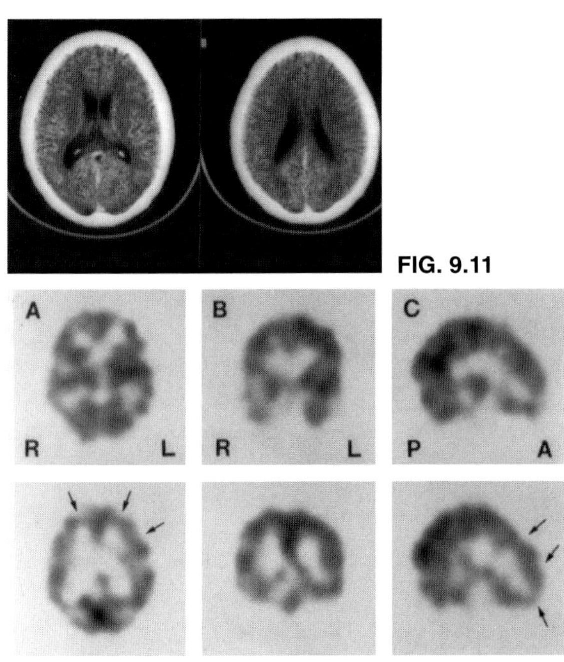

FIG. 9.11

FIG. 9.12

CASE 9-8

Clinical Diagnosis: Major Depressive Disorder

CONTRIBUTOR:	IMAGING DATA:	
Name: Ronald L. Van Heertum, M.D.	**Camera:** GE 400AC/T;STAR II	**Collimator:** High resolution
Institution: St. Vincent's Hospital and Medical Center	**Isotope:** ^{123}I IMP	**Dose:** 3.0 mCi

This 56-year-old man, with a history of major depressive disorder, was referred for evaluation of a severe depression with paranoid ideation but no hallucinations.

The CT scan (Fig. 9.13) and EEG were normal. At the time of the cerebral SPECT study, the patient was receiving amitrip+yline, 50 mg daily.

The cerebral SPECT study (Fig. 9.14) in the transaxial **(A),** coronal **(B),** and sagittal **(C)** planes revealed a decrease in tracer deposition most marked in the frontal lobes.

Published with permission: ***Adv Functional Neuroimaging*** **1988;1:4–11.**

Teaching Point:

As the preceding two cases illustrate, the pattern seen in major depressive disorders is quite different from that noted in acute psychoses such as schizophrenia. The relative decrease of tracer uptake appears to correlate with the severity of the depression.

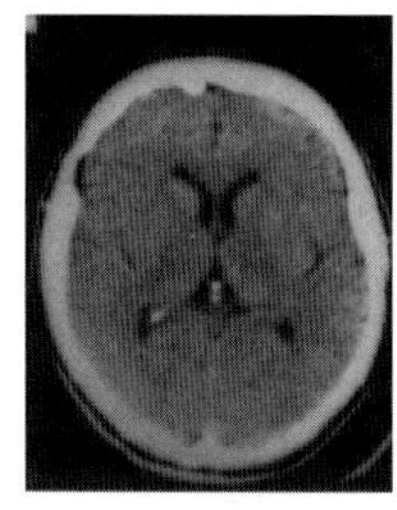

FIG. 9.13

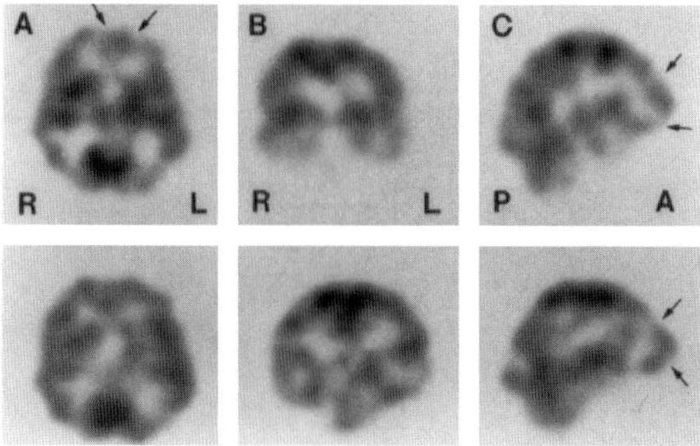

FIG. 9.14

CASE 9-9 Clinical Diagnosis: Bipolar Disorder—Depressed

CONTRIBUTOR:	IMAGING DATA:	
Name: Ronald L. Van Heertum, M.D.	**Camera:** Picker Prism 3000	**Collimator:** Ultra-high resolution, fan beam
Institution: Columbia-Presbyterian Medical Center	**Isotope:** ^{99m}TC HMPAO	**Dose:** 21.3 mCi

This 30-year-old Caucasian man was referred for evaluation of severe depression.

CT scan was reported to be within normal limits.

HMPAO SPECT (Fig. 9.15) in the transaxial **(A),** coronal **(B)** and sagittal **(C)** planes revealed a global decrease in radiotracer uptake that was most marked in the frontal lobes.

Teaching Point:

Cerebral SPECT may be helpful in the evaluation of patients with mood disorders, in particular depression.

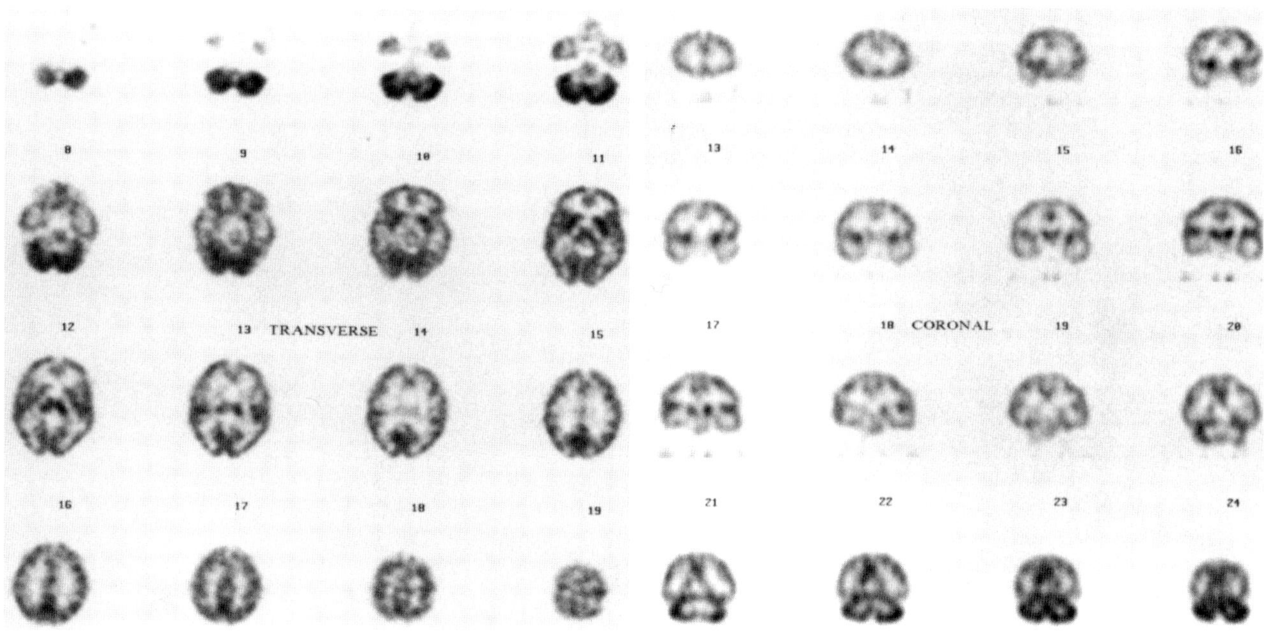

FIG. 9.15A **FIG. 9.15B**

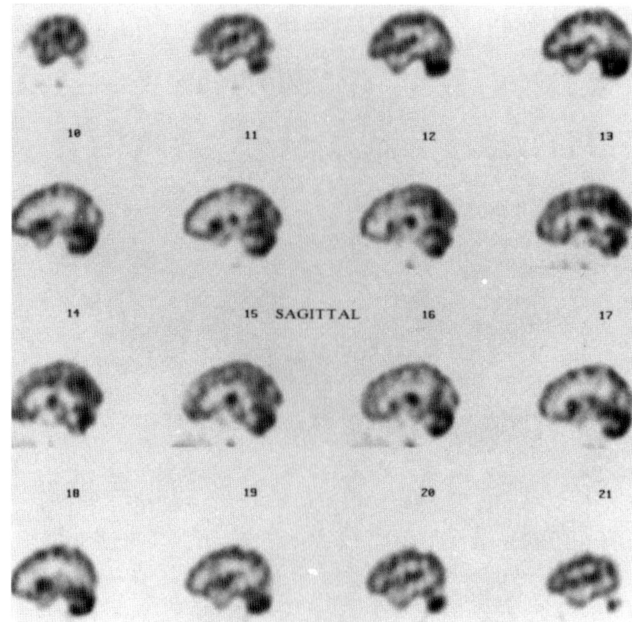

FIG. 9.15C

CASE 9-10

Clinical Diagnosis:

Acute Psychosis After Acute Head Trauma

CONTRIBUTOR:	IMAGING DATA:	
Name: Ronald L. Van Heertum, M.D.	**Camera:** GE 3000 XCT	**Collimator:** Ultra-high resolution
Institution: St. Vincent's Hospital and Medical Center	**Isotope:** ^{99m}TC HMPAO	**Dose:** 19.5 mCi

This 25-year-old man was referred for evaluation and treatment following two attempted suicide episodes. Six months prior to admission, he had sustained a severe traumatic brain injury at the time of a fall from a 3-story building. At that time the patient was found to have a left frontal lobe hematoma, which was evacuated during emergency craniotomy. Over the past several months, the patient was noted to be increasingly delusional, suffering from insomnia and experiencing auditory hallucinations.

A follow-up CT scan (Fig. 9.16) revealed a craniotomy defect in the left frontal region with an underlying area of focal hypodensity corresponding to the site where the left frontal intracerebral hematoma had been evacuated.

An HMPAO SPECT study (Fig. 9.17), in the transaxial **(A),** coronal **(B),** and sagittal **(C)** planes, revealed absent radiotracer activity in the left posterior frontal lobe. The area of absent tracer activity, which extended deep into the adjacent white matter, was significantly larger than the site of the evacuated hematoma noted on CT scan.

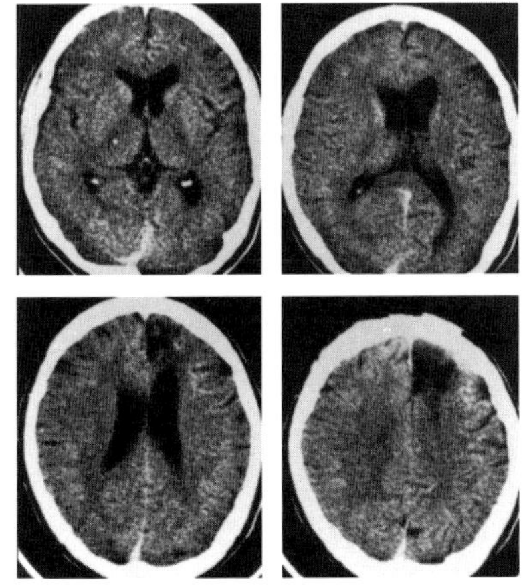

FIG. 9.16

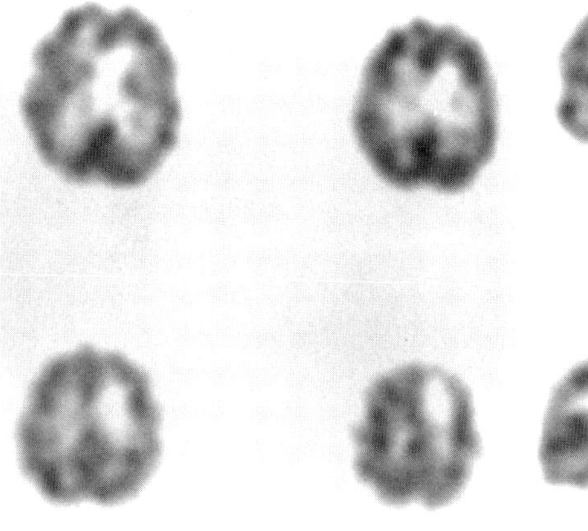

FIG. 9.17A

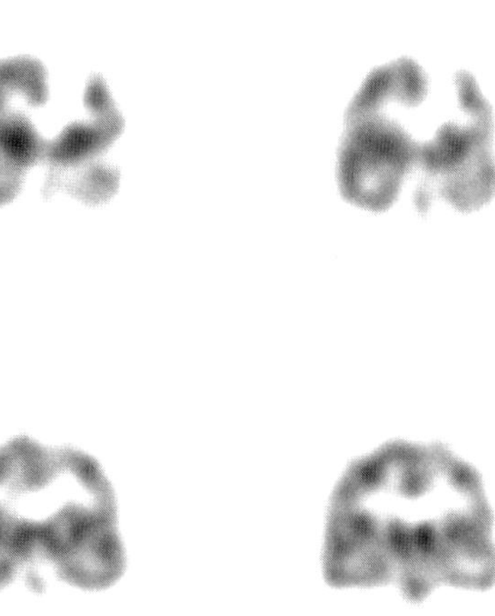

FIG. 9.17B

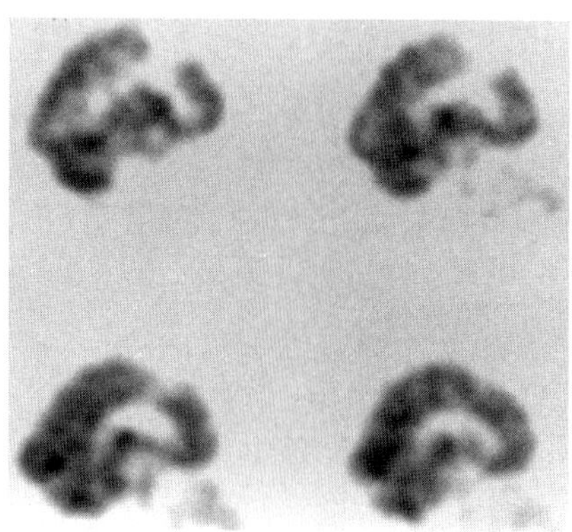

FIG. 9.17C

CASE 9-11 Clinical Diagnosis: Normal Visual Activation Paradigm

CONTRIBUTOR:	IMAGING DATA:	
Name: Thomas C. Hill, M.D.	**Camera:** Strichman SME 810	**Collimator:** High resolution
Institution: Deaconess Hospital	**Isotope:** ^{99m}Tc ECD	**Dose:** 20 mCi

This 43-year-old right-handed normal male volunteer was studied at baseline with eyes open, ears unplugged, in a dark room sitting at a computer console, during a visual activation with full-field visual stimulation (flashing checkerboard).

Baseline ethyl cysteinate dimer (ECD) SPECT study (Fig. 9.18A) in the transaxial plane *(top)* reveals a normal tracer distribution. Activation ECD SPECT (Fig. 9.18B), in the transaxial plane *(bottom)*, injected at the time of visual stimulation revealed enhanced radiotracer uptake primarily in the region of the visual cortex.

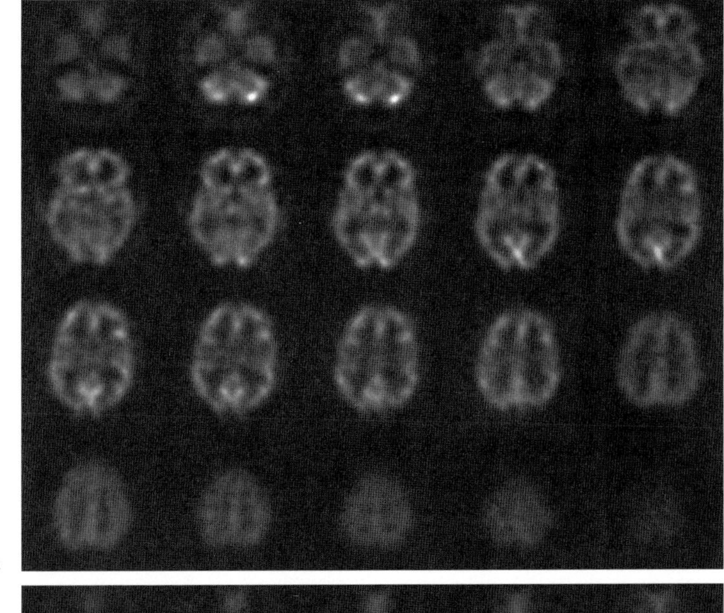

A

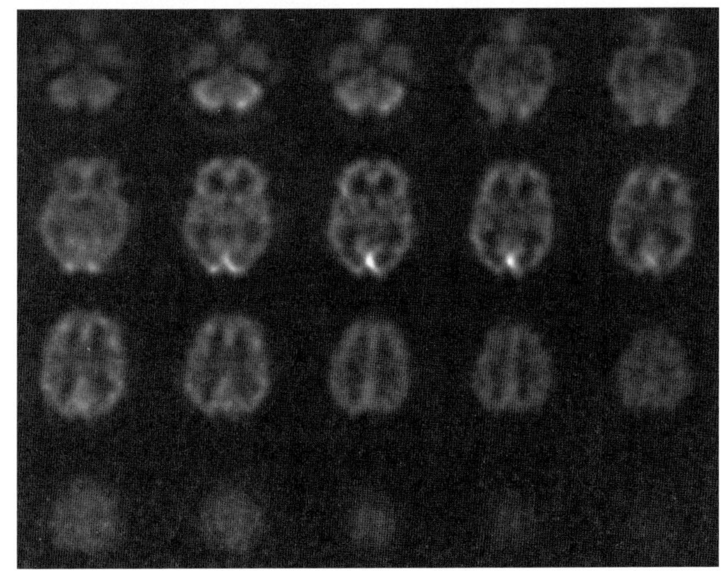

B

FIG. 9.18A-B

Cerebral SPECT Imaging, Second Edition,
edited by R.L. Van Heertum and R.S. Tikofsky.
Raven Press, Ltd., New York © 1995.

CHAPTER 10

Miscellaneous Disorders

Ronald L. Van Heertum and Ronald S. Tikofsky

In addition to cerebrovascular disease, dementia, epilepsy, head trauma, and psychiatric disorders, cerebral SPECT imaging may prove to be useful in a wide variety of other disease states. These disorders include anoxic states, toxic encephalopathy, tinnitus, and brain tumors. Brain tumor imaging, in particular, is currently proving to be a particularly popular technique. Brain scintigraphy using ^{99m}Tc pertechnetate was until the mid-1970s the only imaging technique for studying brain tumors (1). These procedures were eclipsed by the introduction of computed tomography (CT) and magnetic resonance imaging (MRI). However, CT and MRI do not always differentiate recurrent tumor from necrosis. Nuclear medicine's role in the evaluation of brain tumors has been reactivated by the advent of SPECT imaging with ^{99m}Tc sestamibi, ^{201}Tl chloride. The ability of agents such as ^{201}T1 and ^{99m}Tc sestamibi (MIBI) used with SPECT to help resolve these questions is now well documented (2–10). Mountz et al. (11) provide an excellent review of this subject. Taken together, the results of these studies show that ^{201}T1 SPECT brain imaging of brain tumors can aid in:

1. Differentiating high- from low-grade gliomas
2. Directing biopsy to the site of highest tumor burden
3. Evaluating for recurrent tumor vs. postsurgical or radiation changes (sequential follow-up scans can be used to assess efficacy of therapy)
4. Assessing for residual tumor following therapy (Is tumor shrinking as the result of radiation or chemotherapy? Is there a significant decrease in activity and tumor debulking?)

R. S. Tikofsky: Department of Radiology, Section of Nuclear Medicine, Medical College of Wisconsin, Milwaukee, Wisconsin 53226.

R. L. Van Heertum: Department of Clinical Radiology, Columbia University College of Physicians and Surgeons, and Department of Nuclear Medicine, Columbia Presbyterian Medical Center, New York, New York 10032.

Using a dual-isotope technique, Schwartz et al. (12) reported that their technique correlated with the pathologic findings in 14 of 15 cases studied. Their findings for ^{201}T1 are similar to those reported by others. Patients with high ^{201}T1 uptake in treated tumor beds had local tumor recurrence, and those with low uptake showed only radiation changes and no evidence of solid tumor. However, in those patients with an intermediate level of ^{201}T1 uptake in the tumor bed, ^{99m}Tc hexamethylpropyleneamine-oxime (HMPAO) uptake permitted a differentiation of patients with active tumor from those whose tumors were not active. Schwartz et al. (12) suggest that this dual-isotope procedure can be useful in distinguishing sites of potential tumor growth from radiation changes in patients undergoing therapy for malignant glioma. Not all imaging systems are capable of dual-isotope SPECT imaging. An alternative procedure that yields similar results is to perform the ^{201}T1 imaging first; when it is completed, inject the HMPAO and reimage at approximately 1 1/2 to 2 hr post-HMPAO injection. Processing of the thallium and HMPAO data is carried as appropriate for the imaging system being used.

In addition to assessing tumor recurrence and response to therapy, it is also important to determine if radiation or chemotherapy produces necrotic changes in cortex, or if there are other cortical changes resulting from treatment. These effects, typically seen as reduced cortical uptake of HMPAO, reflect one of two conditions. One reflects necrosis of cortex. As cortical tissue becomes necrotic it will take up less tracer. The second factor leading to reduced cortical uptake is diaschisis. In this case the reduced tracer uptake is a result of the complete or partial destruction of pathways that have been damaged by the tumor or the effects of treatment. Thus the use of dual agents such as HMPAO in conjunction with ^{201}T1 SPECT imaging can provide significant clinical information regarding tumor recurrence and the secondary effects of damaged pathways to cortex or treatment.

Interpretation of ^{201}T1 images is usually based on visual inspection of the images. Accumulation of ^{201}T1 provides the best correlation with clinical status. The more avid the uptake of ^{201}T1 the greater the likelihood of a high-grade tumor or tumor recurrence. Some efforts have been made to quantitate ^{201}T1 results of tumor imaging with SPECT (3,9). The indices developed by these research teams suggest that it is possible to use the measures described to classify brain tumors. Jinnouchi et al. (8) have developed a quantitative system using delayed uptake indices to classify meningiomas. They found that high accumulations of ^{201}T1 occurred in all types of meningiomas, but that retention rates change as a function of histological type, with a high retention rate being indicative of malignant potential of the meningioma. For those who will interpret ^{201}T1 images, but who wish a somewhat simpler method of quantitation, Schwartz et al. (12) describe three major categories of uptake based on a ^{201}T1 lesion-to-scalp ratio: (a) high—lesion-to-scalp ratio ≥ 2; (b) moderate—lesion-to-scalp ratio $=1–2$; and (c) low—lesion-to-scalp ratio ≤ 1. With experience it is possible to assess visually how avidly the tracer is taken up by the tumor.

As oncologists and neurosurgeons become increasingly aware of the value of SPECT imaging to assess the recurrence of brain tumors and efficacy of treatment, there will be an increase of referrals to nuclear medicine to perform this type of study.

REFERENCES

1. Biersack HJ, Grunwal F, Kropp J. Single photon emission computed tomography imaging of brain tumors. *Semin Nucl Med* 1991;21:2–10.
2. Mountz JM, Stafford-Schuck K, McKeever PE, Taren J, Beierwaltes WH. Thallium-201 tumor/cardiac ratio estimation of residual astrocytoma. *J Neurosurg* 1988;68:705–709.
3. Kim KT, Black KL, Marciano D, et al. Thallium-201 SPECT imaging of brain tumors: methods and results. *J Nucl Med* 1990;31:965–969.
4. O'Tuama LA, Treves ST, Larar JN, et al. Thallium-201 versus technetium-99m-MIBI SPECT in evaluation of childhood brain tumors: a within-subject comparison. *J Nucl Med* 1993;34:1045–1051.
5. Ueda T, Kaji Y, Wakisaka S, et al. Time sequential single photon emission computed tomography studies in brain tumor using thallium-201. *Eur J Nucl Med* 1993;20:1318–1145.
6. Oriuchi N, Tamura M, Shibazaki T, et al. Clinical evaluation of thallium-201 SPECT in supratentorial gliomas: relationship to histologic grade, prognosis and proliferative activities. *J Nucl Med* 1993; 34:2085–2089.
7. Tonami N. Editorial: thallium-201 SPECT in the evaluation of gliomas. *J Nucl Med* 1993;34:2089–2090.
8. Jinnouchi S, Hosi H, Ohnishi T, et al. Thallium-201 SPECT for predicting histological types of meningiomas. *J Nucl Med* 1993; 34:2091–2094.
9. Mountz JM, Rosenfeld SS, Li Y. Utility of 201-T1 and 99m-Tc-sestamibi SPECT for early determination of malignant brain tumor chemotherapy efficacy. *J Nucl Med* 1993;34:206P(abst).
10. Hoh CK, Khanna S, Harris GC, et al. Evaluation of brain tumor recurrence with T1-201 SPECT studies: correlation with FDG PET and histological results. *J Nucl Med* 1992;33:867 (abst).
11. Mountz JM, Deutsch G, Kuzniecky R, Rosenfeld SS. Brain SPECT: 1994 Update. In: Freeman LM, ed. *Nuclear medicine annual 1994.* New York: Raven Press: 1994; 1–54.
12. Schwartz RB, Carvalho PA, Alexander E III, Loefller JS, Folkerth R, Holman BL. Radiation necrosis vs high-grade recurrent glioma: differentiation by using dual-isotope SPECT with ^{201}T1 and ^{99m}Tc-HMPAO. *AJNR* 1992;12:1187–1192.

CASE 10-1 Clinical Diagnosis: Cystic Astrocytoma: Post-Treatment

CONTRIBUTOR:	IMAGING DATA:	
Name: Donald Fox, M.D. and Caesar Mayo, M.D.	**Camera:** Spectrum 150DT	**Collimator:** High resolution
Institution: San Jose Imaging Center	**Isotope:** ^{123}I IMP	**Dose:** 3.0 mCi

This 61-year-old man was referred for evaluation of increasing confusion. Previously, he had undergone a craniotomy for a cystic astrocytoma of the left temporal lobe. The surgery was followed by radiation and chemotherapy 3 weeks prior to his referral for SPECT studies.

The last follow-up MRI study (Fig. 10.1) showed a diffuse increase in signal intensity throughout the left temporal lobe. This finding was thought to be most consistent with progressive changes attributable to the radiation therapy.

An IMP cerebral SPECT study (Fig. 10.2) in the transaxial **(A),** coronal **(B),** and sagittal **(C)** planes showed decreased tracer deposition in the left temporal lobe. The findings were thought to be consistent with postradiation therapy changes in the left temporal lobe.

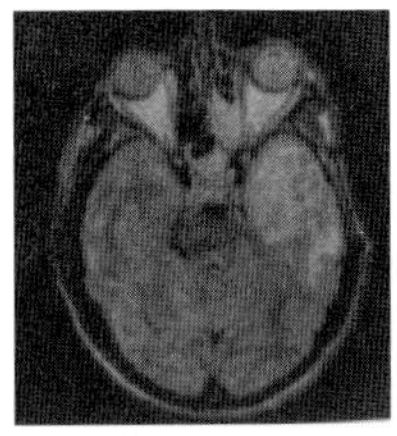

FIG. 10.1

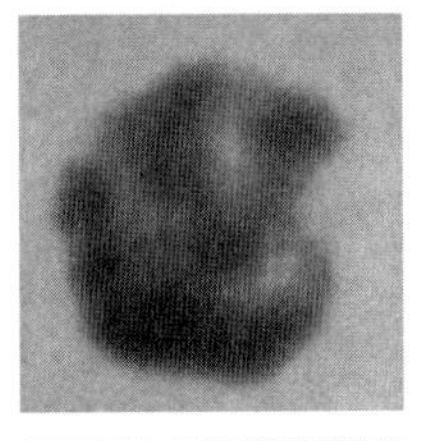

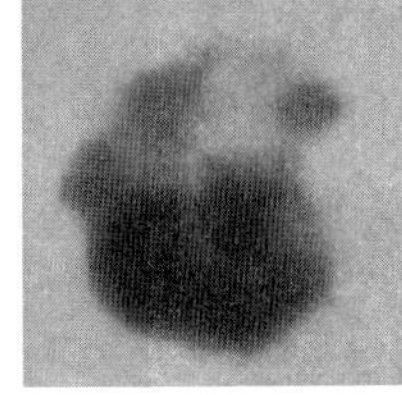

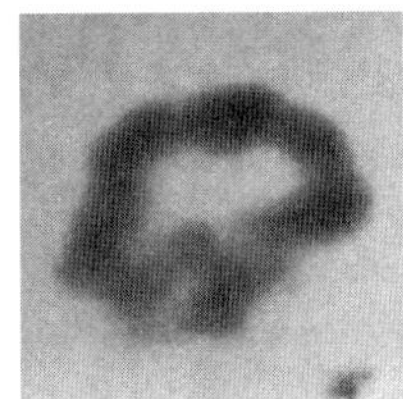

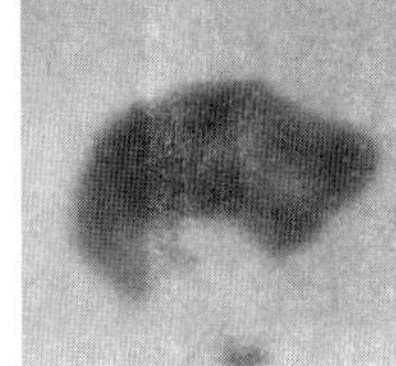

FIG. 10.2

CASE 10-2 Clinical Diagnosis: Astrocytoma

CONTRIBUTOR:	IMAGING DATA:	
Name: Robert S. Hellman, M.D. and Ronald S. Tikofsky, M.D.	**Camera:** GE Neurocam	**Collimator:** High resolution
Institution: Medical College of Wisconsin	**Isotope:** ^{201}Tl Chloride ^{99m}Tc HMPAO	**Dose:** 3.0 mCi **Dose:** 31.3 mCi

This 34-year-old woman with a known right occipital lobe astrocytoma that had been resected and treated with irradiation 6 years prior to admission was referred for evaluation of increasing drowsiness and headaches.

A CT scan showed an enhancing tumor mass at the site of the original lesion. A follow-up MRI scan (Fig. 10.3) revealed a significant increase in size of the right occipital and periventricular tumor compared with the prior CT scan.

A ^{201}Tl SPECT study (Fig. 10.4), in the transaxial plane, revealed intense increased thallium uptake deep in the right hemisphere. This finding is consistent with viable tumor deep in the right hemisphere extending superiorly into the region of the right corpus callosum.

An HMPAO study (Fig. 10.5) in the transaxial plane revealed extensive regions of absent activity in the right temporal, parietal, and occipital regions. In addition, absent tracer uptake was seen in the deep subcortical regions, particularly the right thalamus corresponding to the deep right hemispheric mass identified on MRI and thallium SPECT. A mild decrease in the posterior right frontal lobe radiotracer activity, possibly secondary to prior radiation therapy or diaschisis, was also noted.

Teaching Point:

Combined ^{201}Tl and ^{99m}Tc HMPAO SPECT studies are frequently more helpful than single SPECT imaging studies with either compound.

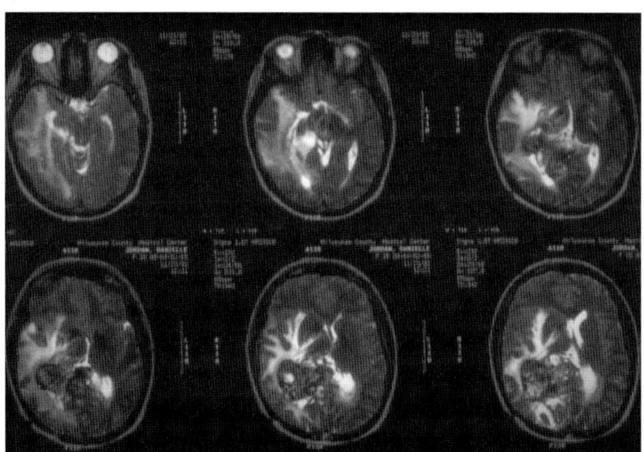

FIG. 10.3

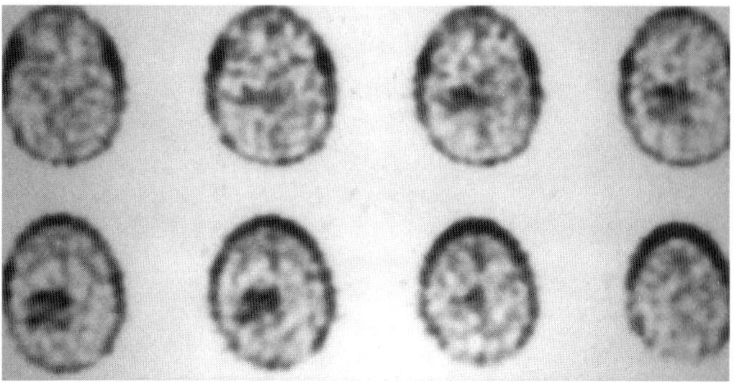

FIG. 10.4

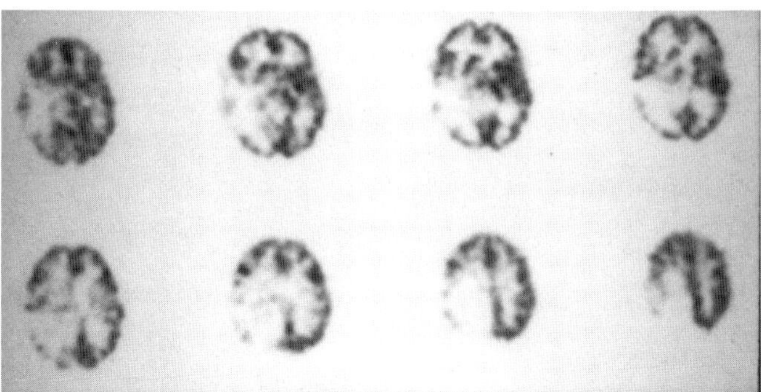

FIG. 10.5

CASE 10-3

Clinical Diagnosis: Recurrent Astrocytoma: Grade III/IV

CONTRIBUTOR:

Name: Robert S. Hellman, M.D. and Ronald S. Tikofsky, M.D.
Institution: Medical College of Wisconsin

IMAGING DATA:

Camera: GE Neurocam
Isotope: ^{201}Tl chloride ^{99m}Tc HMPAO

Collimator: High resolution
Dose: 3.1 mCi
Dose: 32.0 mCi

This 59-year-old woman was referred for evaluation following surgical reopening of a right parietal craniotomy with microsurgical excision of a recurrent glioblastoma multiforme.

A follow-up T1 and T2 weighted MRI study (Fig. 10.6) revealed a lesion in the right thalamus as well as a right temporal parietal mass that had increased in size when compared with prior studies. In addition, a vascular malformation was evident in the left temporal-parietal lobe.

A thallium SPECT study (Fig. 10.7) in the transaxial plane showed foci of increased activity in the right temporal-parietal region and the right thalamus that were felt to represent recurrent tumor.

An HMPAO SPECT study (Fig. 10.8), in the transaxial plane revealed a postsurgical decrease in tracer on the right side and a focus of increased activity in the right parietal temporal region corresponding to the area of abnormality on MRI. Follow-up thallium and HMPAO SPECT studies (Fig. 10.9) showed intense focal increased uptake of HMPAO and thallium in the right posterior temporal lobe secondary to recurrent tumor.

Teaching Point:

In this case, thallium SPECT was helpful in localizing the sites of recurrent tumor.

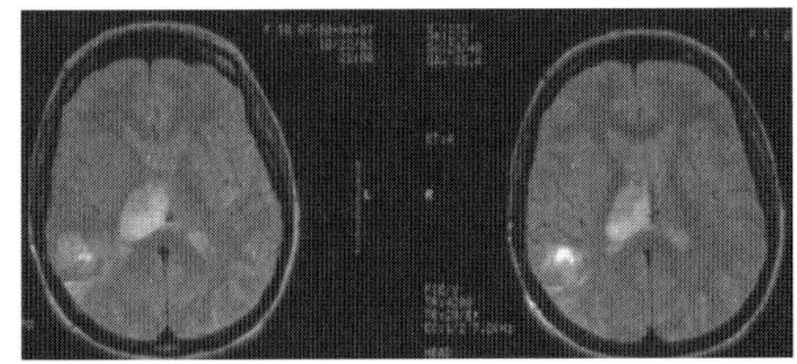

FIG. 10.6A

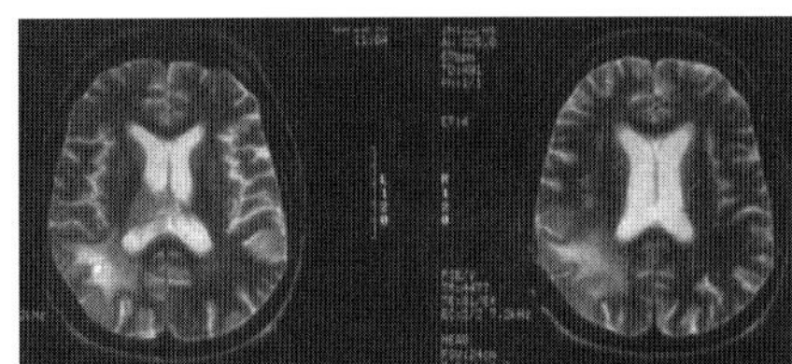

FIG. 10.6B

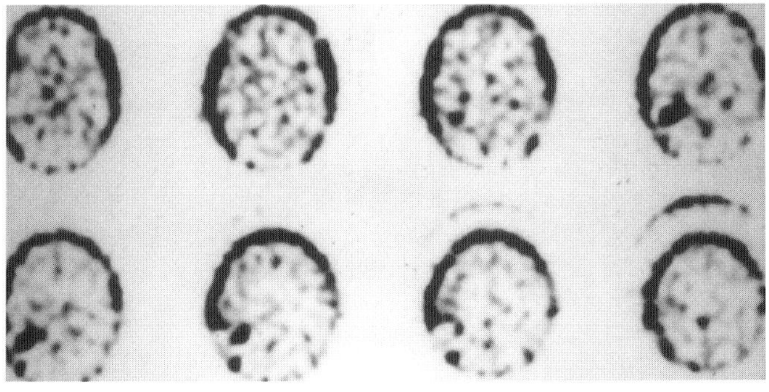

FIG. 10.7

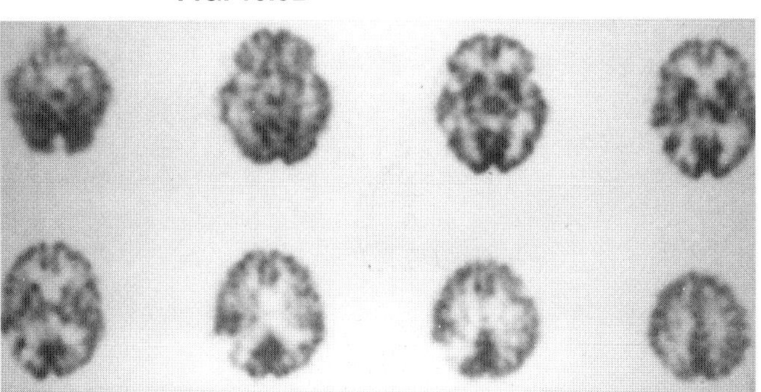

FIG. 10.8

CASE 10-4

Clinical Diagnosis:
Left Frontal Meningioma

CONTRIBUTOR:	IMAGING DATA:	
Name: Ronald L. Van Heertum, M.D.	**Camera:** GE Neurocam	**Collimator:** Ultra-high resolution
Institution: Columbia-Presbyterian Medical Center	**Isotope:** ^{99m}Tc HMPAO	**Dose:** 21.0 mCi

This 75-year-old man with a known left frontal meningioma was referred for evaluation after several episodes of imbalance (unsteadiness).

An MRI study (Fig. 10.9), pre- **(A)** and post- **(B)** gadolinium injection, revealed an enhancing 3-cm meningioma, in the inferior-lateral aspect of the left frontal lobe that was connected to the meninges by a small stalk.

An HMPAO SPECT study (Fig. 10.10) in the transaxial plane revealed focal increased radiotracer uptake in the left inferior frontal meningioma.

Teaching Point:

^{99m}Tc HMPAO tracer uptake in meningiomas may vary. In general, however, the tracer concentration in these lesions tends to be avid.

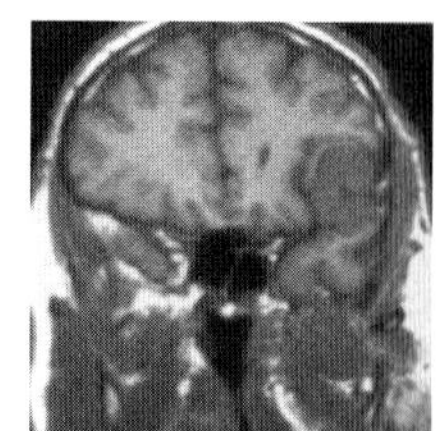

FIG. 10.9A

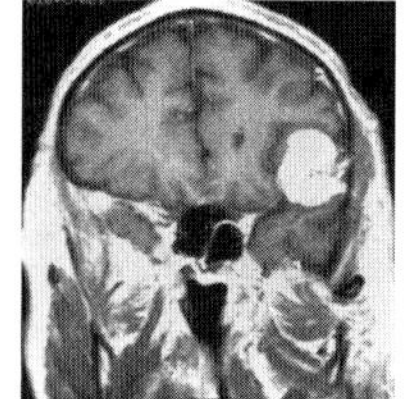

FIG. 10.9B

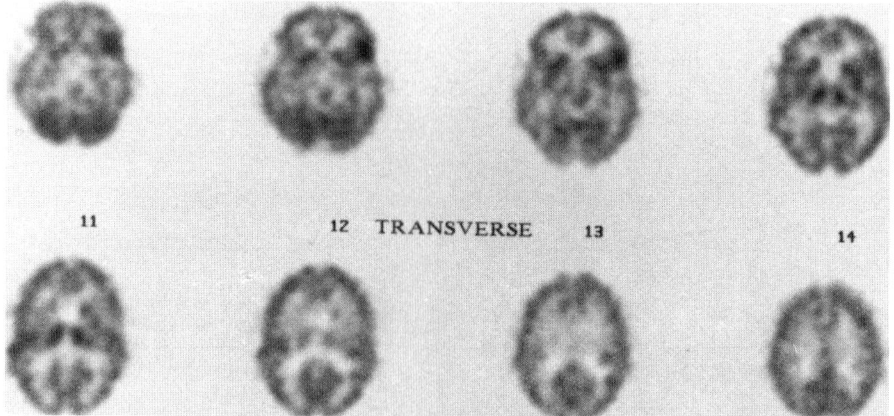

FIG. 10.10

CASE 10-5

Clinical Diagnosis: Falyx Cerebri Meningioma

CONTRIBUTOR:	**IMAGING DATA:**	
Name: Ronald L. Van Heertum, M.D.	**Camera:** GE-3000 XCT	**Collimator:** Ultra-high resolution
Institution: St. Vincent's Hospital and Medical Center	**Isotope:** ^{99m}Tc HMPAO	**Dose:** 20.0 mCi

This 66-year-old woman presented complaining of a progressively increasing "pressure sensation" involving the right side of her head.

A skull series revealed a large predominantly lytic lesion in the right frontal bone with sclerotic margins.

A MRI examination (Fig. 10.11), in the axial **(A)** and coronal **(B)** planes, revealed a large lobular mass with intra- and extracranial components most consistent with a meningioma arising from the falx cerebri.

An HMPAO SPECT study (Fig. 10.12) in the coronal **(A)** and sagittal **(B)** planes revealed radiotracer uptake in the mass seen on the MRI study.

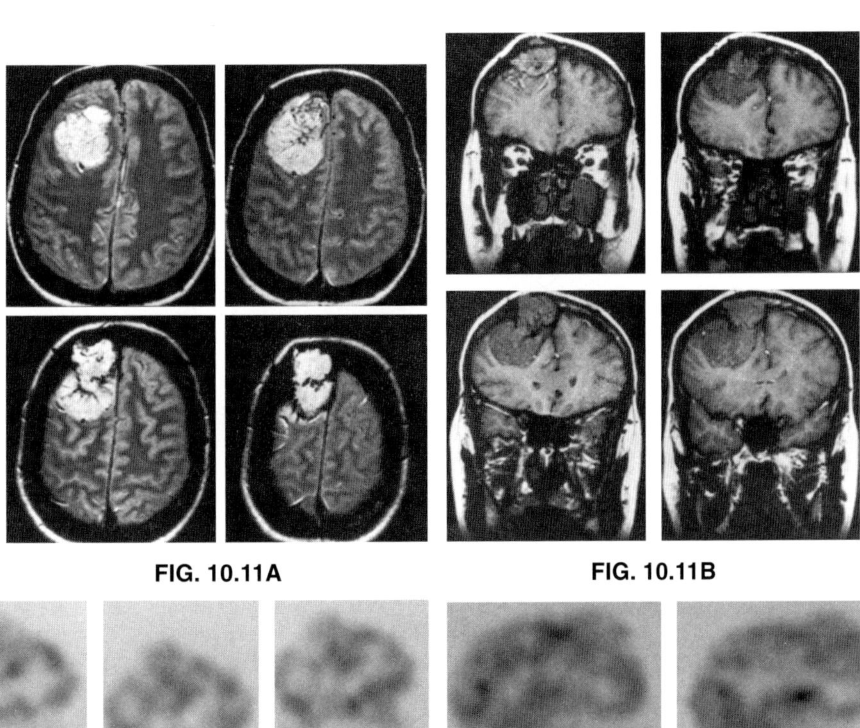

FIG. 10.11A

FIG. 10.11B

FIG. 10.12A

FIG. 10.12B

CASE 10-6

Clinical Diagnosis:
Anoxic Encephalopathy

CONTRIBUTOR:	IMAGING DATA:	
Name: Ronald S. Van Heertum, M.D.	**Camera:** GE 400 AC/T;STAR II	**Collimator:** High resolution
Institution: St. Vincent's Hospital and Medical Center	**Isotope:** ^{123}I IMP	**Dose:** 3.0 mCi

This 76-year-old woman had sustained an anoxic encephalopathy at the time of a cardiac arrest. Despite vigorous attempts at cardiopulmonary resuscitation, the patient remained severely obtunded at the time of referral.

An IMP cerebral SPECT study (Fig. 10.13) in the transaxial **(A),** coronal **(B),** and sagittal **(C)** planes revealed a marked decrease in tracer deposition throughout the cerebral cortex. This was most marked in the occipital, parietal, and frontal lobes as well as the periventricular white matter. The brain stem and cerebellum were relatively spared.

Teaching Point:

This pattern is typically seen in patients who have sustained a severe anoxic episode.

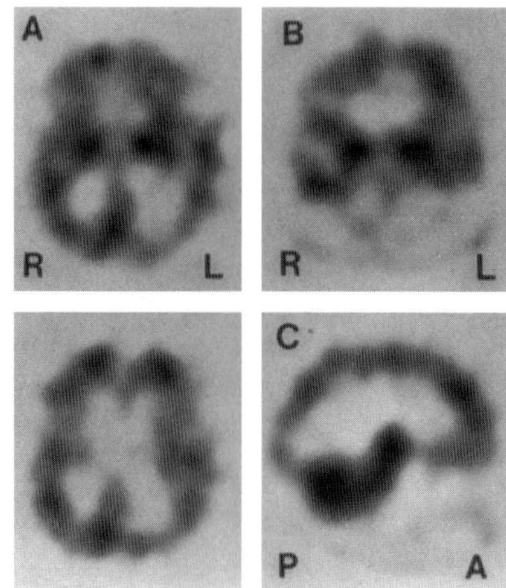

FIG. 10.13

CASE 10-7

Clinical Diagnosis:

Toxic Encephalopathy

CONTRIBUTOR:

Name: James Mountz, M.D., Ph.D.
Institution: University of Alabama Hospital

IMAGING DATA:

Camera: Adac dual-headed Genesys
Isotope: ^{99m}Tc HMPAO
Collimator: High resolution
Dose: 25 mCi

This 52-year-old woman presented with progressive symptoms of insomnia, headaches, and dizziness of 6 years' duration. During this period she also complained of malaise, memory loss, and weakness. The patient said that these symptoms were related to her work environment, where she was exposed to oils, coolants, solvents, fumes, and vapors. These symptoms abated when she was not at work. Neurologic examination showed episodic numbness, dizziness, poor balance, jerky motions or extremities, and a positive Romberg test. Her serum manganese level was very elevated, at 4.8 ng/mL.

An HMPAO SPECT study (Fig. 10.14) in the transaxial plane revealed reduction of tracer uptake in the basal ganglia (body of the caudate nuclei) and thalami. These findings were felt to be related to a toxic encephalopathy.

A repeat study obtained a year after the patient abstained from plant work showed significant improvement in tracer uptake to these regions. At that time, the patient's clinical status had improved significantly.

Teaching Point:

Although there appears to be a strong relation between the manganese level and reduced tracer uptake in the basal ganglia and thalamus, such findings may also be related to other environmentally toxic substances in the patient's workplace.

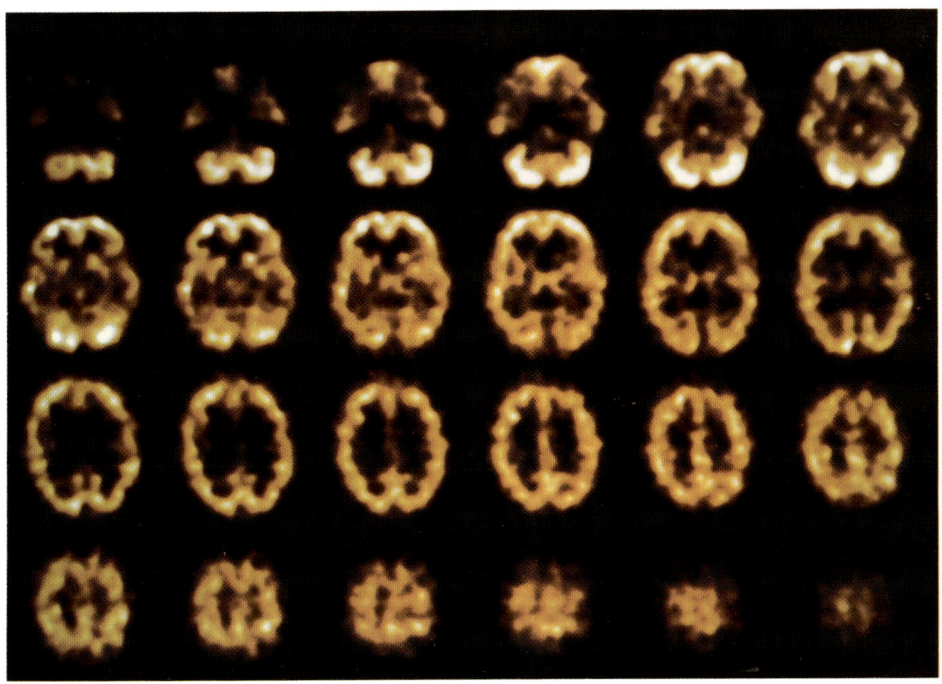

FIG. 10.14

CASE 10-8

Clinical Diagnosis: Severe Disabling Tinnitus

CONTRIBUTOR:

Name: Abraham Schulman, M.D. and Arnold M. Strashun, M.D.
Institution: SUNY Health Sciences Center at Brooklyn

IMAGING DATA:

Camera: Trionix Triad
Isotope: ^{99m}Tc HMPAO
Collimator: High resolution
Dose: 25.0 mCi

This 44-year-old man with known severe disabling tinnitus of approximately 3 years' duration was referred for further evaluation. The patient's symptoms were persistent since ear cleaning for wax removal. The tinnitus was characterized as bilateral, but was greater in the left ear, with a "hiss" and "tea kettle" quality; it was constant in duration, with a tinnitus intensity index of 7 on a scale of 0 to7 (7 maximum). The patient additionally noted intermittent ear blockages (left greater than right) and episodes of dysequilibrium. He also noted a past history of major depression with hospitalization on two occasions and a sleep disorder. The patient's tinnitus gradually increased in severity with an associated loss of hearing but no additional signs of neurologic disease.

Neuropsychological testing revealed a question of cognitive impairment and borderline visual spatial dysfunction.

A CT scan revealed mild diffuse cortical atrophy.

An HMPAO SPECT study (Fig. 10.15), in the transaxial **(A),** coronal **(B),** and sagittal **(C)** planes, revealed reduced radiotracer activity in the bilateral inferior frontal as well as the mesial and midposterior temporal (left greater than right) regions. Overall the subcortical regions were relatively spared.

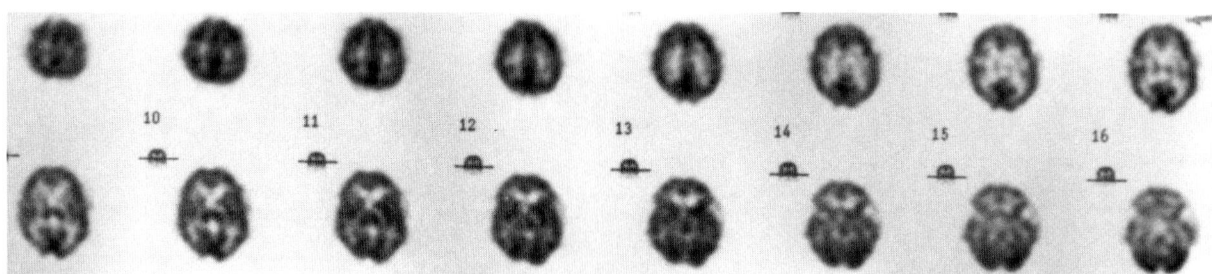

FIG. 10.15A

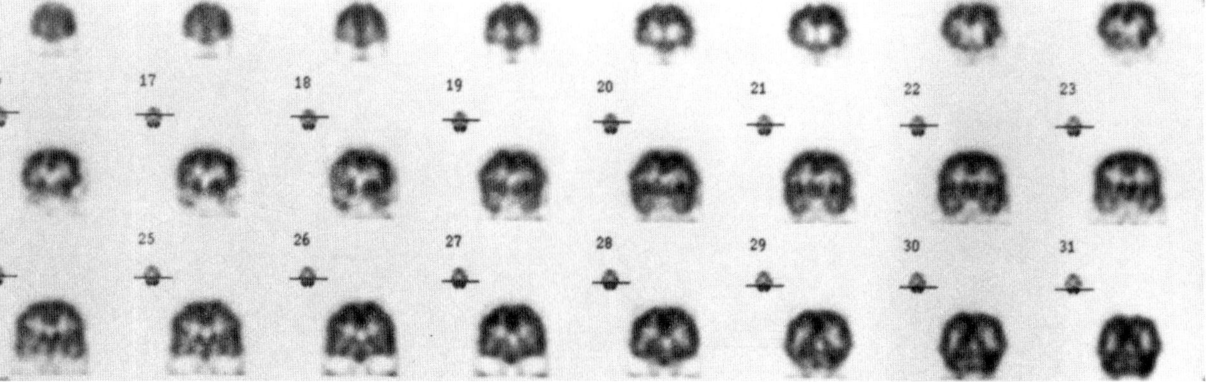

FIG. 10.15B

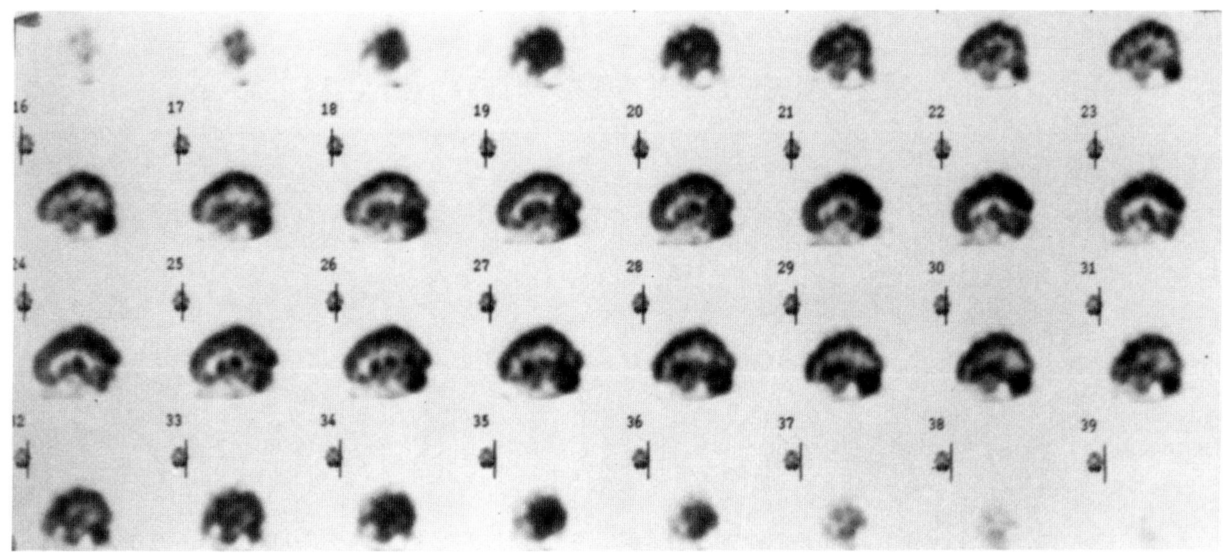

FIG. 10.15C

CASE 10-9 Clinical Diagnosis: Central Type Tinnitus

CONTRIBUTOR:	IMAGING DATA:	
Name: Abraham Schulman, M.D. and Arnold M. Strashun, M.D.	**Camera:** Trionix Triad	**Collimator:** High resolution
Institution: SUNY Health Sciences Center at Brooklyn	**Isotope:** ^{99m}Tc HMPAO	**Dose:** 25.0 mCi

This 72-year-old man presented with tinnitus that had increased in intensity over the past year. The tinnitus was described as a "high ring" in both ears of constant duration and fluctuating intensity. The tinnitus intensity index was 6 on a 0 to 7 scale (7 maximum). The patient noted an associated bilateral hearing loss (left greater than right), early memory dysfunction, and positional dysequilibrium. Subsequent workup identified the tinnitus to be predominately central in type with a bilateral cochlear component (left greater than right) and a presumptive clinical diagnosis of a secondary endolymphatic hydrops on the left.

A head CT scan was reported to be negative.

An HMPAO SPECT study (Fig. 10.16) in the transaxial plane revealed an overall decrease in cortical radiotracer activity than was most marked in the bilateral frontal, temporal, and right parietal lobes and to a lesser degree subcortically.

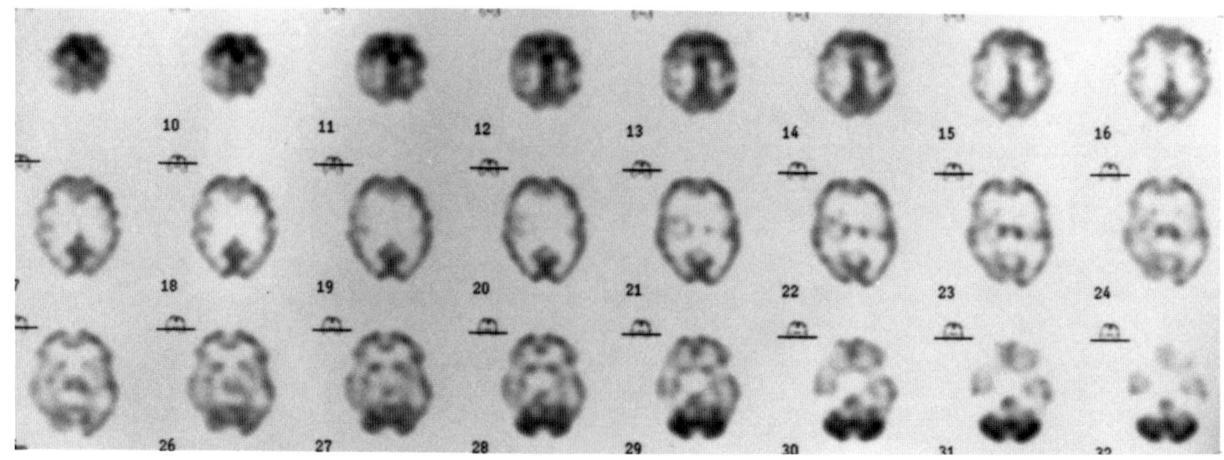

FIG. 10.16

Subject Index